Caregiving on the Periphery

McGILL-QUEEN'S/ASSOCIATED MEDICAL SERVICES STUDIES IN THE HISTORY OF MEDICINE, HEALTH, AND SOCIETY

SERIES EDITORS: S.O. FREEDMAN AND J.T.H. CONNOR

Volumes in this series have financial support from Associated Medical Services, Inc. (AMS). Associated Medical Services Inc. was established in 1936 by Dr Jason Hannah as a pioneer prepaid not-for-profit health care organization in Ontario. With the advent of medicare, AMS became a charitable organization supporting innovations in academic medicine and health services, specifically the history of medicine and health care, as well as innovations in health professional education and bioethics.

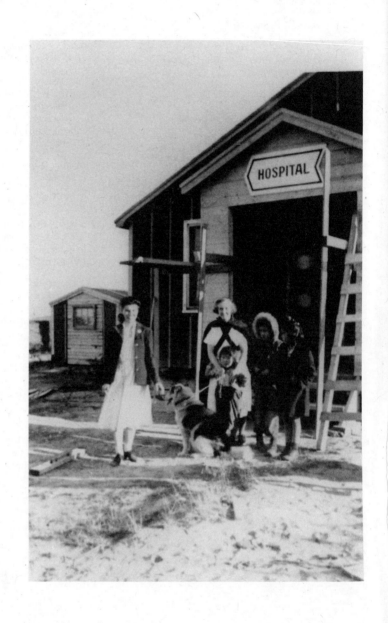

Caregiving
on the
Periphery

Historical Perspectives on Nursing and Midwifery in Canada

EDITED BY MYRA RUTHERDALE

McGILL-QUEEN'S UNIVERSITY PRESS
Montreal & Kingston · London · Ithaca

© McGill-Queen's University Press 2010

ISBN 978-0-7735-3675-3 (cloth)
ISBN 978-0-7735-3676-0 (paper)

Legal deposit second quarter 2010
Bibliothèque nationale du Québec

Printed in Canada on acid-free paper that is 100% ancient forest free
(100% post-consumer recycled), processed chlorine free.

This book has been published with the help of a grant from the Canadian Federation
for the Humanities and Social Sciences, through the Aid to Scholarly Publications
Programme, using funds provided by the Social Sciences and Humanities Research
Council of Canada.

McGill-Queen's University Press acknowledges the support of the Canada Council for
the Arts for our publishing program. We also acknowledge the financial support of the
Government of Canada through the Book Publishing Industry Development Program
(BPIDP) for our publishing activities.

Library and Archives Canada Cataloguing in Publication

Caregiving on the periphery : historical perspectives on nursing and midwifery
in Canada / edited by Myra Rutherdale.

(McGill-Queen's/Associated Medical Services Studies in the history of
medicine, health and society ; 36)
Includes bibliographical references and index.
ISBN 978-0-7735-3675-3 (bnd)
ISBN 978-0-7735-3676-0 (pbk)

1. Nursing–Canada–History. 2. Midwifery–Canada–History.
I. Rutherdale, Myra, 1961– II. Series: McGill-Queen's/Associated Medical
Services studies in the history of medicine, health, and society ; 36

RT6.A1C385 2010   610.73'0971   C2009-907142-8

This book was designed and typeset by studio oneonone in Sabon 10.3/14

Contents

Acknowledgments

This book came together because of the goodwill and patience of the contributors. Their efforts to understand the history of caregiving on the periphery are greatly appreciated. My colleagues at York University's Department of History also deserve my gratitude.

With any collection like this, so much of the work is in the hands of a highly competent editorial team. At McGill-Queen's University Press, it was a pleasure to work with the incomparable Kyla Madden, deputy senior editor, and Joan McGilvray, co-ordinating editor. Thanks also to Eleanor Gasparik, who did an outstanding job on copy-editing. Two anonymous readers provided very useful comments and suggestions for revisions. In addition, I thank the Aid to Scholarly Publications Programme, which provided the financial assistance to make this book possible.

I take sincere pleasure in thanking my family and in acknowledging my good fortune to belong to such a great one. My son, Andrew, my husband, Robert, and my mother-in-law, Jean, have been so helpful with this book and all of my academic efforts to date. Over the years, Jean provided several wonderful stories about her nurse training at the Toronto General and her career as a nurse in the 1940s and 1950s. Rob, as always, encouraged me to stay the course and offered much love along the way. And our son, who has grown up with much 'history talk,' is to be thanked for bringing such joy to our lives. He has also become very good at coming up with great titles! Thanks, Andrew.

Caregiving on the Periphery

Introduction

MYRA RUTHERDALE

I remember one night when I was called to help a new mother
with a cranky infant. Although this is natural for a new baby, I
felt nervous and agreed to meet the mother at the health centre.
(There is no ambulance service for local people; they must find
their own way to the health centre.)

When I arrived, the child was breathing but lethargic. We
had delivered this baby three weeks earlier and it was healthy.
Its heart rate was 60 (120–160 is the norm for this age), which
meant that we had to begin CPR immediately. I knew that the
medivac plane would not arrive for hours. I started an IV, administered oxygen and flicked the baby's heels for the next eight
hours, while I monitored its cardiac status. Sweat ran down my
arms as I tried to reassure the mom that everything would be
okay. I did not let her know that I was petrified. We were all
relieved when Pat O'Connor arrived with the medivac plane.
The child was taken to the University of Alberta hospital in
Edmonton with a diagnosis of RSV, a respiratory infection that
is fatal to infants. I am thrilled to report that little Naiya recovered and is a healthy youngster today.[1]

This is how Donna Hawes recalled one memorable night spent in the
community of Taloyoak (formerly Spence Bay). A trained nurse from
Alberta, Hawes had only just begun her Arctic nursing career when

she encountered Naiya in the summer of 1994. This narrative account exemplifies the kinds of histories that are explored in this book. All nurses and midwives working in rural or in northern Canadian communities at that time would have been able to identify with the way Hawes felt that night. Hawes realized immediately that the baby was in jeopardy, but the resources at her disposal in this small 'peripheral' community limited her choice of action. She knew there was no way to evacuate the child until many hours later, but she had to reassure the baby's mother that the child would be fine even though she herself felt unsure. Perhaps, too, there was a language barrier to overcome with the help of an interpreter. As the only nurse on duty, Hawes was on her own: she had to draw on her knowledge and training to do her best to save the baby. Similar hours of anxiety and hope were shared by the midwives and nurses featured in this book, those who cared for patients in Aboriginal and re-settler communities, in patients' homes, or in nursing stations across Canada throughout the nineteenth century and much of the twentieth.

This collection – the first of its kind in Canadian historiography – gathers together essays on divergent experiences that include those of Ontario and Western Canadian Mennonite midwives, Labrador nurses, northern Ontario Red Cross nurses, Yukon Aboriginal student nursing assistants, an Anglican Sister in the 1885 Northwest Rebellion, and an Alberta-born nurse working along the Alaska Highway in the late 1940s. The geographical and chronological range is extensive; so, too, are the life stories that unfold. Yet these essays reveal many similarities faced by midwives and nurses involved in dispensing health care in circumstances that some people might have considered extraordinary. Insight is provided into the women's work for women, for families, and for community members in the outposts and outports, in the diverse social spaces of rural health care delivery far from large urban centres and traditional hospitals.[2] The many European languages these women spoke ranged from Low German to Russian; some tried to communicate in Cree or Inuktitut and often used interpreters to translate Aboriginal languages. Cultures and regions varied, but explicit across these papers is the fact that each location demanded that health care providers (in the cases revealed here, midwives and nurses) take the initiative. They had to demonstrate creativity and courage in situations not encountered in southern and urban hospital

settings. For instance, the traditional hierarchical relationships between doctors and nurses did not exist in the same way in rural or
northern communities and these nurses and midwives often found
themselves doing what was traditionally considered doctors' work.

While the concept of isolation was critical to the mental cartogra-
phies of several of the nurses and midwives featured in this book, the
term *isolation* must be interrogated. Certainly, seen from the perspective of the early twenty-first century, Toronto seems far from isolated.
But from the point of view of one midwife, whose house sign in 1810
read "Isabella Bennet, midwife from Glasgow," the small community
of York, with 700 inhabitants, no doubt seemed like an isolated or
peripheral outpost.

Isolation, as Mary Jane McCallum has recently argued, is a term
that tended to be overused by policy-makers and by caregivers themselves. It often referred to Aboriginal communities but it could be
used to describe any community outside the metropolis. As McCallum
argues, "'Isolation' is not a naturally occurring geographical feature,
but is made historically through relations of power. By approaching
the history of health services to Aboriginal people as part of a broader
effort to reorder and control landscape according to colonial impera-
tives, we can better understand why concepts of isolation informed
medical journalists' impressions of Aboriginal health."[3] Isolation is in
itself a construction. The inhabitants of communities described as such
did not necessarily see them that way. But the idea of isolation or
periphery provides a critical backdrop to many of these chapters, as
it does to our understanding of Canadian medical history.

Location is a critical dimension in the geography and history of
nursing, but this book also serves as a reminder of ways in which
Canadian identity and ideas of nationhood can be closely tied to the
history of health care, and perceptions of success in that realm. Long
before the federal government took an active role in health care provision through medicare and programs like the Indian and Northern
Health Services, women were active caregivers. Sometimes they served
only within their own communities, but often they went beyond those
boundaries. And frequently, women were recognized for their service.
The medal granted to Hannah Grier Coome for her work during the
Northwest Rebellion and British Columbia's official recognition of
Amy Wilson during the diphtheria outbreak of 1949 are two examples

of how the state officially celebrated nurses' work. In other ways, too, the histories of nursing and midwifery are tied to nation formation. Kathryn McPherson has demonstrated how popular representations and social memories of nursing were reflected in the 1926 National War Memorial in Ottawa, and Margaret MacDonald argues that idealized images of the pioneer midwife are still prominent in the collective identity of Canadian midwives.[4]

The role of nurses in state formation, from the time of Confederation onward, was reinforced when nurses were employed by provincial or federal governments to spread the gospel of public health among both Natives and newcomers and were thus implicated in the state's reform agenda. Because of Canada's colonial history – and in the twentieth century, the propensity for the south to try to colonize the north (what two writers here call *internal colonization*) – medicine and colonialism became inextricably linked. These essays make clear that the modernizing aspects of medicine sometimes clashed with localized or indigenous traditions. The intricate relationships between medicine and colonization are underscored by Australian historian Alison Bashford, who focuses her research on the conflation between empire and health: "Even as medicine and public health brought desirable new effects in terms of better individual health and public works, they were instruments through which indigenous men and women were managed by missions and government. Colonial public health and sanitary reform also aimed to change conduct and personal habits at the most intimate levels."[5] The attempt to assert authority over Aboriginal communities is conveyed by several authors in this collection, but so, too, are the ways that indigenous medicine endured and that nurses and midwives created their own priorities.

Historiography

This book, unlike others in this field, probes the meaning of women's midwifery and nursing work in contexts that have tended to be overlooked by many historians. While it is unique, it also fits into a burgeoning historiography on the social history of medicine in Canada. The history of health care across Canada has received considerable recent attention. Within the last few years, books have been published on the history of general hospitals, medical research, aging in British

Columbia, and birthing in Canada, and an important new study has recently been produced on the history of the treatment of people with spinal cord injuries.[6] Even though some of this work has proceeded without what historian of medicine Peter Twohig has labelled a "historiographical net," the variety of medical history topics has expanded, as has the number of scholars engaged in questions concerning the Canadian social history of medicine.[7]

Well before this current spate of scholarly activity, historians of medicine and health care had asked questions about women's activism as patients, health care providers, and policy-makers. The histories of women doctors and nurses alike, received attention in two edited collections published during the early 1990s. Each book – *Delivering Motherhood*, edited by Katherine Arnup, Andrée Lévesque, and Ruth Roach Pierson, and *Caring and Curing*, edited by Dianne Dodd and Deborah Gorham – has provided conceptual frameworks for understanding the roles women have played in shaping their own health care experiences, as well as those of others.[8] A more recent collection of essays, *Women, Health and Nation* edited by Georgina Feldberg, Molly Ladd-Taylor, Alison Li, and Kathryn McPherson, provides a useful comparison of Canadian and American women's health policies and practices after 1945.[9] Together, these three collections have moved us closer to understanding the complexities, the struggles, and the passions that have contributed to Canada's health care system from the turn of the twentieth century to today.

The history of nursing itself has benefited from this new historiography, and has also expanded. Cynthia Toman's *An Officer and a Lady* details the experiences of 4,000 nurses who served Canada during the Second World War. The bonds created and the new spaces carved out for women during this masculinist military endeavour, argues Toman, shifted gendered expectations, yet also exhorted women to be both 'officers' and 'ladies.'[10] Women's nursing efforts in the battlefield have been part of nursing since its inception with Florence Nightingale's foundational efforts during the Crimean War. Nursing has also had close ties to mission work, yet that nursing aspect has sometimes been ignored. Sonya Grypma's *Healing Henan* adds to our understanding of the international movement of Canadian nursing into China, and of the changes that took place in nurses' practice throughout the sixty years of work at the Presbyterian missions in the province of Henan.[11]

Both Toman's and Grypma's books mark some of the new directions in Canadian nursing historiography, but the most significant work
in the field remains Kathryn McPherson's *Bedside Matters: The Transformation of Canadian Nursing, 1900–1990*. Each scholar who contributed to this collection has acknowledged her gratitude to McPherson
for her path-breaking efforts. Her work situates nursing history at the
nexus of three important historiographies. First and foremost – and undoubtedly influenced by American historian Susan Reverby's *Ordered
to Care: The Dilemma of American Nursing, 1850–1945* – McPherson
locates nursing within the context of labour history.[12] Nurses had to
struggle to maintain adequate wages and to establish satisfactory working conditions. Secondly, she makes the case that while male nurses
practised alongside the female majority, nursing itself was often socially
defined as women's work, and that a feminist perspective helps to situate nursing history within women's history. Thirdly, McPherson places
nursing history firmly within the context of the social history of medicine, a field that has sometimes rejected the importance of nursing, giving
preference instead to a 'scientific' and masculinist medical model.

Although McPherson is sensitive to the way racial barriers were
erected in the nursing profession, and particularly the ways in which
whiteness was played out, our collection extends her discussion to highlight the critical dimensions of race and ethnicity in communities where
nurses practised. These geographical locations and the ways that race
shaped them are critical to this collection. Historians of midwives and
nurses are constantly confronted with issues surrounding race and ethnicity. Cynthia Toman and Meryn Stuart have recently argued, "there is
a need for more work on race and ethnicity, and its role in the history
of nursing. Too few studies use race as a concept of analysis or actively
consider whiteness as a determinant in our history."[13] From conceptu-
alizing meanings of 'whiteness' to interrogating British ethnicity to
querying cultural understandings of Mennonite tradition to unravelling
relations between Natives and newcomers in Aboriginal communities,
this book demonstrates that race mattered in the practice of midwifery
and nursing.

Kathryn McPherson argues that throughout the twentieth century
the practice of medicine was increasingly institutionalized and situated
within hospitals. That is true, of course, for the majority of Canadians, but our book looks at encounters that took place beyond those
more common settings. We are interested in settings that were con-

siderably distant from the typical hospital context. Nursing stations, along with community centres, school gyms, patients' homes, church basements, and traplines, were among the many spaces converted to sites of medical practice.

Autonomy is another important area of consideration in nursing historiography, and also central to McPherson's work. How independent were nurses and midwives in their everyday working environments and how did this autonomy shape notions of professionalism or ideas about occupational identity and integrity? In agreement with American nursing historians like Barbara Mellosh, McPherson describes public health nurses as independent women who had a fair amount of autonomy in their working conditions.[14] Simultaneously, she recognizes that these nurses were conscious of carrying out the agenda of the state, or as Kari Delhi puts it, they were "both products and producers of social and state regulation."[15] This is certainly true in some cases, but as most of the authors here acknowledge, the question of autonomy was complex, and it varied according to circumstance and necessity.[16] Midwives and nurses had to be flexible and innovative. They may have received instructions from far-off headquarters, but they were the ones on the ground facing situations that had to be negotiated on an individual basis.

The nursing-state relationship has been central to discussions in the new international historiography of nursing as well. Recently, Joan E. Lynaugh compiled a list of eight issues that should be at the heart of the agenda for gathering international perspectives on nursing history. She lists nursing-state relations as the top priority and claims that this category has proven to be "endlessly fascinating and constantly changing."[17] The other key criteria in her list include religious influences, economics and nursing, social welfare, gender, scientific thinking, medical changes, and nursing knowledge. She also recommends that research should continue to be undertaken on the international aspects of both race and ethnicity, and on the implications of technology on nursing experiences.

Pushing nursing history beyond national borders has shed light on themes of education, standardized training, and professionalization, as Anne Marie Rafferty has shown in *The Politics of Nursing Knowledge*, and can tell us about the mobility of skilled midwives and nurses who moved beyond their native lands.[18] The potential for travel while working is demonstrated in Catherine Ceniza Choy's *Empire of Care:*

Nursing and Migration in Filipino American History, which makes the case that Filipino women realized a nurse's cap could become their passport.[19] Similarly, nursing historians Margaret Shkimba and Karen Flynn argue that borders opened for the women in their study; the 'White' British and 'Black' Caribbean nurses who migrated to Canada following the Second World War.[20] Shkimba and Flynn discuss the race politics encountered by these two sets of nurses to reveal that the White British nurses often suffered more racism than did their counterparts from the Caribbean. Flynn's research, along with that of Agnes Calliste, on Black nurses in Canada provides an important backdrop for this book.[21] Cross-cultural encounters are highlighted here, as are questions about who is the 'other,' the 'outsider' with respect to access to both health care and the medical professions themselves. These new directions in nursing history point to the potential of demonstrating the international interconnectedness of experience during the growth of nursing as a profession, but they also render explicit the theme of race and ethnic relations within the history of nursing.

The history of midwifery in Canada, and internationally, has also been the focus of renewed scholarly attention. This has coincided with a resurgence of midwifery in Canada. The first collective attempts at writing the history of midwifery in Canada were made during the 1980s, when some scholars were suggesting that midwifery had all but disappeared, mainly due to various turf wars with doctors.[22] New certification programs and colleges of midwifery have prompted reconsideration of midwifery's history in Canada. According to Cecilia Benoit and Dena Carroll, "Individual midwives have for the most part been courageous healers, willing to attend birthing women when no nurse or doctor was at hand and tend to the sick or victims of accident or injury, despite difficult working conditions and little or no economic reward."[23] They argue that it was this willingness to help out that led to the high social standing of midwives in their communities. However, this status did not necessarily translate into 'formal recognition' at least not until recently.

Representative of the new directions in midwifery scholarship is the recently published *Reconceiving Midwifery*, a collection of essays mainly concerned with the post-1945 era. One of the most self-reflective articles provides an interesting explanation about who had been neglected in those earlier studies of midwifery. Lesley Biggs discusses her earlier work and acknowledges her changed perspective:

In rereading my early work in light of the many developments
that have taken place within feminist scholarship, I have become
aware of the *absence* of the stories of different groups of women.
That is, I have become concerned not so much with what I said,
but what I didn't say. There is, for example, in my article no
mention of Aboriginal midwifery; it is as if the history of midwifery began with the arrival of the settlers. In addition almost
all of the sources cited are by commentators of English origin.
What were the views of Irish immigrants who settled during
this time period, or of the other European immigrants who
came later?[24]

Like women's history in general, the histories of both midwifery and
nursing have gained much from a more inclusive perspective. Biggs
was not alone in leaving minority groups out of her earlier work. Her
new analysis has produced a multi-dimensional tapestry of midwife
experiences, one that centres not on the dominance of the "neighbour
midwife" but rather concludes that, historically, Canada has witnessed
the emergence of several types of midwives: "In the rewriting of the
history of Canadian midwifery, we do not necessarily have to reject the
concept of the neighbour midwife outright, since she too represents a
set of experiences, but they are only part of the story. We need, then,
to research and write the stories of the many other women, from different racial, cultural, ethnic, and class positions, drawing these lyrics
together, celebrating the multiple rhythms and accepting the discor-
dant beats."[25] Such a perspective is useful for both the history of nursing and the history of midwifery in Canada.

This book attends to the diversity of experience across several regions
and almost two centuries. While a historical perspective informs all of
these essays, this text is multi-disciplinary, with contributions from
scholars in departments of nursing, women's studies, geography,
Native studies, and history. However, as the chapters remind us, locating sources on midwifery and nursing can be a challenge. The unique
and groundbreaking approach adopted by Laura Thatcher Ulrich in
A Midwife's Tale highlights that looking outside of the conventional
archival records can bring a deepened understanding of the many caregiving tasks carried out by midwives.[26] In an effort to provide a balanced
interpretation, the authors have used a wide range of sources including
city directories, census data, autobiographies, biographies, letters, news-

paper articles, contemporary magazines and journals, oral interviews, and government documents. Such sources can hardly sit silent when they speak of moments, like those of Nurse Hawes at Taloyoak, that are actually part of a much larger pattern of outpost nursing and midwifery through the shifting eras of colonialism, post-colonialism, and changing medical practice.

The Chapters

Part One: The Multifaceted Lives of Midwives (Chapters 1 to 3)

Like other women's history projects, the stories of midwives and nurses can sometimes only be revealed after very careful digging. In the first chapter, for example, the author identifies the lives of nineteenth-century Toronto midwives through the excavation of city directories and census material. Occasionally, only fragments – or as Linda Kealey puts it, "fragmented autobiography" – remain. These bits and pieces of life writing force the historian to read between the lines for meaning and to give voice to experiences that were no doubt shared by many women in several different geographical contexts. Finding sources is even more challenging when looking for evidence about women who did not have the opportunity to learn how to write. Although they often looked after bodies from before birth until after death, working class women, Aboriginal women, and first-generation immigrants to Canada rarely left written sources. However, interviewing family members – as Marlene Epp did – can help to recover at least some of the narratives. The first three chapters in this collection make important methodological contributions: through their use of unique sources, they each provide an analysis of the multifaceted tasks of midwives and nurses who were either working class, immigrants, or both.

Judith Young's exploration of midwives and nurses in nineteenth century Toronto adds much to our understanding of the multi-dimensional nature of early caregiving. Her careful analysis of primary sources suggests that midwives, and later monthly and sick nurses, came from working-class backgrounds and were often widows, and that the wages enabled them to carve out a living, support family members, and pay rent for their housing in Toronto's working-class neighbourhoods. Her essay highlights the fluidity, too, of job categories.[27] Those who were once midwives eventually may have become monthly nurses, able to sustain themselves on wages earned for post-partum care. As the century progressed and the city of Toronto grew, more opportunities for private nursing arose and at least some of the women who were earlier registered as midwives appeared in the official records by the 1880s as "sick," "monthly," or "private" nurses. By 1891 only one registered midwife remained. Their demise was not because of a turf war with doctors, as has been traditionally argued – although that could have mattered for some. Many became nurses, though often their caregiving roles had yet to be formalized. In part, as Young so ably demonstrates, midwives reinvented themselves to meet the growing demands for multifaceted care and to fit into the newly devised professionalizing categories of nursing.

It does not take a tremendous leap of logic to imagine how essential the Toronto midwives were to the burgeoning neighbourhoods in which they served. Much like the Mennonite women of Marlene Epp's study, they no doubt cared for all manner of illness, often because they were seen as women who had medical knowledge. They were valued community members who came to represent a sense of cultural cohesion along with local history. Not only did Epp's midwives assist in the delivery of thousands of babies, they also looked after other medical matters. One Mennonite midwife, Katherina Born Thiessen, remembered that she was often called upon because she was known for "expertly delivering babies, setting bones, diagnosing illnesses and prescribing remedies for everything from lung disorders to skin cancer, and also saving lives through emergency surgery." Mennonite midwives also served as local undertakers, standing as they did on the "confluence of life and death."

Epp deepens our understanding of the critical and multifaceted role played by Mennonite midwives. Focusing her attention on their "vocational importance within the social, familial, and religious life of immigrant, rural settlers" provides us with a richly textured portrayal of immigrant life and women's networks that we cannot otherwise see. These women held power within the community because of the trust and confidence of their patients and the newly bereaved.

Power could also emanate from passing on received wisdom. The boundary between official and unofficial training was often crossed in the context of midwifery. Some midwives learned at the feet of their mothers, while others trained formally at schools in England and continental Europe. Some Mennonite midwives took lessons from Aboriginal women about local herbs and curatives. Others studied chiropractic, and sent away to Europe for new medical textbooks. Myra Bennett (née Grimsley), the subject of Linda Kealey's chapter, was trained as a nurse and certified by the Central Midwives Board in England. Once in Newfoundland, she seemed to take much pleasure from introducing 'traditional' midwifery techniques to young women in her community of Daniel's Harbour.[28]

By paying close attention to the fragments of Bennett's life, Kealey reinforces ways in which the work of community midwives can be characterized as "occupational pluralism." Bennett's duties included immunization, surgery, dentistry, and pediatrics, as well as school visits and public health. She also raised children, kept the books for her husband's merchandising business, and entertained all those who visited Daniel's Harbour and wanted to chat over a cup of tea. Not only that, she was seen as the community disciplinarian, since mothers sent their daughters to her to be "straightened out." Kealey also underscores how the occupation of nursing/midwivery could allow one to gain social status. Like the women in Young's study, Bennett had a working-class background, having been born and raised in East London where her father worked at "several trades." In leaving England and answering the call for an outpost nurse/midwife, Bennett was taking her first steps toward constructing a new identity. Apart from the appeal of adventure and the possibility, as Kealey puts it, of "exploring the margins of empire," Bennett's voyage to Daniel's Harbour represented the opportunity for her to become a new person. She was a professionally trained authority figure to be categorized with other professionals like the local schoolteacher. She appears to have even taken on an upper middle-class British accent. Both geographic and social mobility shaped Bennett's life as an outpost nurse and midwife in mid-twentieth-century Newfoundland.

Part Two: Writing Their Own Lives: Life Writing in Nursing History
(Chapters 4 to 6)

As the historian of medicine Sasha Mullally has argued, life writing can tell us much about "the contemporary preoccupations of the writer," as well as the author's own self-reflexivity: "Historians now understand the many ways that life writing in general, and autobiography and biography in particular, are historically contingent on both the literary milieu of the individual author, as well as the political understandings about the importance of 'the self' and 'individual' at any given point in our cultural past."[29]

Approaching the histories of nursing and midwifery from the perspectives of biography, autobiography, and other forms of life writing – if done with caution – can bring us closer to understanding the day-to-day experiences of both the women under consideration and their patients in the communities in which these women worked. We can also gain insight into the motivations behind women's entry into their occupations. The individual, the everyday, and the countless small acts of life that women wove together created patterns over time that allow us to reach conclusions about how the midwives' and nurses' personal and professional lives blended. As Linda Kealey makes clear, the contours of Bennett's life were shaped not only by her desire for adventure but also by a sense of duty and calling. The conflation between the notion of a calling and women's medical work should not be underestimated.

This is especially evident in the life of Hannah Grier Coome, an Anglican nursing sister who served during the Northwest Rebellion of 1885. For her, spirituality and nursing service were one. As Elizabeth Domm clearly demonstrates, Coome's experiences as a young girl growing up in an eastern Ontario parsonage and later as a young woman influenced by the deaconesses in England led her almost inevitably to a life of religion and medicine. As conscious as she was of the new nursing roles carved out by Florence Nightingale, she was as ready to serve her country at a battlefront when needed as she was to enthusiastically take up parish nursing later on. Her self-sacrifice and practicality were demonstrated in a number of ways, but cutting off her hair suggests what Domm sees as her desire to set an example for the other nurses, and also to recognize the reality of western travel and living conditions. At her makeshift hospital in Moosejaw, Coome ran a tight and, equally important, clean ship. She was frugal with her funds and smart in her nursing techniques. Although hired to look after soldiers who were fighting for the "government side," she also looked after the First Nations people in the area, befriending some of them along the way. In the end, her work was officially acknowledged, as attested to by her service medal, which honoured all those who served the government. Coome represents the type of women explored in Ruth Compton Brouwer's path-breaking study *New Women for God*.[30] In her independence, Coome sought out a sphere of work for herself and also opened doors to other women who wanted to serve Christ and heal bodies.

Throughout the nineteenth century, nursing increasingly went hand in hand with spiritual or mission work. It became a viable option for women who wanted to maintain both their respectability and their independence. Within the confines of religious institutions women like Coome created occupational lives and built their own communities of workers. They cloaked themselves and their bodies – either literally or figuratively, and sometimes both – in nursing/religious veils. They claimed a place for themselves within various public spheres, including Toronto neighbourhoods, Western Canadian rebellion sites, and resettled communities and outports all across Canada. Embodiment and occupation were intricately linked. Their bodies represented the kinds of work they were engaged in and gave them authority in their various communities.[31]

The ways these communities formed and the complexities within them varied substantially. The Mennonite midwives of Marlene Epp's study would have encountered patients with experiences that were significantly different than those of patients in Bennett's world. Nonetheless, in order to understand how midwives and nurses carried out their daily duties, and how their various patients received them, it is necessary to know where they fit within the settlements they worked in. What were their neighbours like? How did these newcomer nurses and midwives imagine their own communities? What racial tensions or class hierarchies did nurses have to negotiate?

These are some of the questions posed by Mary-Ellen Kelm in her careful study that links space, place, and, more importantly, race to the experiences of one missionary nurse, Margaret Butcher, who worked in the village of Kitamaat from 1916 to 1919. Butcher's letters form the central evidence in Kelm's rendering of her world. As a nurse in the Methodist Elizabeth Long Memorial Home, a residential school that opened in 1896, Butcher sought connections in her community and along the coast. What became increasingly important for her was less one's whiteness than one's Englishness. She was comfortable and felt a sense of belonging with those from her home country, or at least those who acted 'English,' but she felt a sense of loss for those 'English' men who married Haisla or other Aboriginal women. Englishness, too, was tightly constructed. Like other missionary/nurses, she also yearned for England and took comfort in various reminders of 'English behaviour,' or English landscape. As Kelm so cleverly puts it: "declaring someone or something 'English' was Butcher's way of claiming that person or place as familiar, valuable, as belonging to her white world."[32] Above all, Butcher was told in no uncertain terms that no matter what, the main thing was that she must do her best to fit in.

All of the women in this study – whether recently arrived midwives walking the streets of Toronto to visit from house to house or nurses at work in outport Newfoundland or on the coast of British Columbia – had to 'fit in' to a new cultural environment so that they could continue with their duties. Many were part of a cluster of skilled, later professional, elite who moved into small communities and clung together to celebrate cultural or religious occasions. And, like many women who went uninitiated in the outdoor life, Butcher found opportunities to test herself against the elements – sometimes unsuccessfully. The real significance of Butcher's letters is that they show us how an 'ordinary' nurse/missionary participated in the colonial process that dispossessed Aboriginal peoples of their land.[33] Ironically her participation was intended not as an act of conquest but as one of nurturance, healing, and helping. Kelm's essay brings us closer to understanding the kinds of connections created in the new towns and settlements that became homes to many of the nurses and midwives that we meet in each of the chapters of this book.

Learning more about individual nursing experiences usefully complicates any ideas we might have about the sameness of women's experiences or the uniform nature of all mission nurses. Coome and Butcher were as different as chalk and cheese, yet they had similar goals and objectives. These two biographical accounts add to nursing history by making explicit the connections between nursing and the

promotion of nation and colonialism. Through their religious institutions, both women were, interestingly, serving the needs of the state
and at the same time working through in their own minds the ways
that race and gender shaped their opportunities.

After the Second World War, it was more common for nurses to
seek secular work through governmental departments or non-govern-
mental organizations. The essay by Myra Rutherdale examines, through
autobiography, the experiences of Amy Wilson, a nurse who worked
along the Alaska Highway for the federal Department of Health's
Indian and Northern Health Services Branch. Like Coome's biography
and Butcher's letters, Wilson's autobiography is especially important
for the light it casts on individual experience. Her life story stands in
stark contrast to those of many women who, during the 1950s, stayed
at home to raise children in the new post–Second World War suburbs.

In *No Man Stands Alone*, Wilson describes how she was willing to
go on an adventure, eager to take up her position as the "Alaska
Highway Nurse." According to Rutherdale, Wilson's independence,
developed through years of public health nursing in small Alberta
communities, served her well. She was keen to travel aboard whatever conveyance was necessary to reach her patients, and did not
refrain from mixing with the old trappers and various other northern
men that she met in the course of her duties. In fact, as Rutherdale
argues, Wilson preferred the company of men, adopting a 'fraternal
mode' of expression in her life writing. While Wilson found comfort
in a circle of newcomers that included many men, she also enjoyed
learning about Aboriginal medicine. Here lies the main contribution
of Rutherdale's work. We are aware of the disruptions caused by colonization, but how newcomers in Aboriginal communities actually
sought to learn from their new associates is often neglected. Wilson
was curious about and respectful toward Aboriginal medicine. Careful note is made in this essay that Wilson recorded details about the
cures used and saw the value in much that was Aboriginal. This is not
to overstate Wilson's admiration for native medicine, but only to
balance the assumption that Westernized medicine was a closed
system with no room for negotiation.

A distinct quality shared by all of the women in the first two
sections of this book – from Young's nurse/midwives to Bennett and
Wilson – was the extent of their independence. None were constrained

by hospital hierarchies. For the most part, they worked in small communities, either on their own or with a partner.[34] As such, they were away from the gaze and critique of supervisors, and certainly worked less frequently with doctors. This is not to say that race, gender, and other constraints, exclusions, and professional anxieties did not exist in smaller institutions or tiny communities. They simply had to confront problems on their own more often. And in some interesting ways, all of these women could be considered travellers and their writing, in particular that of Wilson, could be categorized as travel writing. As recent studies of gender and travel writing have made clear, women's modes of expression in this genre vary greatly according to context and are contingent on whether women were liberated by or suffered from the mobility expressed in their narratives, and on whether they sought to construct themselves or others as exotic. The multiplicity of travel and writing experiences and the level of 'narrative authority' ultimately contributed to how gender, identity, and experience were shaped.[35]

Part Three: Regulating Nurse Training and Professional Boundaries
(Chapters 7 and 8)

As the essays in this book make clear, race, class, and gender must be carefully interrogated within the matrix of nursing history. The chapter by Laurie Meijer Drees adds a critical dimension to both nursing and Native/Newcomer historiography. Drees makes the compelling case that the Government of Canada sought to include Aboriginal Canadians in the health care system by offering to train Aboriginal women to fill various positions. Those in charge of the Indian and Northern Health Services Branch frequently made statements attesting to their efforts: "Every effort is made to hire Indians and Eskimos. About 15% of the staff are from these ethnic groups. There are as yet no Indian or Eskimo physicians, but there are a few fully trained and registered public health nurses and many more native ward aides. The male native staff serves mainly as technicians, maintenance men, drivers, etc. although in 1961 the first Indian Sanitarian qualified."

Aboriginal nurses were educated and hired; however, they tended to take work in "Indian hospitals." Although the program worked to enhance opportunities for Aboriginal peoples, it seemed at best haphazard and often parsimonious. As Drees points out, efforts to recruit nursing students were limited. Instead, there was a focus, especially starting in the 1960s, to encourage Aboriginal peoples to enter the lower ranks of the health care hierarchy. The limitations of the program were sustained because of the enduring racism that prevailed in the minds of many Canadians. The idea that Aboriginal peoples had only a partial capacity for employability was still believed by some as late as the 1960s.[36]

Like Epp's chapter on midwives, Drees' also highlights one of the fascinating areas that require more attention in the histories of nursing and midwifery: the role of "unofficial" training. Drees offers the example of Muriel Innes, a young woman from the Cowessess First Nation who was dropped off by her father at the Lac La Ronge nursing station. There, the nurses "informally" trained her as a nursing aide. This enabled her to acquire a paid position in Prince Rupert. Women's unofficial work as role models or mentors, especially in communities without training institutions, is an important theme in this book, and one that can potentially contribute much to our understanding of both medical and women's histories.

Given the geographic locales of the chapters in this book, from early Toronto to various outports, outposts, small prairie settlements, and northern Ontario towns, the concepts of 'official' and 'unofficial,' 'formal' and 'informal' are particularly useful. What constituted official training? Were the Aboriginal women who helped Mennonite midwives officially trained, or were the Native women encountered by Amy Wilson formally educated? Were midwives official? Is the term meant to indicate 'Western' or imply that medicine is only official if sanctioned by institutions under the guidance of 'scientific men'? Heidi Coombs-Thorne claims that the Grenfell nurses in her chapter are to be understood within the context of "an informal medical environment."

For Coombs-Thorne, the distinction between formal and informal is in part what first attracted many of the women to the Grenfell nursing stations in Newfoundland and Labrador. After all, for Nurse Dorothy Jupp, and others like her, the informal aspect of the work was intricately linked with independence. She contrasted the formal confines of a hospital with the independence of running a nursing station. The outpost nurse had a huge variety of tasks, both medical and non-medical. As one Grenfell nurse recalled, about running a nursing station: "you've got the whole town on your doorstep and you either sink or swim."

But, the independence and the ability to go beyond what may have been viewed as traditional nursing duties presented a professional and personal challenge to many of the Grenfell nurses as well as nurses who worked in similar situations, particularly in northern locations. Boundaries, both geographic and professional, were tested in these communities. Sometimes, too, as Coombs-Thorne so clearly articulates, nurses came into conflict with those accustomed to maintaining strict boundaries within the hierarchical structure of the medical profession. Occasionally, doctors felt a bit uncomfortable with such independent women telling them what their intentions were. The confidence gained in handling their own nursing stations, with all the attendant problems, allowed them to look differently at their own careers and take control of their own destinies.

Part Four: Northern Nursing, Natives, and Newcomers
(Chapters 9 to 11)

The question of autonomy was central to Red Cross nurses in northern Ontario. Jayne Elliott's perspective on this issue is similar to that of Coombs-Thorne, but she recognizes that independence was a double-edged sword because of increased workload and increased responsibility. She demonstrates that the desire expressed by outpost nurses to be independent was complicated by the personal relationships between nurses, community members, supervisors, and local physicians.[37] Negotiation between all of these parties became the key to the successful operation of the Red Cross stations. Elliott's case study provides a unique contribution because of its revealing depiction of the northern Ontario setting and its careful scrutiny of the structure of the Red Cross nursing program.

Elliott shows clearly the anxiety felt by nurses when their supervisors visited from Toronto to inspect the stations and to ensure the nurses were up to standard. The nurses were also aware of the need to maintain their dignity and respectability among their community members and patients. Their behaviour was carefully scrutinized. Even more challenging though were their relations with doctors. Like the Grenfell nurses, they were admonished not to overstep their professional boundaries, but they also had to compensate for doctors who were incapable or make excuses for those who had, as one nurse in

Elliott's study put it, "regular bouts" or, as another nurse said, "one bad fault." Gender power dynamics had to be negotiated and in their desire to provide for their patients, sometimes nurses, and ultimately their charges, lost out to stubborn or errant doctors. At times, too, the patients themselves could not adapt to the programs being suggested by middle-class, urban, educated nurses. These tensions, Elliott cautions, must not be overlooked when coming to terms with the experiences of outpost nurses.

Whether working for the Methodist mission in northern British Columbia, the Red Cross in northern Ontario, the Indian and Northern Health Services Branch in provincial and territorial norths, or for the Department of Public Health in northern Saskatchewan, southern nurses in northern communities often brought with them their own sense of proper decorum, hygiene, and appropriate behaviour. This cultural baggage was part of who they were as white, middle-class professional women. Sometimes it conflicted with their settler neighbours, who they may have deemed as rather "rough," or with Aboriginal peoples, who they periodically saw as in need of "citizenship work." Their program for reform could be harsh; the cultural conflict could be intense. The tensions caused by the introduction of nurses in northern Saskatchewan communities are strikingly rendered by Lesley McBain. The ambiguities are suggested in her conclusion when she states that the nurses were both "hegemonic and beneficial." The complicated nature of the encounter is offered by one of the supervisors in McBain's essay, who in writing to an outpost nurse made explicit the awkward nature of the enterprise: "your approach to the nutrition problem in the north seems so wise. It seems so unreasonable to expect those people to accept our way of life. Much more sensible to improve their own way of life. It is too bad that more persons do not have your attitude." The notion is that Aboriginal peoples needed change, but of course they could never be 'White.' This is similar to the government's program to educate Aboriginal health care workers: in essence, the policy was to educate Natives, but only to a certain level.

Elliott and McBain both raise the point that although northern nurses appeared to be independent in their nursing stations, they were in fact constrained by the bureaucratic structures within which they worked and the gendered nature of the medical profession itself. Judith Zelmanovits recognizes these limitations, too, especially when it came

time for northern nurses to fulfill their functions as public health promoters. Like McBain, she finds that the nurses were meant to act as
agents of the state, yet at the same time they came to represent the
needs and interests of their patients: "While it cannot be denied that
nurses were agents of the federal government's policy of internal colonization, much of their work as educators was aimed at undoing or
minimizing the wrongs of the past by halting the spread of infectious
and other diseases introduced to isolated communities from the 'outside.'" The difficulties entailed in their public health work brought
many nurses face to face with the fact that the teaching material they
were given and the preparation they received for their work were simply inadequate. The tragic impact of tuberculosis and the belief in the
germ theory moved the government to encourage public health education, yet the nurses themselves found that they had to be creative in
their efforts to carry out this work, and sometimes, out of necessity,
they entirely disregarded government directives.

+++

The essays collected here emphasize the complex roles shared by
nurses and midwives throughout the past two centuries of Canadian
history. They shed light on individual experiences and demonstrate how
women performed what they saw as their duty in looking after the bodies of the ill and needy. Their patients came first, whether they were
newly arrived immigrants in Toronto, sick Inuit in Arctic communities,
or new settlers in Newfoundland's outport communities. At the same
time, nursing and midwifery provided respectable occupational opportunities for women long before they were accepted into other areas
of work. Along with being able to earn an income, health care providers
were able to travel and experience adventures. In fact, many women
claimed that the desire for adventure was why they signed up for work
with the Grenfell mission or why they went to northern Canada.

Independence is one of the key themes that binds these chapters
together and, as Veronica Strong-Boag asserted, the histories of nurses
and midwives tell us much about women's history.[38] Equally important, this book lays a foundation for understanding how midwives and
nurses were often caught between their patients, their own consciousness, and the larger bureaucratic structures that underpinned health
care services. Nurses and midwives confronted the gender hierarchy of

the health care profession and often, through a process of negotiation, came out of their battles having won the day. They tested the professional and gendered boundaries and revealed their fluidity.

The generation of scholars represented here has come of age during a time when historians began to take seriously the place of gender, race, and class in the making of Canadian society. Bringing these issues to bear on medical history has proven fruitful. This book will open further avenues of research and interpretation, and will contribute to the ongoing conversation about the histories of midwifery and nursing and their critical place in Canadian history.

NOTES

1 Karen Scott and Joan Kieser, eds., *Northern Nurses: True Nursing Adventures from Canada's North* (Oakville: Kokum Publications, 2002), 43.
2 This book builds on the recent work of nursing historians who have started to probe the history of outpost nursing, including Jayne Elliott, "Blurring the Boundaries of Space: Shaping Nursing Lives at the Red Cross Outposts in Ontario, 1922–1945," in *Canadian Bulletin of Medical History/Bulletin canadien d'histoire de la médecine* 21 (2004): 303–25; Nicole Rousseau and Johanne Daigle, "Medical Service to Settlers: The Gestation and Establishment of a Nursing Service in Quebec, 1932–1943," in *Nursing History Review* 8 (2000): 95–116; Laurie Meijer Drees and Lesley McBain, "Nursing and Native Peoples in Northern Saskatchewan: 1930s–1950s," in *Canadian Bulletin of Medical History/Bulletin canadien d'histoire de la médecine* 18 (2001): 43–65. See also Dianne Dodd, Jayne Elliott, and Nicole Rousseau, "Outpost Nursing in Canada," in Christina Bates et al., *On All Frontiers: Four Centuries of Canadian Nursing*, 139–52 (Ottawa: University of Ottawa Press, 2005).
3 Mary Jane McCallum, "This Last Frontier: Isolation and Aboriginal Health," in *Canadian Bulletin of Medical History/Bulletin canadien d'histoire de la médecine* 22 (2005): 109.
4 Kathryn McPherson, "Carving Out a Past: The Canadian Nurses Association War Memorial," in *Histoire Sociale/Social History* 29 (Nov 1996): 417–29; Margaret MacDonald, "Tradition As a Political System in the New Midwifery in Canada," in Ivy Lynn Bourgeault et al., *Reconceiving Midwifery*, 46–66 (Montreal & Kingston: McGill-Queen's University Press, 2004).
5 Alison Bashford, "Medicine, Gender and Empire." In Philippa Levine, ed., *Gen-*

der and Empire: Oxford History of the British Empire Companion Series, 117 (Oxford: Oxford University Press, 2004). See also Alison Bashford, *Imperial Hygiene: A Critical History of Colonialism, Nationalism and Public Health* (London: Palgrave MacMillan, 2004).

6 David Gagan and Rosemary R. Gagan, *For Patients of Moderate Means: A Social History of the Voluntary Public General Hospital in Canada, 1890–1950* (Montreal & Kingston: McGill-Queen's University Press, 2002); W.G. Godfrey, *The Struggle to Serve: A History of the Moncton Hospital, 1895–1953* (Montreal & Kingston: McGill-Queen's University Press, 2004); Alison Li, *J.B. Collip and the Development of Medical Research in Canada: Extracts and Enterprise* (Montreal & Kingston: McGill-Queen's University Press, 2003); Megan J. Davies, *Into the House of Old: A History of Residential Care in British Columbia* (Montreal & Kingston: McGill-Queen's University Press, 2003); Wendy Mitchinson, *Giving Birth in Canada, 1900–1950* (Toronto: University of Toronto Press, 2002); Geoffrey Reaume, *Lyndhurst: Canada's First Rehabilitation Hospital for People with Spinal Cord Injuries, 1945–1998* (Montreal & Kingston: McGill-Queen's University Press, 2007). It is worth noting that most of these books have been published under the McGill-Queen's Associated Medical Services Studies In The History of Medicine, Health and Society Series.

7 Peter L. Twohig, *Labour in the Laboratory: Medical Laboratory Workers in the Maritimes, 1900–1950* (Montreal & Kingston: McGill-Queen's University Press, 2005), 15.

8 Katherine Arnup et al., eds., *Delivering Motherhood: Maternal Ideologies and Practices in the 19th and 20th Centuries* (London and New York: Routledge, 1990); Dianne Dodd and Deborah Gorham, *Caring and Curing: Historical Perspectives on Women and Healing* (Ottawa: University of Ottawa Press, 1994); Kathryn McPherson, *Bedside Matters: The Transformation of Canadian Nursing, 1900–1990* (Toronto: Oxford University Press, 1996). See also Wendy Mitchinson and Janice Dickin McGinnis, eds., *Essays in the History of Canadian Medicine* (Toronto: McClelland and Stewart, 1988). There is still a gap in terms of the history of women doctors in Canada, but there are several popular books including Carlotta Hacker, *The Indomitable Lady Doctors* (Toronto/Vancouver: Clarke, Irwin & Company Limited, 1974); Margaret McCallum, *Emily Stowe* (Toronto: Grolier Limited, 1989).

9 Georgina Feldberg et al., *Women, Health, And Nation* (Montreal & Kingston: McGill-Queen's University Press, 2003).

10 Cynthia Toman, *An Officer and a Lady: Canadian Military Nursing and the Second World War* (Vancouver: University of British Columbia Press, 2007).

11 Sonya Grypma, *Healing Henan: Canadian Nurses at the North China Mission, 1888–1947* (Vancouver: University of British Columbia Press, 2007).

12 Susan Reverby, *Ordered to Care: The Dilemma of American Nursing, 1850–1945* (New York: Cambridge University Press, 1987).

13 Cynthia Toman and Meryn Stuart, "Emerging Scholarship in Nursing History," in *Canadian Bulletin of Medical History/Bulletin canadien d'histoire de la médecine* 21, 2 (2004): 227.

14 Barbara Mellosh, *"The Physician's Hand": Work, Culture and Conflict in American Nursing* (Philadelphia: Temple University Press, 1982).

15 Keri Delhi, "Health Scouts for the State: School and Public Health Nurses in Early Twentieth Century Toronto," in *Historical Studies in Education* 1, 2 (1990): 260.

16 For further elaboration on the role of public health nurses, see Meryn Stuart, "'Half a Loaf is Better than No Bread': Public Health Nurses and Physicians in Ontario, 1920–1925," in *Nursing Research* 41 (January–February, 1992): 21–7; Meryn Stuart, "Shifting Professional Boundaries: Gender Conflict in Public Health 1920–1925." In Dianne Dodd and Deborah Gorham, eds., *Caring and Curing: Historical Perspectives on Women and Healing in Canada*, 49–70 (Ottawa: University of Ottawa Press, 1994); "Ideology and Experience: Public Health Nursing and the Ontario Rural Child Welfare Project, 1920–25," in *Canadian Bulletin of Medical History/Bulletin canadien d'histoire de la médecine* 6 (1989): 111–31; Sharon L. Richardson, "Frontier Health Services for Children: Alberta's Provincial Travelling Clinic, 1924–1942." In Cheryl Krasnick-Warsh and Veronica Strong-Boag, eds., *Children's Health Issues in Historical Perspective*, 479–507 (Waterloo: Wilfrid Laurier University Press, 2005).

17 Joan E. Lynaugh, "Common Working Ground." In Barbara Mortimer and Susan McGann, eds., *New Directions in the History of Nursing: International Perspectives*, 195 (Oxford: Routledge, 2005).

18 Anne Marie Rafferty, *The Politics of Nursing Knowledge* (London: Routledge, 1996). See especially chapter 4.

19 Catherine Ceniza Choy, *Empire of Care: Nursing and Migration in Filipino American History* (Durham: Duke University Press, 2003).

20 Margaret Shkimba and Karen Flynn, "'In England we did nursing': Caribbean and British nurses in Great Britain and Canada, 1950–70." In Barbara Mortimer and Susan McGann, eds., *New Directions in the History of Nursing: International Perspectives*, 141–57 (Oxford: Routledge, 2005).

21 Karen Flynn, "Experience and Identity: Black Immigrant Nurses in Canada, 1950–1980." In Marlene Epp et al., *Sisters or Strangers?: Immigrant, Ethnic and*

Racialized Women in Canadian History, 381–98 (Toronto: University of Toronto Press, 2004); Karen Flynn, "Proletarianization, Professionalization, and Caribbean Immigrant Nurses," in *Canadian Woman Studies* 18 (1998): 57–64. See also Agnes Calliste, "Women of 'Exceptional Merit': Immigration of Caribbean nurses to Canada," in *Canadian Journal of Women and the Law* 6, no. 22 (1993): 85–102.

22 See especially, Lesley C. Biggs, "The Case of the Missing Midwives: A History of Midwifery in Ontario from 1795–1900." In Katherine Arnup et al., eds., *Delivering Motherhood: Maternal Ideologies and Practices in the 19th and 20th Centuries*, 20–35 (London and New York: Routledge, 1990). For a response to Lesley Biggs, one which argued that the doctors in Ontario were less threatened by midwives than they were worried about regulating the "irregular" doctors, see J.T.H. Connor, "Larger Fish to Catch Here than Midwives: Midwifery and the Medical Profession in Nineteenth-Century Ontario." In Dianne Dodd and Deborah Gorham, eds., *Caring and Curing: Historical Perspectives on Women and Healing in Canada*, 103–34 (Ottawa, University of Ottawa Press, 1994). For an earlier piece on the history of midwifery and the early tensions between midwives and nurses, see S. Buckley, "Ladies or Midwives? Efforts to Reduce Infant and Maternal Mortality." In Linda Kealey, ed., *A Not Unreasonable Claim: Women and Reform in Canada, 1880s–1920s*, 131–49 (Toronto: The Women's Press, 1979).

23 Cecilia Benoit and Dena Carroll, "Canadian Midwifery: Blending Traditional and Modern Practices." In Christina Bates et al., *On All Frontiers: Four Centuries of Canadian Nursing*, 41 (Ottawa: University of Ottawa Press, 2005).

24 Lesley Biggs, "Rethinking the History of Midwifery in Canada." In Ivy Lynn Bourgeault, Cecilia Benoit, and Robbie Davis-Floyd, eds., *Reconceiving Midwifery*, 18 (Montreal & Kingston: McGill-Queen's University Press, 2004).

25 Ibid., 38.

26 Laura Thatcher Ulrich, *A Midwife's Tale: The Life of Martha Ballard, Based on Her Diary 1785–1812* (New York: Knopf, 1991).

27 For more on the variety of titles given to caregivers, see Judith Young and Nicolle Rousseau, "Lay Nursing From the New France Era to the End of the Nineteenth Century (1608–1891)." In Christina Bates et al., *On All Frontiers: Four Centuries of Canadian Nursing*, 11–27 (Ottawa: University of Ottawa Press, 2005).

28 For histories of midwifery and nursing in the Atlantic provinces, see C. Benoit, "Mothering in a Newfoundland Community: 1900–1940." In Arnup, *Delivering Motherhood*, 173–89; C. Benoit, "Midwives and Healers: The Newfoundland Experience," in *Healthsharing* 5, 1 (1983): 22–6; Gordon H. Green, *Don't Have*

Your Baby in the Dory: A Biography of Myra Bennett (Montreal: Harvest House, 1974); Douglas O. Baldwin, *She Answered Every Call: The Life of Public Health Nurse Mona Gordon Wilson (1894–1981)* (Charlottetown: Indigo, 1997).

29 See Sasha Mullally, "History, Memory and Twentieth-Century Medical Life Writing: Unpacking a Cape Breton Country Doctor's Black Bag." In E.A. Heaman et al., *Essays In Honour of Michael Bliss: Figuring the Social*, 437 (Toronto: University of Toronto Press, 2008).

30 Ruth Compton Brouwer, *New Women For God: Canadian Presbyterian Women and Indian Missions, 1876–1914* (Toronto: University of Toronto Press, 1990).

31 While Coome was a Protestant Anglican, the same can be said for Catholic women who occupied lay nursing roles from the early contact period. See such works as Robert Lahaisie and Noél Vallerand, *La Novelle-France, 1524–1760* (Outremont: Lanctøt Editeur, 1999; Toronto: The Women's Press, 1987). For the nineteenth-century and women's expanding roles within the Catholic Church, see Marta Danylewycz, *Taking the Veil: An Alternative to Marriage, Motherhood, and Spinsterhood in Québec, 1840–1920* (Toronto: McClelland and Stewart, 1987).

32 For a good understanding of the meanings of "whiteness," see Ruth Frankenberg, *White Women, Race Matters: The Social Construction of Whiteness* (Minneapolis: University of Minnesota Press, 1993). See also Mathew Fry Jacobson, *Whiteness of a Different Colour: European Immigrants and the Alchemy of Race* (Cambridge: Harvard University Press, 1999).

33 On the history of colonization in British Columbia, see Adele Perry *On the Edge of Empire: Gender, Race and the Making of British Columbia, 1849–1871* (Toronto: University of Toronto Press, 2001).

34 The ways in which imperial expansion opened employment opportunities for some women, especially white middle-class women, is just beginning to be explored. Mission histories point this out. See, for example, Myra Rutherdale, *Women and the White Man's God: Gender and Race in the Canadian Mission Field* (Vancouver: UBC Press, 2002). See also Angela Woollacott, *To Try Her Fortune in London: Australian Women, Colonialism, and Modernity* (New York: Oxford University Press, 2001). See also Lisa Chilton, *Agents of Empire: British Female Migration to Canada and Australia, 1860s–1930* (Toronto: University of Toronto Press, 2007). For nursing history, see Helen Gilbert, "Great Adventures in Nursing: Colonial Discourse and Health Care Delivery in Canada's North," in *Jouvert* 7 (2003): http://social.chass.ncsu.edu/jouvert. See also Susan Nestel, "(Ad) Ministering Angels: Colonial Nursing and the Extension of Empire in Africa," in *Journal of Medical Humanities* 19, 4 (1998): 257–77; Margaret

Jones, "Heroines of Lonely Outposts or Tools of Empire: British Nurses in Britain's Model Colony: Ceylon, 1878–1948," *Nursing Inquiry* 2, 3 (2004): 148–60.

35 For an excellent and diverse collection of scholarship on gender and travel writing see Kristi Siegel, *Gender, Genre and Identity in Women's Travel Writing* (New York: Peter Lang, 2004).

36 Naturally there were women who had broken down barriers. Charlotte Edith Anderson Monture and Jean Cuthand Goodwill, two Aboriginal women who trained as nurses are discussed in Christina Bates et al., *On All Frontiers: Four Centuries of Canadian Nursing*, 86 and 116 (Ottawa: University of Ottawa Press, 2005).

37 An interesting narrative of the life of an outpost nurse is provided in Gertrude LeRoy Miller, *Mustard Plasters and Handcars: Through the Eyes of a Red Cross Outpost Nurse* (Toronto: Natural Heritage Books, 2000).

38 Veronica Strong-Boag, "Making A Difference: The History of Canada's Nurses," in *Canadian Bulletin of Medical History/Bulletin canadien d'histoire de la médecine* 8 (1991): 231–48.

Part One

The Multifaceted Lives of Midwives

1

+ + + + +

"Monthly" Nurses, "Sick" Nurses, and Midwives: Working-Class Caregivers in Toronto, 1830–91

JUDITH YOUNG

In the nineteenth century, before the advent of the trained nurse, nursing for pay was carried out by a diverse group of working-class women,
and occasionally by men.[1] The status of the untrained nurse in society
was undoubtedly that of a servant, but historians have debated the
degree of skill with which she practised, and her level of respectability.[2] Many details of the life and work of these early caregivers remain
elusive. This essay uses Toronto as a case study to explore the diversity
of women who practised as nurses in the nineteenth-century city, a
diversity that ranged from one who was an 'expert' though informally
trained practitioner to one who was decidedly ignorant and unsavoury.
Nineteenth-century nurses worked in a society where governments,
whether municipal, provincial, or territorial, assumed very limited
responsibility for the care of the sick. Families with the means looked
after sick members in the home; the less fortunate relied on aid from
charitable organizations and grudging help from state institutions such
as the hospital and asylum. Toronto's only general hospital did not
receive secure provincial funding until 1874.[3]

I highlight the fluid nature of nursing roles during the period, and
the changing definition of *nurse* over time. In the nineteenth century,
the term *nurse* was equally applied to those caring for the sick, to
women who provided postpartum care (who might be midwives),
and to those looking after children. Few nurses appeared in the records
of early Toronto, but as the city grew from small garrison town to

industrialized metropolis, nursing emerged as a reputable trade for working-class women.[4] When trained nurses came onto the scene – in Ontario, during the last quarter of the nineteenth century – the transition from untrained nurse to professional was less than seamless and the two groups co-existed well past the turn of the century.

British historian Barbara Mortimer has provided a useful model for investigation of early nurses. As working-class women, nurses have left little in the way of personal documents,[5] but by combining information from various sources, the careers of some can be followed over time. Mortimer searched public records for data on "domicilliary" nurses in mid-Victorian Edinburgh and found several had not insubstantial careers.[6] Using information from the Canadian census and Toronto city directories,[7] I look at the range of women who provided nursing care in nineteenth-century Toronto. I discuss the class background, marital status, ethnicity, and living arrangements of nurses who worked independently in Toronto. Where did they fit into the system of health care at the time, and how did they compare with nurses working in Toronto hospitals and asylums? Significant in nineteenth-century nursing was the role of the *monthly*, also known as the *ladies'*, *nurse*, an individual who cared for a new mother and infant for one month following the birth. Midwives come into the picture because some worked as monthly nurses and their role, particularly from mid-century, appeared inextricably linked with that of nurses. The title of *sick nurse* is self-explanatory and, although the term appeared only occasionally in the records, does help to differentiate nineteenth-century nursing work. Women caring for children were also called *nurse* and, in arriving at numbers of private nurses, I have excluded these workers.[8] I also limit my discussion to lay nurses. The first Catholic sisterhood reached the city at mid-century, but these women constituted a special group of nurses whose work, with its social service dimension, appears quite different from that of the nurses I discuss.[9]

Early Midwives in the Town of York

In 1815, York (Toronto) had existed for barely two decades, a "small undistinguished village" of 700 inhabitants clustered in wooden houses overlooking the harbour.[10] But the town's position as capital of Upper

Canada ensured growth and immigrants arrived steadily. Although physicians and midwives settled in York, as a pioneering society, the majority of its citizens relied on their own resources in time of illness or injury. Self-medication was popular and until the mid-1800s, care of the sick was part of the "domestic economy" with medicines and herbs essential household commodities and advice and help freely sought from relatives and neighbours.[11] The services of a doctor might be sought for difficult or protracted illness and that of a midwife in time of childbirth.

Possibly the first midwife in York was the wife of the King's Printer who, in 1810, placed a sign on her house: "Isabella Bennet, midwife from Glasgow."[12] Later, in the *Colonial Advocate*, a York paper, Bennet informed the public of a change of address.[13] In 1829, also in the *Advocate*, Mrs Sarah Tebbutt announced that she was an experienced midwife from England, that she "refers to Dr Widmer" and that she would be setting up practice in York.[14] Dr Christopher Widmer, an early York physician, was a medical leader in the town, so a significant ally.[15] Physicians were yet to stake their claim to superiority in obstetrical care and were generally accepting of reputable midwives. Widmer, as well as working with local midwives, supported midwifery training. As head of the York Medical Board he proposed a lying-in hospital that would serve destitute immigrants and "be made subservient to the instruction of students and midwives."[16]

An early York charitable organization, The Female Society for Relief of Poor Women in Childbirth, employed the services of a midwife. Founded in 1820 by a group of the town's more advantaged women, the society, in its first report, recorded that seventeen women had been assisted "with comfortable clothing of all kinds, a midwife, and Physician (if required) and the best nourishment."[17] This seems to indicate that a midwife was more likely to be present for deliveries, and a doctor only in case of difficulties. For the destitute sick there was the General Hospital, erected in 1820 but not opened for nine years due to lack of operating funds.[18] A dispensary under the direction of Widmer formed part of the hospital's services. Female nurses would have been hired as hospital staff but we know nothing of them at this time. If there were private nurses in the town, they remained invisible in this early era.

Midwives and Hospital Nurses in the
Developing City, 1833–50

As the city transformed from small town to a centre for trade that attracted larger numbers of immigrants, the increasing health care needs
of the population provided opportunities for women's work. The independent midwife, respected by her community, can be considered at
the top of a hierarchy of health care workers. The hospital nurse most
likely came from the lowliest ranks of the working class. In 1834, York
became the incorporated city of Toronto, a town of just over 9,000 people. Politically, the next few years were turbulent,[19] but despite the city
briefly losing its status as the provincial capital, business and commerce
grew steadily in Toronto in this pre-industrial phase of growth.

The first city directory, published in 1833, recorded two midwives,
M. McAul and Mrs Bennett, in the street listings.[20] There is no record
of nurses but midwives may have fulfilled a nursing role. The diary of
Martha Ballard, an early nineteenth-century midwife in New England,
showed that she acted as midwife, made sick calls, and dispensed herbs
and pills.[21] Of the two early Toronto midwives, McAul did not remain
in the city. A midwife named Margaret McCaul, advertising in the
Brockville Chronicle in September 1835, considered that her "long experience and good reputation in Toronto" would make her popular
with women in Brockville. In contrast to the mobile McCaul, Bennett
appeared to have a long career in Toronto, if we assume that the individual in the 1833 directory was indeed the Isabella Bennet who hung
up her shingle in 1810 and who advertised in the *Colonial Advocate*
in 1828. She continued to be listed in each directory up to 1846.

No more than two midwives appeared in city directories during the
1830s and '40s though other women likely practised in the town. As
there was no licensing, anyone could call herself a midwife and some
may have fallen into the category of the "helpful neighbourhood
woman"[22] who had no need to advertise. Certain midwives had special credentials. Mrs Mahon, listed as a midwife in 1843,[23] advertised
her arrival from Dublin two years earlier in several issues of the *Christian Guardian*. In her advertisement, Mahon notified the public of her
twenty years' experience "with the higher and lowlier classes of
ladies": she would "cheerfully attend any calls" and assured potential clients that they would be truly satisfied with her "real knowledge,

experience and attention."[24] Mrs Miller, another Irish midwife, announced in the 1850 directory that she was from Dublin.[25] This was a way of indicating experience and perhaps some formal or informal training, a possibility in a city such as Dublin. From the early eighteenth century many European cities had established lying-in hospitals and these institutions trained both midwives and medical students.[26] Midwives in Toronto who were recent immigrants from Great Britain or Ireland could have had some formal training. Mortimer described the availability of a three-month course at the Edinburgh Maternity Hospital.[27] A similar program existed in Montreal at the Lying-in Hospital. Staffed by physicians from McGill University, the program offered training to both medical students and "any woman desirous of acquiring an acquaintance with the duties and practice of Obstetrics."[28] It is obvious that well-trained midwives existed. Thus, although it is important to acknowledge that many practised without benefit of instruction, it is equally significant that others could be considered skilled and knowledgeable. Some of these found their way to Upper Canada and Toronto.

It is difficult to know how well midwives were accepted in Toronto and if they earned a decent living. In an urban setting they were certainly competing with doctors who, as the century progressed, increasingly attended births. The number of physicians in Toronto went from fifteen in 1833 to twenty-nine by 1850, though not all of these were in general practice.[29] Doctors did complain of competition from midwives and 'quacks' when they were unable to make a decent living.[30] According to historian Wendy Mitchinson, around mid-century, midwives were charging two dollars as opposed to the usual physician's fee of five dollars for a delivery. Moreover, midwives stayed longer and probably helped with household chores, so for the less wealthy they were more cost effective.[31] From the diary of Captain William Johnson of Georgina, Ontario, we learn that in 1832 he paid five dollars to a Mrs Elwes to attend at the birth of his daughter,[32] a sum that would have included care following delivery.

According to city directories, Toronto midwives lived in working-class areas in the centre of town. The fact that none had husbands listed at the same street address likely indicated that they were, in fact, widows eking out a living. As working-class women, they would have to make their own way around the city, not an easy task without public

transportation. In the 1840s, Toronto streets were "wretchedly" paved
and the sidewalks were made of wooden planks where nails could
become loose, making walking treacherous.[33] Drinking was endemic
and inebriates wandering the streets posed a special danger for women
whose work necessitated that they move about the city. March Street,
where midwife Bennett lived, was known as "a thoroughfare of ill
repute." A change of name to Lombard Street was intended to "elevate" its reputation but it remained filled with dwellings "for the most
part of the wretched class."[34] It is hard to imagine that Bennett, a long-
time resident, was prosperous; however, she did belong to a small
group of independent women workers. No doubt, midwifery, even if
the work was irregular, was more rewarding than charring, taking in
washing, or working as a live-in servant – the limited options for a
working-class widow. The reputable midwife also had the satisfaction
of being a person of some standing in her community.

Very little is known of Toronto hospital nurses in the 1830s and
'40s, but the occasional portrait that emerges is unflattering. Available
descriptions refer to nurses in makeshift isolation hospitals, so it is difficult to know if regular staff at the General Hospital or at the Lunatic
Asylum were as inept. In city directories, little information is given
about nurses in public institutions. We learn only that Toronto General, in 1850, had an average of 100 patients and "about one nurse
to every ten patients"[35] – if accurate, a very good ratio for the time.
Matron and nurses were housed in the hospital, still in its original
1820 location on King Street. The Asylum, in 1846, still occupied the
premises of the former city jail and, at that time, had three nurses and
five "keepers" on its staff.[36]

The decades of the 1830s and '40s were characterized by an influx
of immigrants and significant outbreaks of cholera. Each year, the
breakup of ice heralded the arrival of immigrants and increased the likelihood of the spread of disease. Like most Victorian cities, the sanitary
arrangements in Toronto were appalling. The bay suffered from an
accumulation of filth and debris piled up on the ice through the winter:
in April 1832, a writer to the *Canadian Freeman* deplored the condition of the bay and suggested that an alternative source of drinking
water be found.[37] This concern proved prophetic as that summer a
cholera epidemic killed 400 people. When a second cholera epidemic
occurred two years later, a temporary hospital was set up close to the
General but there were many problems equipping it and procuring suit-

able nurses.[38] Charles Sheward, the surgeon appointed to administer the hospital, complained that the nurses "were so unfit in every respect to assist him, that unless others were hired, his health must be sacrificed."[39] Lack of fitness may have indicated inadequate skill and dedication, poor personal qualities, or all of these. While sympathizing with Sheward in his plight, it is not hard to imagine the extreme difficulty and danger of caring for cholera patients in makeshift, badly equipped surroundings. Given the dangerous, poorly paid work, nurses most likely were recruited from among the lowest classes and the most desperate families; lacking experience and instruction, it is not surprising they were totally inadequate for the job. Sick immigrants and epidemics continued to strain the city's resources through the 1840s. Although the sheer numbers of sick and starving immigrants were much less than in Quebec City and Montreal, Toronto had many newcomers arriving on its shores and suffered outbreaks of typhus and further cholera epidemics in the 1840s. A citizen, many years later, recalled seeing great numbers of Irish immigrants ill with what was called "emigrant fever," and considered fatal. They were "lying on beds or stretchers in rows of sheds, open at the sides," that had been erected on land adjacent to the General Hospital.[40] Nursing was likely rudimentary.

There is evidence that it was difficult, particularly in special times of need, to find sufficient nurses to care for sick people.[41] This could have been due to the difficulty of the work or, as nurses came from the working class, to the general shortage of servants. Nurses hired to care for the indigent in the General Hospital and for the insane in the Asylum were most likely from the lower echelons of the working class. Although the work of a servant in a private house was hard, the servant's life was probably preferable to living and working in the asylum or hospital – and less dangerous to health and well-being. By contrast, the independent midwife represented the upper level in a hierarchy of female health care providers. The trained midwife was capable of providing care according to the best knowledge of the time, and some had the support of physicians. The experienced though untrained midwife could, if she was skilful, build up a practice by gaining a good reputation in the community. By 1851, the population of Toronto had reached 30,000. Immigrants from Britain and Ireland predominated and, from their ranks, came the majority of women who were to work as nurse or midwife in the city in the next few decades.

Monthly Nurses and Sick Nurses:
Private Nursing, 1850–70

As the population and wealth of the city grew, it seems apparent that
a demand was created for private nursing. Although Toronto was not
fully industrialized until the 1870s, the '50s and '60s saw considerable
expansion of manufacturing while, at the same time, railway development linked the city more easily with other centres. As the Toronto
population grew, women outstripped men in number, a reversal of earlier times; this meant that an increasing number of women were seeking work.[42] The names of five monthly nurses can be found in the
Toronto directory of 1850,[43] the first year that private nurses appeared
in these records.[44] By the time of the 1861 Canadian census, there were
likely nineteen nurses in private work in Toronto,[45] although the
directory of the same year yielded only six names. The reason for this
discrepancy may be that the census, with its detailed record of each
household, captured nurses working casually as well as full-time, while
the directory listed only those who professed nursing as their major
occupation. What is evident is that by 1861, with a special listing in
the "Professional and Trades" section of the city directory, nurses were
identified as individuals offering special services to the public.

Nurses in mid-nineteenth-century Upper Canada struggled to carve
out a role that was sometimes complementary to and sometimes independent of other practitioners. They were part of a divergent array of
health care providers that also included regular physicians, druggists,
midwives, and a variety of non-regular medical practitioners.[46] As the
century progressed, physicians gained greater public approval through
innovations such as anaesthesia and physician management of obstetrics, and their numbers grew.[47] Middle-class women increasingly
looked to physicians for care in childbirth and this created fierce competition with midwives. It is perhaps not surprising that as physician
power and prestige grew, some midwives chose monthly nursing as an
alternative to midwifery, perhaps even masking their midwifery services
behind the title of nurse.

The Monthly Nurse

The term *monthly nurse* appeared interchangeably with *ladies'* or
lady's nurse in city directories and in the census; both terms indicated

a nurse who specialized in caring for mother and infant for one month postpartum. At mid-century, this appeared to be the most usual type of private work and it seems probable that it was through monthly nursing that the private nursing market developed in Toronto. Some midwives were known to prefer monthly nursing because each case provided four weeks of steady earnings.[48] From mid-century, the names of nurses appeared more frequently than midwives in the Toronto directories.

Some Toronto nurses may have initially combined the role of midwife and monthly nurse. For example, Mrs Scott of Richmond Street West was recorded in the 1861 directory as both a monthly nurse and a midwife.[49] In the census of the same year, most likely the same Mrs Scott was enumerated as a nurse living in St Andrew's Ward (which included Richmond Street). A forty-six-year-old widow born in Ireland, she was living in a one-storey frame house with her children Annie, a tailoress aged fifteen, and Ian, a fourteen-year-old printer. William Scott, sixty-three years old, had died the previous year of consumption.[50] Lacking a male breadwinner, a widow relied on the wages of her children to supplement her own work in order to make ends meet. In the case of Scott, she was also ensuring that her children learned a skilled trade. Mrs Elizabeth Miller of Adelaide Street moved freely between the roles of nurse and midwife. Listed as a midwife in the 1861 directory,[51] she was recorded in the census as a nurse living alone on Adelaide Street in a one-storey frame house. Irish-born, she was a fifty-year-old widow.[52] Subsequently, she appeared in the directory at the same address, but as a ladies' nurse[53] then later still just as a nurse.[54] It is possible that some women listed themselves as nurses but continued to practise midwifery. This seems more likely after 1865 legislation required midwives to be licensed.[55]

What were the specific duties of the monthly nurse? To gain some knowledge we can turn to the Victorian manual *Beeton's Book of Household Management*, first published in Britain in 1861. Best known as a recipe book, the manual included advice on the duties of servants, the management of the sick room, the rearing of children, and the medical treatment of disease.[56] It was a popular book and could have been brought to Toronto by middle-class immigrants or have been sent from England.[57] According to Isabella Beeton, desirable qualifications of the monthly nurse were that she be "scrupulously clean and tidy in her person; honest, sober, and noiseless in her movements; she should possess a natural love for children, and have a strong nerve in case of emergencies."[58] Age was important, with women between thirty and fifty years considered to have the required maturity but sufficient stamina to be on duty day and night. The nurse was expected to be observant, to notice problems or illness in her charges, and, if a doctor was called upon, to carefully follow his instructions. Problems with breastfeeding were considered one of the greatest challenges of the monthly nurse and she was advised to encourage the infant to feed frequently and, if necessary, to know how to keep the breasts "well drawn" to prevent inflammation. It is easy to see how the knowledge gained by an experienced midwife would be useful in fulfilling the duties of the monthly nurse. With regard to strictly domestic tasks, the nurse was expected to keep her patient's room clean and tidy, to empty slops promptly, and to help with laundry. Mrs Catherine Cole may have typified the monthly nurse of 1860s Toronto. A widow, she appeared first in the 1866 city directory as a ladies' nurse[59] and was subsequently listed for six years. From the 1871 census we learn that she was English-born and fifty-four years old. On the night of the census, she was enumerated in the home of a twenty-nine-year-old barrister, his wife, and new infant.

The Sick Nurse

Use of the term *sick nurse* was only occasionally employed in the Toronto public records.[60] Most women, if they were not designated as a monthly nurse, were simply titled *nurse*. Mary Ginn, according to the 1861 census, was a fifty-seven-year-old widow of English birth living in a one-storey frame house in central St John's Ward. She could read and write. The household included her daughter, thirty-one years, a dressmaker; an eleven-year-old girl (a family member); and a male lodger (a tanner). Widowhood may have sent Ginn into nursing since her return recorded the previous year's death of a sixty-five-year-old male in the household; it is after this that she first appeared as a nurse in the city directories.[61] Ginn was still working at age sixty-eight. Ann Lilley, a sixty-year-old widow of Scottish birth, was described as a sick nurse in the 1871 census[62] but did not advertise herself in the city directories.

The duties of the sick nurse can be ascertained from a variety of sources, such as *Beeton's Book of Household Management*, the writings of Florence Nightingale, and articles by contemporary physicians. Beeton anticipated that an experienced nurse would be hired in case of serious or lengthy illness, though she addressed her remarks to all women who might be called upon to care for the sick.[63] She was obviously a great admirer of Nightingale and, in her directives concerning ventilation, cleanliness, diet, and order in the sick room, quoted freely from Nightingale's *Notes on Nursing*. In her book, Nightingale advised on the personal conduct of the nurse, on the importance of keen, accurate observations, and on ways the patient could be helped to gain health and strength. She particularly urged the nurse to follow a doctor's orders and to avoid "amateur physiking."[64] To gain knowledge of procedures the nurse might be expected to perform we can turn to contemporary physicians.

Nurses were expected to provide assistance to the physician with procedures such as bloodletting, to give medications and therapeutic diets as ordered, and to carry out treatments such as poultices, enemas, and douches. Case studies in the *Canadian Lancet* indicated something of physician expectations. In describing an "unusual" postpartum case, a physician in 1872 noted that he relied on the attending nurse to administer medication every four hours, to give enemata, warm poultices, vaginal washes, and specific strengthening nourishment.[65] The nurse in this particular case was lauded as skilful in her observations and in calming the patient. In a further *Lancet* article, a physician discussed the use of "hot water injections in uterine disease." He considered that this treatment was "best done by an intelligent nurse."[66] As Canada had no programs for the training of nurses at the time, these physicians were most likely relying on the skills of a paid, experienced but untrained nurse. It is possible that a nurse could have gained experience in a hospital, but it is more likely that she acquired therapeutic knowledge from physicians in the course of her private work.

Toronto private nurses in the mid-Victorian period were usually middle-aged or older working-class widows. According to census information, the majority were literate and there is only the occasional record of a private nurse who could not read and write.[67] The majority lived in the well-populated inner city wards, some with their families,

some in boarding houses. For women living alone, boarding made
financial sense as nurses slept away from home when on a case. Although certain careers can be traced over more than a decade, the
names of nurses in the directories varied considerably from year to year.
This is not surprising given the often transient nature of working-class
life and the fact that work, for the married or widowed woman, had to
be adapted to family demands through the life cycle. It is hard to know
what type of status nurses had as workers in Toronto, or what kind of
living they made. It was unlikely that they attained the degree of mod-
est prosperity that Mortimer indicated for some of her Edinburgh
nurses. Edinburgh was a city known particularly for its medical training and practice and, therefore, a place where the more ambitious nurse
had opportunity to expand her skills and to gain clients. Toronto was
still a relatively small, mainly pre-industrial city with as yet poorly
developed hospitals and medical training. Yet some women did make
a living from private nursing. Exact numbers are hard to pinpoint, but
between 1850 and 1870 private nurses clearly emerged in Toronto as
a small but significant group of women workers.

Expansion of Nursing in the Industrialized City,
1870–91

Continuity and change can be traced among Toronto nurses as their
numbers grew in the decades of the 1870s and '80s. By 1891 the city's
population was 181,000 while the number of nurses that can be
counted in independent private work reached approximately 148, a
higher growth rate than that of the population. The significant increase
from twenty years earlier[68] can only be partially attributed to the
advent of the trained nurse. Although trained nurses had moved into
private work by the late 1880s, they remained a minority. Essentially,
the profile of the majority in the private workforce was the same as
in earlier decades.[69] This is in contrast to the picture presented in the
hospitals of the city. At first, expansion of institutions created jobs
for untrained workers,[70] but as training schools were established,
young probationers quickly replaced many of the existing workers.
The decade of the 1880s ushered in a period of transition for Toronto's
nurses at a time when rapid industrial growth meant "the scale of the

city and the texture of its life were radically transformed."[71] New jobs in health care were in part the result of new health and medical needs created by industrialization. But many nurses continued to service the domestic health care market, providing a range of service to poor and rich alike.

A Career for Widows: Private Nurses in Toronto

For most of the 1870s and '80s, private nursing in Toronto remained the domain of untrained women, the majority of them widows. Reverby observed that "widowhood was often the pathway into nursing,"[72] and throughout the decades of the nineteenth century, apart from their working-class status, widowhood stood out as the single most common factor among Toronto nurses. As a monthly nurse or sick nurse, a widow could draw on her experience of raising a family, whereas a career as a midwife required more specialized skills. In Toronto, the number of widows in earlier decades was particularly high, and although the proportion declined, it remained significant. In 1881, out of forty-three private nurses, twenty-six had lost a spouse; in 1891, despite the entry of young, single graduates into the market, a little over 50 per cent remained widows.[73] In the general population, Toronto consistently had more than three times as many widows as widowers.[74] According to historian Bettina Bradbury, widowers were much likelier to remarry – often to younger, single women less worn out by hard work and child rearing.[75] Working-class widows needed a means of support and, from my evidence, nursing provided, for some, a useful "survival strategy."[76]

Rosanna Baillie, a forty-five-year-old monthly nurse, was, at the time of the 1871 census, in the home of a physician and his wife who had just had a new baby.[77] This family was well able to afford a nurse as their household included four servants. We do not know when Baillie was widowed. She did have children as we later learn that she was living, first with a twenty-nine-year-old single son, a carpenter, and then with a married daughter.[78] According to the 1891 census, she was still wage-earning. The nursing career of Elizabeth Fidge can be traced from 1878 to 1895. A forty-nine-year-old widow in 1881, she was head of a household that included two children, fifteen and twenty-one years old, both wage-earning.[79] Later in her career, with children no doubt away from home, Fidge found it more convenient to board. A small percentage of nurses had a husband living.[80] Irish-born Anne Guidock lived with her Québécois husband, a labourer; a daughter aged sixteen, a dressmaker; and a school-aged son.[81] Very few of the early private nurses were single women but Elizabeth Williamson stands out, as it was possible to trace her career from 1877 to 1891. She was variously recorded as a nurse and as a ladies' nurse and remained living alone on Nassau Street, a working-class area of the inner city.[82]

In histories of nursing, the nineteenth-century untrained nurse was invariably portrayed as a mature woman. Data on the Toronto private nurses generally supported this view, with the majority being middle-aged. The ages of institutional nurses tended to be more widely divergent. In contrast to British statistics, where a considerable number of older nurses remained in the work force, there was very little evidence of nurses still working at seventy years of age. Why Toronto should be different from England is a matter for conjecture. Toronto's private nurses came from Ireland, England, or Scotland. Up to 1881 all but a very few were immigrants. Initially, the Irish predominated but by 1881 the English made up more than half. At mid-century, Irish-born residents were the single largest ethnic group in Toronto,[83] but from the 1860s, English immigrants predominated, as they had early in the century; the private nurse population reflected this change. There may have been nurses among other small ethnic groups in the city but if so, they were not identified in the census.

Nurses remained overwhelmingly working class. We know this from their living circumstances and the occupations of their daughters, sons, and husbands. Among the few husbands who were still living, we find a cook, a watchman, a labourer, and a tailor. Daughters were seamstresses, milliners, book folders, and housemaids, and sons were carpenters, labourers, furniture finishers, and butchers. Although the families of some nurses were of the unskilled working class, family members of a significant number were in the skilled trades. Daughters were more likely to be dressmakers than servants; many sons were in trades and a few were clerks.

By 1891 nurses lived throughout Toronto's twelve wards but the majority were centrally located in working-class neighbourhoods. Some moved frequently, the stability of home ownership being unlikely among the working class. As with many working-class people, the earnings of older children helped the family economy. Kate Rogers, widowed at quite a young age, had five children living at home when she was enumerated in 1881. With three children earning, as well as herself, she was able to keep her two daughters aged fifteen and eleven in school.[84] The nineteenth-century nurses of Toronto were mostly literate. There was only the occasional record of a nurse who was unable to read and write, a fact that challenges the way they are often presented in nursing history.

We do not know a great deal about the relationship between untrained private nurses and physicians. The *Canadian Lancet*, which commenced publication in the 1860s, only occasionally mentioned nurses.[85] Given a nurse's position, it is unlikely that, without formal training, she posed a threat to physicians. Her work involved personal care and household duties and, with regard to medical treatments, she was urged from mid-century to refer to the physician and to carefully carry out his instructions. In 1883, the *Lancet* announced a Directory for Nurses "under the auspices" of the Toronto Medical Society. The Directory was to be open day and night so that "persons in want of a nurse will always know where to apply."[86] As there were very few graduate nurses in Ontario at the time, the Directory must have relied on untrained nurses.

A Postscript on Midwifery in Toronto

Six midwives can be identified in the 1881 Toronto census but ten years later the name of only one, Mrs Hannah Woods, a forty-two-year-old Irish-born widow, can be found.[87] Prior to 1865 midwives in the province did not require a license, but according to historian J.T.H. Connor, even when the exemption from licensing was removed, unlicensed midwives were pursued less vigorously than individuals falsely representing themselves as physicians. However, midwives were placed in a legal "grey area."[88] Connor argued that the "demise" of midwifery was due to a variety of forces, not just pressure from physicians. He named as contributing factors the "ambivalence" of Victorian society toward midwifery as well as the inability of Ontario midwives to organize and arrange training programs.[89] Wendy Mitchinson concurred with Connor's multiple-causation theory,[90] though Lesley Biggs placed the elimination of midwifery squarely on the shoulders of the doctors who, she considered, in pushing for licensing, created terms it was impossible for midwives to fulfil.[91] Whatever the cause, with only one midwife identified in the 1891 census, they seem to have all but disappeared from city practice. As in earlier decades, some midwives continued to work as nurses. Mary O'Loughlin, recorded as a midwife in 1881, appeared in city directories up to 1886 as a nurse. Adelaide Newman, also a midwife in 1881, was recorded as a sick nurse ten years later.[92] We do not know if these women continued to attend deliveries along with their nursing work.

Toronto Hospital Nurses

Toronto General remained the only general hospital in the city until the last decade of the nineteenth century. At mid-century, according to historian J.T.H. Connor, nursing duties at the hospital were similar to those of a household maid. In the "pecking order," nurses warranted slightly higher pay than the washerwoman but less than the orderly, and employment, dependent as it was on patient numbers, could be transitory.[93] Toronto General had a very checkered early history due to frequent financial woes and warring medical factions, but also due to unsuitable staff. An 1855 inquiry into complaints about the hospital noted abuse by some staff, in particular Mrs Donelly, a nurse, who was rough and drank on duty.[94] As part of their duties in the new 1856 hospital, nurses were urged to behave with "tenderness and propriety" toward their charges.[95] At the time of the 1871 census, Toronto General had a matron and five nurses living on the premises. Ranging in age from eighteen to forty-six years, the nurses were a mix of English, Irish, and Scottish immigrant women, and two were widows.[96] For accounts of these nurses we must rely on Charles Clarke, medical superintendent, and Mary Agnes Snively who became lady superintendent in 1884.[97] Of staff in the 1870s, Clarke later recalled that two or three were said to be experienced, the rest "raw and uncultured ... [but] good enough girls." Eliza, an older woman, kept the patients in order at night but was not considered a good nurse.[98] Snively described the untrained nurses as mostly illiterate and "some intemperate."[99] Her comments on illiteracy are not exactly borne out by census information: in 1861, three out of eight nurses could not read or write; from 1871, all nurses at the General Hospital were recorded as literate. The charge of intemperance more likely holds, as excessive use of alcohol was common at all levels of Victorian society. Living conditions at Toronto General were rough. Nurses slept on straw beds on the wards and had meals in the basement. Pay was nine dollars per month, though if an employee gave up the daily beer allowance, wages were increased by one dollar.[100] Personal details of most nurses are lacking, but something is known of Margaret Davis, one of sixteen nurses at the General in 1881. A middle-aged widow,[101] she continued to work at the hospital after the nursing school was introduced in 1881 and was seen as a link between the 'old-time nurse' and the new. In a short obituary, which appeared in the newly published *Canadian Nurse* in 1905, Davis was described as lacking professional instruction but able to do "good work" according to her abilities, as a person who possessed "good common sense, loyalty and discipline."[102]

In 1871, the Toronto Lying-in Hospital had one nurse and a matron, both middle-aged widows, while the Provincial Lunatic Asylum employed twenty-three young women as nurses, along with male "keepers." The Hospital for Sick Children, newly established in 1875, was run by a Ladies' Committee that sought respectable, God-fearing women as nurses. Hiring and keeping staff was not always easy. As working-class women, nurses frequently had obligations to their own families. The Ladies' Committee tried to solve this problem by allowing some nurses to keep older dependent children with them at the hospital.[103] In 1881, the small hospital had two nurses, a forty-three-year-old Scottish-born widow and her eighteen-year-old daughter, as well as a matron and one servant to care for the twelve patients.[104] The nurses bathed, fed, and dressed the children, treated wounds and sores, rolled bandages, supervised play, and taught bedtime prayers. Most of the children had orthopaedic conditions and their splints and braces must have made daily hygiene difficult. The Ladies' Committee valued their workers and provided comfortable accommodation for them close to, but away from, the hospital.

Nurse Training Introduced in Toronto

By the end of the 1870s, Toronto, and most of Canada, had fallen behind Britain and the United States with regard to changes that were occurring in nursing.[105] The introduction of nurse training programs

was part of the expansion and reorganization of hospitals, which came
with developments in surgery and medicine,[106] but was also in response
to the work of philanthropic groups, particularly those of women.
Formal nurse training was intended not only to improve the care of the
sick but also to provide a suitable career for middle-class women.
Canada's first nursing school was started in 1874 in St Catharines,
Ontario; however, it was small and, by 1880, had only produced a
handful of graduates. In January 1879, the *Canadian Lancet* announced the establishment of a Training School for Nurses at the
Toronto General Hospital but it took another two years before the
school opened its doors.

When the nursing school opened, the seventeen untrained nurses at
Toronto General were offered places if they agreed to remain for two
years and then undergo an oral examination. Five agreed to these conditions and gained certificates two years later.[107] Early training school
standards were not high, but I consider that the successful transition of
these women does indicate a degree of competence and potential on
their part.[108] Not all the old-time nurses were dismissed – for example,
Margaret Davis remained at the General. However, she may have been
an exception since, when training schools were introduced,[109] most
untrained nurses in the hospitals were quickly replaced by young
trainees.[110] This change occurred much more slowly in private nursing.

Private Nursing in 1891

From the late 1880s graduate nurses entered private nursing in
Toronto.[111] In the early years, they constituted a relatively small group
but their arrival on the scene likely caused a rivalry with the existing
group of private nurses. No regulations defined practice and the title
nurse could be assumed by anyone. According to Susan Reverby in her
discussion of Boston private nurses,[112] the untrained practitioner
received less money than the trained. Although Toronto wages were
likely less, Boston graduates in the 1890s charged fifteen to eighteen
dollars a week while untrained nurses received five to ten dollars
less.[113] Job functions could be the same for both groups. Untrained
nurses were more likely to carry out postpartum care, since graduates
were less willing to undertake the domestic labour that this work involved. The old-time nurses had fewer inhibitions about performing

domestic chores and were comfortable with their place as members of the skilled working class.[114] In the 1891 census, at least seventeen Toronto nurses were named as ladies' nurses. Physicians in Toronto continued efforts to provide the names of nurses available for private work.[115] In 1890, a Directory for Nurses, with Dr W.H. Peplar as registrar, was located in an office at the College for Physicians and Surgeons of Ontario.[116] Many of the nurses on its books would still have been untrained. Some physicians were known to support the older nurses for less well-to-do patients because their services were more affordable than those of the new graduates.

It is evident that through the 1880s there was a considerable increase in the number of nurses in Toronto. During this time, the profile of nurses in the city was beginning to change as trained nurses entered the field, though this change was less dramatic in private work than in the hospitals. The majority of nurses in private work in 1891 were still widowed or married working-class women, and private nursing, without formal training, remained a practical way for them to earn a living.

+++

The nineteenth-century untrained nurse could be any one of a range of working-class women – from the highly respectable, intelligent practitioner to one who was both ignorant and uncaring. While acknowledging that some nurses were disreputable, it seems likely that many of the women carrying out nursing in Toronto were of the respectable working class, seeking to earn an honest living when it was difficult for women to obtain decent-paying work. In the words of Anne Summers, many were "neither unskilled nor unkind, just unrefined."[117] Through the decades of 1830 to 1890, Toronto nurses and midwives worked in a changing environment as the city evolved from a small colonial town to a centre of industry that was part of a self-governing nation. During this time capitalism and industrialization transformed the city and created a prosperous middle class that sought additional services for the home. In increasing numbers, working-class women offered their services as nurses. Their chief motivation was most likely survival not an altruistic desire to aid mankind, but as women without benefit of wealth or formal training, they took advantage of opportunities that came with the growing city.

According to the nineteenth-century Canadian census, nursing came under the occupational category of domestic and personal service. As long as nurses remained untrained, their position in a middle-class household was unambiguous and clearly that of a servant. Independent, private nurses were most commonly mature, working-class widows, or married women, possibly with some experience gained in the 'old country' but unregulated and without what we would consider formal training. We know that at least from the 1860s, most of them could read and write. Some used the 'professional' strategy of advertising to notify the public of their trade. In Toronto, it was midwives who initially advertised their services, then monthly nurses – some of whom were midwives – and finally general nurses who cared for the sick. It is difficult to discuss nineteenth-century nurses without including midwives as available evidence suggests that roles were fluid and midwives worked as monthly nurses or switched from midwife to nurse as their career progressed. This was probably because after 1865 unlicensed midwives were practising illegally in Ontario. There was certainly strong evidence from the Toronto records that, as the city grew, the number of midwives diminished and those remaining either practised as nurses or continued to deliver babies cloaked in the title of nurse.

Historians of women and work have explored the effect of waged work on women's work. Clearly, the advent of industrial work and, later, service work offered many women important alternatives to the domestic labour that had characterized women's labour options of the past. Still, historians recognize that many of the new waged jobs for women were extensions of female domestic labour and, as such, were often devalued and underpaid. The emergence of nursing as a paid work option must be seen as part of this process.

During the course of the nineteenth century, nursing developments occurred in the open market in health services. Growth of the city created an increasing number of working women but also a prosperous class who sought paid nursing services in the home. With restrictions on midwifery, women turned to private nursing and this form of caregiving became the most common type of paid nursing work. Until hospitals were seen to provide 'scientific' care and a suitable environment for middle-class patients, nursing in the home remained the predominant mode of care for all but the most disadvantaged. By the last decade of the century, there was a mix of trained and untrained nurses in Toronto. As the major caregiver in hospitals, the old-time nurse was quickly replaced but the inevitability of her disappearance from the private arena was less certain at this stage. In 1891 the majority of private nurses continued to practise as they had in previous decades – without formal education – while a few made the transition to graduate status. Though it is possible to gain some understanding of the women working as nurses in Victorian Toronto, much remains unknown about this elusive group.

NOTES

I should like to acknowledge the significant help given by Kathryn McPherson, Department of History, York University, Toronto, Ontario, in guiding the research and writing on which this essay is based. I also thank the anonymous reviewers for their suggestions for revision of this article.

1 I focus exclusively on female nurses. Except for male "attendants" at the Provincial Lunatic Asylum, I found no mention of male nurses in the Toronto records until 1895 when four were listed in the city directory. The situation on the east coast (St. John, NB and Halifax) was different and male nurses can be identified in the census for 1871 and 1881, no doubt a reminder of the tradition of male caregivers in the early military hospitals of the region.

2 For accounts of early nurses in Canada see John M. Gibbon and Mary S. Mathewson, *Three Centuries of Canadian Nursing* (Toronto: The MacMillan Company of Canada Limited, 1947) and Joyce M. MacQueen, "Who the Dickens Brought Sarai Gamp to Canada," in *The Canadian Journal of Nursing Research* 21, 2 (Summer 1989): 27–36. Nineteenth-century nurses have received brief mention in Canadian women's labour history. For example, Elizabeth J. Errington, *Wives and Mothers, School Mistresses and Scullery Maids: Working Women in Upper Canada 1790–1840* (Montreal & Kingston: McGill-Queens University Press, 1995) and Marjorie Griffith Cohen, *Women's Work: Markets and Economic Development in Nineteenth Century Ontario* (Toronto: University of Toronto Press, 1988). The inadequate skills of lay nurses are discussed in literature on Canadian epidemics. See Michael Bliss, *Plague: A Story of Smallpox in Montreal* (Toronto: Harper Collins, 1991) and Geoffrey Bilson, *A Darkened House: Cholera in Nineteenth Century Canada* (Toronto: University of Toronto Press, 1980).

3 J.T.H. Connor, *Doing Good: The Life of Toronto's General Hospital* (Toronto:

University of Toronto Press, 2000), 104–5. The secure funding came through the Ontario government's Charity Aid Act of 1874.

4 The term was used by Susan Reverby in her history of the development of American nursing. See Susan Reverby, *The Dilemma of American Nursing 1850–1945* (Cambridge and New York: Cambridge University Press, 1987), 11–21.

5 Elizabeth Innes of Saint John, New Brunswick did leave a diary. Born in 1786, she worked as a midwife and monthly nurse and nursed the sick. Her diary is in the New Brunswick Museum, Saint John.

6 By combining information from the census, city directories, and hospital and insurance records, Mortimer followed the careers of Edinburgh nurses from 1850 to 1870. See Barbara Mortimer, "Independent Women: Domiciliary Nurses in Mid-Nineteenth-Century Edinburgh." In Anne Marie Rafferty, Jane Robinson, and Ruth Elkan, eds., *Nursing History and the Politics of Welfare*, 133–49 (London: Routledge, 1997) and Barbara Mortimer, "Counting Nurses: Nursing in the 19th Century Census," in *Nurse Researcher* 5, 2 (Winter 1997/8): 31–43. See also Anne Summers, "The Mysterious Demise of Sarah Gamp: The Domiciliary Nurse and Her Detractors c. 1830–1860," in *Victorian Studies* 32, 3 (1989): 365–86. Summer's research is focused on London, England.

7 I have utilized the Canadian censuses for 1861, 1871, 1881, and 1891 and the York/Toronto City Directories between 1833 and 1891. Toronto data from the 1851 census has been lost. The nominal records of the Toronto census are on microfilm at the Toronto Reference Library, 789 Yonge Street, Toronto, Ontario. City directories are also in the Reference Library and those from 1833 to 1876 can also be accessed through the Library's website: http://digitalcollections.torontopubliclibrary.ca.

8 My numbers are estimates only. In order to identify nurses in private work, I studied the household. If a nurse was enumerated as the head of a working-class household (or with a husband), she was most likely practising independently. Nurses enumerated with other families were harder to differentiate though some private nurses could be cross-checked in city directories and counted as 'on the job.' Children's nurses (nannies) were, on the whole, young women and the term "nurse girl" indicated a very young nursemaid or childminder (aged from eleven years). Differentiation was made easier in the 1891 census when children's nurses were termed "domestic" in relation to the head of the household.

9 The Sisters of St. Joseph arrived in Toronto in 1851.

10 Edith G. Firth, ed., *The Town of York 1815–1834: Further Documents of Early Toronto* (Toronto: University of Toronto Press, 1966), xviii.

11 Paul Starr, *The Social Transformation of American Medicine* (New York: Basic Books, 1982), 32.

12 J.T.H. Connor, "'Larger Fish to Catch Here Than Midwives': Midwifery and the Medical Profession in Nineteenth-Century Ontario." In Dianne Dodd and Deborah Gorham, eds., *Caring and Curing: Historical Perspectives on Women and Healing in Canada*, 110 (Ottawa: University of Ottawa Press, 1994). Originally quoted in Eric Hounsome, *Toronto in 1810* (Toronto: Coles, 1975), 72.

13 Connor, "'Larger Fish to Catch Here,'" 110.

14 Errington, *Wives and Mothers, School Mistresses and Scullery Maids*, 63.

15 R.D. Gidney and W.P.J. Millar, *Professional Gentlemen: The Professions in Nineteenth Century Ontario* (Toronto: University of Toronto Press, 1994), 23.

16 Firth, *The Town of York 1815–1834*, 237. Letter from Dr Widmer to the Lieutenant Governor, April 1832. When the Lying-In Hospital finally opened in 1848 it provided instruction for medical students but not midwives.

17 Ibid., 227.

18 Ibid., lxii. The building was paid for by surplus funds collected for veterans of the 1812 War. Money was sufficient for a brick building but insufficient to furnish and staff the hospital. It was used as a temporary legislature for several years.

19 Control of local government by the "Family Compact," an elite group of landowners, led to the Rebellion of 1837. A few years later, with the Union of Upper and Lower Canada, the colony was granted more responsible government.

20 George Walton, *York Commercial Directory, Street Guide, and Register, 1833–34*, 20 and 74.

21 Laurel Thatcher Ulrich, *A Midwife's Tale: The Life of Martha Ballard, Based on Her Diary, 1785–1812* (New York: Vintage Books, 1991), 40. During August of 1787, Ballard performed four deliveries, made sixteen 'sick' calls mainly to children, prepared three bodies for burial, and dispensed medication to a neighbour. One of the sick calls was to a male with a wounded leg, another to a boy with a rash.

22 Connor, "'Larger Fish to Catch Here,'" 105.

23 Francis Lewis, *The Toronto Directory and Street Guide for 1843–4*, 51.

24 Connor, "'Larger Fish to Catch Here,'" 110 and 130.

25 J. Armstrong, *Rownsell's City of Toronto and County of York Directory for 1850–51*, 83.

26 Vern L. Bullough and Bonnie Bullough, *The Emergence of Modern Nursing* (Toronto: The MacMillan Company, 1969), 76–7.

27 Mortimer, "Independent Women."

28 Wendy Mitchinson, *The Nature of Their Bodies: Women and Their Doctors in Victorian Canada* (Toronto: University of Toronto Press, 1991), 184–5. Mitchinson noted that training was available to women at mid-century.

29 J. Armstrong, *Rownsell's City of Toronto and County of York Directory for 1850–51*, xxxviii.

30 Mitchinson, *The Nature of Their Bodies*, 169.

31 Ibid., 168–69.

32 Errington, *Wives and Mothers*, 58.

33 W.H. Pearson, *Recollections and Records of Toronto of Old* (Toronto: William Briggs, 1914), 122–3.

34 Henry Scadding, *Toronto of Old*. Abridged and edited by F.H. Armstrong (Toronto: University of Toronto Press, 1996). Complete edition first published in 1873.

35 J. Armstrong, *Rounsell's City of Toronto and County of York Directory for 1850–51*, xxvii.

36 George Brown, *Brown's Toronto City and Home District Directory 1846–7*, 31. The impressive Queen Street Asylum did not open until 1850.

37 Firth, *The Town of York 1815–1834*, 236. The *Canadian Freeman* was a local newspaper.

38 Geoffrey Bilson, *A Darkened House: Cholera in Nineteenth Century Canada* (Toronto: University of Toronto Press, 1980).

39 Bilson, *A Darkened House*, 88. Sheward's comments were addressed to governor Sir John Colborne.

40 Pearson, *Recollections and Records of Toronto of Old*, 120.

41 Bilson, *A Darkened House*, 56.

42 Carolyn Strange, *Toronto's Girl Problem: The Perils and Pleasures of the City 1880–1930* (Toronto: University of Toronto Press, 1995). In 1851 the ratio was 102.7 women to 100 men. This had increased by 1901 to a ratio of 112.5 to 100.

43 J. Armstrong, *Rowsell's City of Toronto and County of York Directory for 1850–51* published in 1850. There is no separate listing of nurses but they can be identified at their street addresses. All lived in the downtown area.

44 Directories were only published intermittently. The next, in 1856, yielded the name of one midwife but no nurses while, in 1859, six nurses were listed but no midwives. The directories were not published annually until 1861.

45 I calculated as follows. Of the eighty-six women recorded as nurses I considered nineteen to be independent private nurses, thirty-nine children's nurses or nursemaids, while twenty-eight worked in institutions.

46 Gidney and Millar, *Professional Gentlemen*, 100.

47 Toronto directories listed forty-six physicians for 1861, including four home-opaths (*Brown's Toronto General Directory for 1861–62*, 328) and fifty-three physicians for 1871 (*Robertson's and Cook's Toronto City Directory for 1871–72*, 305).

48 Mortimer, "Independent Women."

49 W.R. Brown, *Brown's Toronto General Directory for 1861–62*, 258 and 326.

50 Census for 1861, Reel C1101, St Andrew's Ward, Div. 3. No. 121.

51 Brown, *Brown's Toronto General Directory for 1861–62*, 221.

52 Census for 1861, Reel C1101, St Andrew's Ward, Div. 3, No. 189.

53 J.L. Mitchell, *Mitchell's Toronto Directory for 1864–65*, 189.

54 *Mitchell and Co's General Directory for the City of Toronto 1866*, 3.

55 As there were no training programs in Upper Canada, midwives lacked the means of obtaining the necessary qualifications for a license.

56 Isabella Beeton, *Beeton's Book of Household Management* (London: Jonathan Cape Limited, 1968), 1020–2. A first edition facsimile. First published in bound edition 1861.

57 There are two copies of the early edition in the University of Toronto libraries.

58 Beeton, *Beeton's Book of Household Management*, 1020.

59 *Mitchell and Co's General Directory for the City of Toronto 1866*, 145.

60 Sick nurse and the French equivalent, *garde malade*, appear much more frequently in the Montreal censuses.

61 Census for 1861, Reel C1106, St John's Ward, Div. 3.5, No. 69. See also directories for 1862, 1866, 1870, and 1872.

62 Census for 1871, Reel C633, St John's Ward, Div. 3, No. 41.

63 Beeton, *Beeton's Book of Household Management*, 1017–20.

64 Florence Nightingale, *Notes on Nursing: What It Is and What It Is Not* (Philadelphia: J.B. Lippincott Company, 1992), 74. Commemorative edition. First published in London 1859.

65 S.S. Connell, "Case of Catalepsy," in *Canadian Lancet* 4, 7 (March 1872): 308–13.

66 T.A. Emmet, "Hot Water Injections in Uterine Disease," in *Canadian Lancet* 7, 3 (November 1874): 82.

67 Mrs Mary Boys, a forty-nine-year-old monthly nurse born in England, was an exception. She could not read or write and her census schedule was signed by her twenty-one-year-old son, a clerk (Census for 1861, Reel C1106, St John's Ward, Div. 1, No. 98).

68 Although all my numbers are approximate, there were not more than twenty in 1871.

69 Of the 148 private nurses I calculated in the 1891 census, 36 (24 per cent) listed themselves as "trained" or "professional" or could be identified as such from training school records.

70 New institutions included the Hospital for Sick Children, the Andrew Mercer Eye and Ear Infirmary, and the Smallpox Hospital (formerly a House of Refuge). Three Lying-In Hospitals amalgamated in 1869 to form the Burnside Lying-In Hospital. Toronto General remained the only general hospital until St Michael's was opened by the Sisters of St Joseph in 1892.

71 Peter G. Goheen, *Victorian Toronto 1850–1900* (Chicago: University of Chicago Press, 1970), 221.

72 Reverby, *Ordered to Care*, 16.

73 There were 74 widows out of 148.

74 In 1871 the ratio was 627 widowers to 2,304 widows; in 1881, 995 to 3,231; and in 1891, 1,632 to 5,295.

75 Bettina Bradbury, *Working Families: Age, Gender, and Daily Survival in Industrializing Montreal* (Toronto: Oxford University Press, 1993), 184–5.

76 Bradbury lists a variety of jobs including shopkeeping, charring, taking in washing, and taking in lodgers but does not include nursing. See Bradbury, *Working Families*, 197–203.

77 Census 1871, Reel C633, St John's, Div. 2, 12.

78 Census 1881, Reel C13246, Div. C1, 59 and Census 1891, Reel T6372, Div. H6, 100.

79 Census 1881, Reel C13246, Div. D1, 57. See also directories for 1878, 1890, and 1891.

80 Out of forty-three in 1881, seven were enumerated with husbands.

81 Census 1881, Reel C13247, Div. G3, 51.

82 See Might and Taylor, *Toronto Directory for 1877*, 394 and *Toronto City Directory for 1891* (Might's Directory Co.), 1605. See also Census for 1881, Reel C13247, Div. H2, 2 and Census for 1991, Reel T6372, Div. G6, 44.

83 J.M.S. Careless, *Toronto to 1918: An Illustrated History* (Toronto: James Lorimer and Co. Publishers, 1984), 74.

84 Census 1881, Reel C13246, Div. D2, 148.

85 Nurses are mentioned in a few early case studies and, starting in the late 1870s, the question of nurse training is discussed.

86 "Directory for Nurses," in *Canadian Lancet* 15, 5 (January 1883), 159.

87 Census 1891, Reel T6371, Div. E3, 13 and *Toronto City Directory for 1890* (Might's Directory Co.), 1453.

88 Connor, "'Larger Fish to Catch Here,'" 107.

89 Connor, "'Larger Fish to Catch Here,'" 122.

90 Mitchinson, *The Nature of Their Bodies*, 162–75.

91 C. Lesley Biggs, "The Case of the Missing Midwives: A History of Midwifery in Ontario." In Katherine Arnup, Andrée Lévesque, and Ruth Roach Pierson, eds., *Delivering Motherhood: Maternal Ideologies and Practices in the 19th and 20th Centuries*, 20–35 (London and New York: Routledge, 1990).

92 Census for 1881, Reel C13247, Div. G1, 48 and Census 1891, Reel T6370, Div. B1, 4.

93 Connor, *Doing Good*, 50.

94 Ibid., 72. Donelly was also accused of threatening medical students and jumping on a patient. An orderly was also cited as abusive.

95 Ibid., 87.

96 Census 1871, Reel 634, St David's, Div. 4, 58.

97 Charles Kirk Clarke, *A History of the Toronto General Hospital* (Toronto: William Briggs, 1913) and Mary Agnes Snively, "The Toronto General Hospital Training School for Nurses," in *Canadian Nurse*, 1 (March 1905): 7–9.

98 Clarke, *History of Toronto General*, 82.

99 Snively, "The Toronto General Training School for Nurses," 7.

100 Snively, "The Toronto General Training School for Nurses," 7. This was in 1879.

101 Census 1881, Reel C13246, Div. B3, 145.

102 E.C. G[ordon], "Mrs Davis," in *Canadian Nurse* 1 (December 1905): 39.

103 There is a record of at least two nurses allowed to keep older children with them. One highly regarded nurse left in 1877 to be with her very young children in the Orphan's Home. See Judith Young, "A Divine Mission: Elizabeth McMaster and the Hospital for Sick Children, Toronto, 1875–92," in *Canadian Bulletin of Medical History* 11, 1 (1994): 71–90.

104 Census 1881, Reel C13246, Div. D2, 143.

105 The well-known Nightingale School at St Thomas' Hospital dates from 1860. In the U.S., the first nursing school was in 1873 at the Bellevue Hospital, New York. This was quickly followed by eleven more USA schools.

106 Two classic accounts of this change are Charles E. Rosenberg, *The Care of Strangers* (New York: Basic Books, 1987) and Morris J. Vogel. *The Invention of the Modern Hospital* (Chicago: University of Chicago Press, 1980).

107 Snively, "The Toronto General Training School."

108 A similar situation occurred at the Hamilton General Hospital when two nurses already employed at the hospital became the new school's first graduates in 1891. See Marjorie Freeman Campbell, *The Hamilton General School of Nursing 1890–1955* (Toronto: The Ryerson Press, 1956).

109 Prior to 1890, a further four schools were started in Ontario towns and cities and another in Toronto at the Hospital for Sick Children.

110 In the 1891 census all but one of the nurses recorded at the Hospital for Sick Children were trainees who subsequently graduated. The hospital started a training program in 1886.

111 In the Toronto directories, the first graduate nurse I identified in private work was in 1886 (Annie Boyd, a Toronto General graduate). The Toronto General had earlier sent out its students, in the course of their training, to nurse in private homes. This was a common practice in the early schools and provided added income for the hospital.

112 Susan M. Reverby, "'Neither for the Drawing Room Nor for the Kitchen': Private Duty Nursing in Boston, 1873–1920, Women and Health in America," in Judith Walzer Leavitt, ed., 2nd ed., 460–74 (Madison: University of Wisconsin Press, 1999). This article also appeared in the first edition in 1984.

113 Ibid., 465.

114 Ibid., 463–4.

115 The first nurse-run registry in Toronto was set up in 1905.

116 *Toronto City Directory for 1890* (Might's Directory Co.). As the College of Physicians and Surgeons of Ontario rented out rooms in its new building, the directory was not necessarily under its auspices.

117 Anne Summers, "The Mysterious Demise of Sarah Gamp: The Domiciliary Nurse and Her Detractors c. 1830–1860," in *Victorian Studies* 32, 3 (1989), 376.

2

+++++

Catching Babies and Delivering the Dead: Midwives and
Undertakers in Mennonite Settlement Communities

MARLENE EPP

Aganetha Reimer was a community midwife in Steinbach, Manitoba,
until 1938 when, after a hospital was built, her career gradually came
to an end. She had taken a three-week course in birthing and the use
of home remedies from a Minnesota woman, who was summoned to
Manitoba in the late nineteenth century when the need for a midwife
in town was felt "very badly." Reimer assisted at the delivery of almost 700 babies, in one case attending a birth only three days after
giving birth herself. Reimer also functioned as the undertaker, bathing
and clothing the bodies of the dead and helping to arrange their
coffins. In reflecting on Reimer's life, her grandson commented: "It
seems entirely fitting to me that in pioneer times the local midwife
usually served also as an unofficial, behind-the-scenes undertaker.
Who would understand better than a midwife that the squirming,
squalling new human emerging so eagerly from the womb must someday end in the marble dignity of the dead, all care, woes and fleeting
joys gone forever."[1]
For most of human history, women have given birth in their own
homes, either alone or assisted by family members or neighbours, by
lay or professional midwives, or by doctors. In Canada, homebirths predominated until just before the Second World War.[2] Even in Ontario –
where urbanization and industrialization began earlier – more births
occurred at home than in hospital right up until 1938.[3] In rural and
remote areas, hospitalization as a norm for childbirth came even later.

[Prior to the hospitalization and medicalization of childbirth, the community midwife was a central figure in the lives and households of women giving birth.]

[Much of the published literature on midwifery explores reasons and factors in the early twentieth-century decline of lay or trained midwives, or examines midwifery in the context of the medicalization of childbirth. The gradual near-disappearance of baby-catching[4] – prior to its late twentieth-century resurgence and recognition, of course – as a female vocational option is generally [attributed to technological developments that gave preference and prominence to medical-scientific approaches to childbirth as well as institutional hegemony over the regulation of childbirth. As such, the historical and contemporary literature on midwifery frequently focuses on the relationship between midwives and physicians, and often assumes a dynamic of hostility between the two.[5] Such investigations have emphasized a turf-war struggle in which midwives – whether trained formally or informally – and medical school–educated physicians each tried to claim their superior skill in assisting a woman in childbirth. [More recent studies, however, suggest that the dynamic between midwives and doctors was more complex, more variable, and at times mutually beneficial when it came to maximizing support for women in childbirth.[6] In sparsely [settled rural areas, for instance, there may have been more of an alliance between midwives and doctors, as both tried to serve families with high fertility rates over large geographic distances]. Toward the middle of the twentieth century, as the number of midwives began to decline while the number of physicians increased, there was inevitably a period of overlap during which families might have a choice between one or the other. Unless a woman in labour had a particular affinity for a female baby-catcher, or for a male doctor, she [may well have opted for whoever was nearest and likely to arrive first.] Furthermore, for identifiable ethnic or religious minority groups, the cultural identity of a woman's labour attendant may have been a factor of equal, or sometimes greater, consideration, alongside sex and vocational training.

This essay will not address the midwife-physician debate to any great extent. Nor will I add anything substantially new to our understanding of the decline of community lay midwifery during an era of increasing medicalization of childbirth. I do want to address the [role of community midwives in a particular ethno-religious group, the Mennonites, and attempt to give visibility to their vocational importance within the social, familial, and religious life of immigrant, rural settlers. Furthermore, I wish to highlight the fact that in many settings, midwifery was a "many-faceted calling"[7] in which a woman took upon herself a wide range of health care duties. The historiographical emphasis on the dynamic between midwives and ·physicians has focused, for obvious reasons, on the specific skills and tasks that related to childbirth, without addressing the more general role midwives played in cases of illness and injury. Few studies of midwifery really explore the vocational identity of women who were, in some cases, the primary health care provider within a large geographic area, though a recent article about 'lay nursing' in Canada points out that "nursing and midwifery are hard to separate" in accounts of early caregiving.[8] The range of healing skills offered by midwives, as well as their relatively easy movement between the role of 'midwife' and that of 'nurse' is demonstrated by both Judith Young and Linda Kealey in their essays in this volume. In addition to their more well-known functions as birth attendants and village healers, some Mennonite midwives also attended at deathbeds and functioned informally as community undertakers. This study represents an initial exploration into the fascinating confluence of life and death in the vocational roles of midwives in early Mennonite settlement communities.

Even while the much-examined 'decline' of midwifery in Canada was escalating in the first half of the twentieth century, midwives in rural and ethnic communities continued to fulfill an essential semi-public function. In early Mennonite immigrant settlements, whether along the Grand River in southwestern Ontario or on the prairies or, in later eras, on Pelee Island in Lake Erie or in the Fraser Valley of British Columbia, the midwife-healer was a central community figure. Given that many new immigrant groups as well as long-resident ethnic groups in both Canada and the United States retained the services of midwives longer than in so-called 'English' communities, it is actually surprising that there have been few particularized studies of midwives or birth practices within identifiable cultural groups. Exceptions to this in Canada include various studies of childbirth in Newfoundland and within First Nations communities, as well as an oral history of

childbirth as experienced by Mennonite women.[9] In her study of the
professionalization of childbirth in Wisconsin, Charlotte G. Borst
acknowledges that the relationship between midwifery and immigrant
communities was an important one, and hasn't been adequately
explored.[10] And in her survey of childbirth in Canada in the first half
of the twentieth century, Wendy Mitchinson proposes that: "Midwifery lasted longest in cohesive communities that were isolated
from the pressures of modern industrialized society as a result of
geographic or cultural separation."[11] This was certainly true for first-
and sometimes second-generation Mennonite immigrants to Canada.
As further evidence of the linkage between midwifery and cohesive
communities, various studies have noted that immigrant women predominated among midwives in both the United States and Canada
during the era of high migration from Europe in the late nineteenth
and early twentieth centuries. Judith Young, in chapter 1, demonstrates the predominance of immigrant women among midwives in
nineteenth-century Toronto, although all of these were from Ireland,
England, or Scotland as opposed to continental Europe or other
source countries. For some immigrant groups, the practices and functions of community midwives were among a range of cultural and
belief traditions that were maintained, sometimes modified, through
the process of leaving their homeland for new horizons.

[Maintaining 'old country' practices of midwife-assisted births once
in Canada helped ethnic groups like the Mennonites conserve an important sense of group and cultural identity. The fact that Mennonites
settled in rural group concentrations and were, at least in the early
decades, geographically isolated meant that women of necessity relied
for birthing assistance on women within their own group. For nineteenth-century Mennonite immigrants from Russia, vocational midwives also served to reinforce traditional practice in the midst of an
initially unfamiliar environment that required social and economic
adaptation in many other respects. Although there are limited available
sources on the practice of midwifery among Mennonites in nineteenth-
century Russia, one historian has concluded that, "male doctors, professionally trained or self-taught, were rarely called upon to assist with
deliveries. This was the domain of the midwife."[12] At least earlier in the
century, few midwives had specialized training, the only qualifications
for their vocation being that they were female and had assisted at other

deliveries. That community midwives may have been quite plentiful within the Mennonite settlements of southern Russia is implied in the diary of one Mennonite leader whose wife was assisted by four different midwives for five births in an eleven-year period.[13]

Given the tumultuous events of the early twentieth century in the Russian empire and then Soviet Union that brought crisis to Mennonite families and settlements, midwives on occasion found themselves in circumstances that they would never face in Canada. Susanna Epp, trained as a midwife in Prussia in 1906, travelled with four armed men when she was summoned to assist women in labour during the years of the Bolshevik Revolution and civil war and anarchy that followed. In one case, Makhnovite anarchists threatened to shoot her if she didn't assist at a difficult birth or if the mother died. Epp insisted that a witness be present, and although the child was stillborn, she was able to save the mother. Apparently, the Makhnovites then gave her a letter that allowed her to travel unhindered.[14] It is clear that midwives served crucial occupational roles within the Mennonite settlements of Ukraine and, quite possibly, had an even more professionalized status than they would have later in Canada.

Many of the earliest midwives practising on the Canadian prairies received their training and had begun to exercise their vocation while still resident in Russia in the nineteenth and early twentieth centuries, where they sometimes were officially appointed to their positions. One example is Katherina Born Thiessen who went to Germany in 1860 where she received training in midwifery, bone-setting, and naturopathic treatment. After marriage in 1862, she migrated to Kansas in 1874, serving as the 'practical doctor' for the community until the family moved north to homestead in Manitoba eleven years later.[15] Elizabeth Harder Harms, after training for two years in the city of Riga, was certified as a midwife in 1912, and the next year was hired to be the official midwife in Schoenfeld, a village within the Mennonite settlements of Ukraine. When Harms immigrated to Canada in 1925, she continued to practise community midwifery, although her husband did not consider it proper for her to work in a hospital when she was offered such a job.[16] Similarly, Katharina Ratzlaff Epp studied bone-setting and also took a course on obstetrics in Russia in the 1920s. She later entered the school of medicine in Halbstadt in the Mennonite settlement of Molotschna, but was unable to receive a diploma because

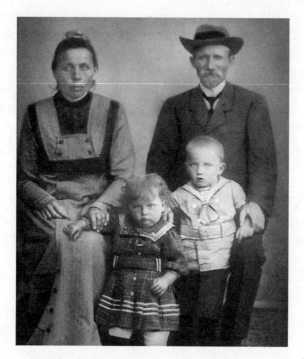

2.1 Sarah Thielman with her family. Thielman was
a midwife who worked in Russia, Saskatchewan, and
Ontario. She recorded over 1,000 births between
1909 and 1941.

of her unwillingness to join the Communist party. When she migrated
to Paraguay in 1930, she continued her varied practice that included
midwifery and nursing, bone-setting, physical therapy, and counselling.
She was called Dr Epp though she had no medical credentials.[17] In such
cases, community recognition and respect of skill surpassed professional certification.

It is difficult to investigate the practice of midwifery within frontier
and early settlement communities, or within somewhat closed immigrant groups, because written records are extremely limited. Those
midwives who did keep a log of births attended often recorded little
more than a date and a name; some were just too busy or considered
their work too informal to do even that. Rare are journals such as that
kept by Sarah Dekker Thielman, a Mennonite midwife who migrated
to Canada from the Soviet Union in 1929. Thielman's record book,

which included descriptions of and treatments for female maladies, and detailed drawings of the female anatomy, also recorded over 1,000 births at which she presided between the years 1909 and 1941. Like in the record book of Myra Bennett, described by Linda Kealey in chapter 3, each of Thielman's entries includes obvious statistical information – date and time of birth, weight and length of infant, for instance – but also details about the mother's temperature, length of contractions, complications of the birth, and name of the father.[18] As other historians have found, the common female vocation of healer or midwife in the pre-industrial era is the most difficult to document, despite its importance to communities.

The Mennonite midwife in late nineteenth- and early twentieth-century Canadian settlement communities functioned much like the early modern European midwife of the fifteenth through seventeenth centuries. Like the early modern midwife, and indeed similar to the Toronto midwives profiled by Judith Young in chapter 1, Mennonite baby-catchers varied widely in their training, skill level, degree of multiple roles, and level of activity. Midwives of the early modern period in Europe shared certain characteristics, which are described by Hilary Marland as follows: "Most were mature women, married or widowed, who started to practice when they had grown-up families, most were trained by some form of apprenticeship, formal or informal, most were of middling status, the wives of artisans, craftsmen, tradesmen or farmers, for whom the practice of midwifery, though not necessarily vital for the family income, was a useful addition."[19] As in the early modern period, many Mennonite midwives performed a multitude of health-related functions other than assisting at childbirth. Because of the diversity of the tasks they performed, traditional – as opposed to professional – midwives were also called "handywomen."[20] The degree of training and expertise they possessed also varied. Some midwives received formal obstetrical training in Russia or Germany prior to immigration, while others took short courses in Canada. The nineteenth-century Mennonite settlers in Manitoba, aware of the vital need for a trained midwife to assist with the numerous births that occurred in the highly fertile community, brought a midwife from a sister community in Minnesota to provide a few weeks of training to several Canadian Mennonite women. Other women trained as apprentices, often working alongside their own mothers who passed along their knowledge. Some women functioned more in the tradition of *Kind-betthelferinnen* – helpers in childbed – who looked after the women in labour until the real midwife arrived, and then remained to offer care after the birth.

Birthing was often the primary, but rarely the only, health service offered by women described as midwives. Women sometimes began their practices by assisting at childbirth, but once their skills and acumen were verified, people would seek them out for other services, such as pulling teeth, tending to injuries, and offering advice and treatment for various maladies. Conversely, in some cases a wider healing practice would gradually incorporate midwifery services. In particular, bone-setting and other chiropractic-related treatments were common accompaniments to a midwifery practice. Few rural midwives within Mennonite settlements were just birth attendants. With trained medical personnel virtually non-existent in early rural immigrant communities, and hospitals and doctors many kilometres away, "the most important medical person in the community was the midwife."[21]

One example of this multi-functionality is Katherina Hiebert who became possibly the first midwife to serve Mennonite pioneer women and their families of southern Manitoba after immigrating herself in 1875. Hiebert received recipes for herbal treatments from neighbouring Aboriginal women and was known to roam the woods and meadows collecting "Swedish bitters, chamomile, and thyme."[22] Assisting French, English, and Mennonite women, she was mainly self-taught, ordering medical books from Germany and the United States as well as receiving advice from Aboriginal women. In a spread-out community of large families, midwives were kept busy and it is said that, "almost every day somebody called for Katherina." Her daughter recalled that, "She was always away, day and night, summer and winter, tending the sick."[23] Katherina Born Thiessen, mentioned above, included in her varied practice "expertly delivering babies, setting bones, diagnosing illnesses and prescribing remedies for everything from lung disorders to skin cancer, and also saving lives through emergency surgery." In her later years, her activity consisted largely of selling "Dr Chase's Patent Medicines."[24] Another trained midwife, Elizabeth Harder Harms, found herself providing a wide array of medical care when she moved to the immigrant community of Yarrow, British Columbia in the early 1930s. She mixed her own pharmaceutical compounds and created a successful remedy to treat a unique infection under the fingernails, caused by strong cleaning solutions, that plagued Mennonite women who worked as domestic help.[25] Barbara Bowman Shuh, an Ontario Mennonite midwife who died in 1937, was known to have inherited the 'gift' of charming, a traditional semi-spiritual folk healing practice, which she used mainly for treating bleeding, burns, and scalds.[26] Sharing both name and vocation with Shuh was her contemporary, Barbara Zehr Schultz, trained in midwifery by her grandfather, but whose skill in herbal medicine and charming went beyond his.[27]

Early Mennonite settlement patterns, at least those that were established in Manitoba and Saskatchewan and, in modified form, in British Columbia, may have enhanced the viability of a midwife's practice, and also allowed the vocation itself to persist longer than elsewhere. On the prairies, Mennonite immigrants initially lived on farms situated in 'street villages' organized within block reserves, settlement patterns that had existed in Russia for over a hundred years prior. The street village was created when ten to thirty families combined their homestead allotments, and then built their homes and barns (the two buildings often connected) closely together along a central road. The surrounding pastureland and fields were then divided or worked commonly.[28] The block reserves meant that, at least in the earliest years, Mennonites lived within geographically and ethnically defined rural enclaves, while the street villages saw rural households located in much closer proximity than was the case in most homesteading patterns. With their 'rural' homes thus situated close together, women could connect easily with their neighbours who were, at least in the early years of settlement, often members of their extended family. In this, the Mennonite women who arrived on the prairies in the 1870s had a distinct advantage over other British and European immigrant settlers. Being able to walk a short distance to one's neighbour and kin undoubtedly allowed for the sharing of advice, household supplies, childcare, and community news in ways that were simply not possible for households separated by several kilometres. This model of settlement may have been a significant factor in alleviating the isolation that was so common for other homesteading immigrant women on the prairies. Knowing that a neighbour or relative was only a short distance away helped to diminish fears of childbirth and illnesses on the frontier. A female culture already nourished by kinship networks was further reinforced by the frequent ritual of childbirth in Mennonite communities.

As Charlotte G. Borst has noted in her study of Wisconsin at the turn of the twentieth century, midwifery in rural areas "resembled more closely the patterns of gender-specific mutual aid that farm women provided for one another than it did an organized, income-producing activity."[29] In these cases, women offered their assistance at childbirth as much out of neighbourliness as because they considered themselves to be vocational midwives. In isolated areas, a "neighbor-midwife" was generally only self-trained and attended a small number of births, usually within her extended family and local community. Yet Borst's conclusion about the small practices of immigrant midwives does not hold true for all Mennonite baby-catchers, some of whom had very prolific careers: for example, Anna Toews who delivered 942 babies, and Sarah Thielman who delivered over 1,000 infants in a thirty-two-year period. However, Borst's observation that most immigrant midwives served their own ethnic group was true also for the Mennonites. The preference for midwives who shared a birthing woman's ethno-religious identity was due to a variety of factors, including language (for Mennonites until mid–twentieth century this meant a German dialect), the likelihood of kinship relationships between the two women, and also shared religious traditions and other cultural customs. In her chapter 5 essay about Margaret Butcher, a nurse-midwife in northern British Columbia, Mary-Ellen Kelm argues that 'Englishness' as equated with 'whiteness' created a sense of belonging for Butcher, vis-à-vis the Aboriginal community in which she worked. While Mennonites were white Europeans, and thus privileged as immigrant settlers, for them the term 'English' was often an all-inclusive label applied to society that existed outside the boundaries of Mennonite communities, and because of their separatist tendencies, was often a derogatory label. As much as possible, Mennonites sought out services – commercial, health care, education, for example – from within their own group, rather than from the 'English,' which could mean any white person who was not Mennonite. Indeed, as recent research has shown, a legal clash between provincial authorities and the Mennonites in Manitoba over the licensing of physicians and midwives was viewed by the Mennonites as the intrusion of 'English' society on their 'way of life' and so they attempted, unsuccessfully, to seek exemption from the prevailing laws.[30]

Even in areas where the traditional settlement patterns had dissolved or were not possible from the outset, rurality itself enhanced the role of the midwife. In the relatively isolated locales frequently preferred by Mennonite settlers, limited access to professional medical care meant that births and other healing services were provided by community midwives out of necessity. One chronicler of Mennonite funeral practices in pioneer settings observed that in villages with less then 500 people, the only 'professional' care for the sick and dying was a "self-trained midwife."[31] Pelee Island in Lake Erie, where several dozen Mennonite families sharecropped tobacco beginning in the mid-1920s, was one community that relied on several midwives for health care, especially during the long winter months when access to the mainland was limited or impossible. My own mother was born on the island with the assistance of Anna Wiebe, who trained as a nurse in Russia and served the islanders for twenty-five years.[32] Similarly, when a small group of Mennonites attempted to establish a remote settlement called Reesor in northern Ontario in 1925, the nearest hospital was in the town of Hearst, twenty-seven miles away and accessible only by a daily train. And, since the "main support needed was at the time of birthing," the small immigrant group soon looked to women within their own community to serve as midwives. One of these was Frieda Isaak, who had prior midwifery experience in Ukraine and whose first delivery in Reesor was a set of twins who were born after a very difficult labour. Isaak, who was called an "angel of mercy," travelled on skis or with dog and sled, with supplies on her back, when called to a childbirth during the long winters of northern Ontario.[33]

In addition to their varied expertise and services in providing health care, midwives quite often held another important function, that of undertaker, which might include certifying deaths and, especially, preparing bodies for burial. Already in Russia, midwifery and the performance of funeral duties were among the few positions for which women received public recognition.[34] While these positions were sometimes held separately, they were more often within a combined vocation. In the southern Manitoba community of Blumenort, the midwife "was, in effect, the village undertaker, and was authorized to sign death certificates."[35] She would also wash the body and cover it with a white pleated fabric that was nailed to the coffin sides.[36] In the Depression-

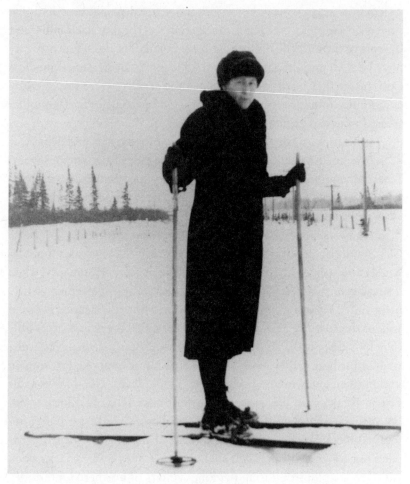

2.2 Frieda Isaak, midwife from Reesor, Ontario. Pictured here on cross-country skis, she was known locally as "an angel of mercy."

era Mennonite settlement at Yarrow, British Columbia, it was "customary for midwives ... to prepare the bodies for burial, which included closing the eyes and tying a scarf under the chin to keep the mouth closed. This had to be done immediately, before rigor mortis set in. They washed the body with alcohol to clean the skin and prevent an odour, then packed the body in ice."[37] Midwives would then dress the bodies in clothing chosen by the family. It was precisely their versatility in healing services that made midwives well suited to deal with the duties of death. Anna Toews, turn-of-the-century midwife in Manitoba, was called to provide official certification of death exactly because of her widespread reputation as "a person with medical knowledge."[38] Since they were called to assist those who were ill, they were often the ones present when death came and, as such, families looked to them to make the necessary physical preparations for burial.

Even when the functions of assisting at births and deaths were not necessarily combined, it was usually women who looked after burials. A Mennonite from rural Saskatchewan, whose parents had given over part of their land for a community cemetery, recalled that, "it was a tradition amongst the Mennonites, brought over from Europe, that each settlement had a few women that acted as mortitions [*sic*] who prepared the body of the dead." Jacob Guenter goes on to describe the services of Justina Goertzen and Gertrude Wiebe, whose functions included "washing, preservation, dressing and wrapping the deceased in linen cloth and placing the body in the coffin." The women were reportedly "well-respected members of the community" who waived their normal fee for the "underprivileged."[39] The source does not indicate whether these particular women were also midwives. While homemade coffins were generally constructed by men in the village, it was the women who completed the inside of the coffin, lining it often with white cotton or linen. Those same village women were also the ones who washed and dressed the body. In some communities, it was very important that the women called upon to prepare the body were not family of the deceased, since it was believed that bad luck would fall to relatives who performed those tasks.[40] In her research on Mennonite burial customs, Linda Buhler remarked that, "without doubt, it was the women in the Mennonite communities who took care of the burial arrangements."[41] Women and children, in particular, were prepared by midwives, though in some communities, it was deemed preferable for male neighbours to wash and prepare bodies of men.[42]

Other examples of a combined vocation include Elisabeth Rempel Reimer who was described as "midwife, nurse, and undertaker." She also had a fur coat– and hat-making business in Russia prior to her immigration.[43] Anna Peters Martens, midwife in rural Saskatchewan at the turn of the century, helped birth 280 babies during her career, but also prepared bodies for burial and maintained a garden of medicinal herbs that she would harvest and dispense to the community.[44] Anna Olfert Fast assisted her mother, who was called to prepare and dress

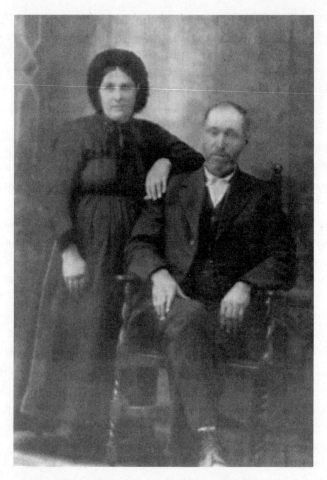

2.3 Anna Peters Martens was both a midwife and an
undertaker in turn-of-the-century Saskatchewan.

bodies for funerals, and became the third generation in her family to
provide this service within her particular Mennonite community.[45] The
roles that women played as undertakers in early settlement communities
in Canada were replicated when conservative factions of Mennonites
migrated to Central and South America in the first half of the twentieth
century. In those regions, female predominance over burial preparations
continued throughout the twentieth century. One woman recalled that
the customs followed in the 1920s in Manitoba were almost identical
to those that were maintained in Paraguay in 1980.[46]

The poetic and romanticized reflection about Aganetha Reimer quoted at the outset of this essay masks, to a certain extent, the hard reality in the close and fundamental connection between birth and death that was central to the vocation of midwives. The practical linkage of birth and death in the varied skills of midwife-undertakers arose not only from questions of expediency and sensibility, that is, the midwife as healer already possessing the supplies and physiological knowledge that were useful for both functions. The collapsing of vocational roles also made explicit, in a kind of pre-modern sense, the close life-cycle ties between birth and death. At a symbolic level, these ties were indicated by the primary role that women in traditional societies carried for "deathwork and mourning."[47] At a concrete level, the linkage indicated the very real possibility of death – for either mother or infant – in childbirth. In eras and geographic locales where hospitals or other medical help was far away, "the midwife alone stood between life and death," as one historian has observed.[48] Or, as an early modern French proverb went, "a pregnant woman has one foot in the grave."[49] Prior to the Second World War, maternal mortality rates in Canada were high[50] – indeed higher than in most other Western countries except the United States – and childbirth-related death was second only to tuberculosis in cause of female deaths. Referring to the late nineteenth and early twentieth century, Nanci Langford says, "Perhaps no other aspect of life on the Prairies endangered women as much as did the birthing of their children." This reality was so great that Langford describes one case of a woman preparing herself for giving birth by also laying out her wedding gown in readiness for her burial.[51] A comprehensive one-year survey conducted beginning in mid-1925 found a rate of 6.4 maternal deaths per thousand live births in Canada; more specifically, 1,532 women died in childbirth in that one-year period.[52] Interestingly, there were notable ethnic differences in statistics on maternal mortality. For instance, Russian-Canadian women (which possibly included Mennonite immigrants from Russia) had a rate of 8.4.[53] Given such circumstances, midwives had to be prepared for death as fully as they had to be prepared for birth.

The fear of death in childbirth was heightened in rural, isolated areas, where assistance by either midwife or physician or both was far away. Katherine Martens, in her oral history of childbirth in Mennonite communities, notes that if sex and death are difficult to talk

about, childbirth, carrying associations of both, may be even more
secretive. Martens notes that for the twentieth-century women in her
collection of stories, "Even in normal birth and delivery, there is a
sense of moving into the unknown that some of the women ... associate with death."[54] As this statement might suggest, the nexus between
life and death in the context of childbirth held certain religious con-
notations as well, which, for European midwives of the early modern
period, was possibly more concrete. Writing about eighteenth-century
France, historian Jacques Gélis observed that midwives were called to
assist at births and also to attend to the laying out of the dead: "By
presiding at births and preparing people for their last journey, the midwife held both ends of the thread of life," he noted.[55] One 1745 British
midwife issued a bill for the following three services: "midwifery,
washing linen, and laying out the dead child in its coffin."[56] The possibility that birth might be quickly followed by death, of infant or
mother or both, meant that in earlier eras, such as sixteenth-century
Europe, or in seventeenth- and eighteenth-century New France, a priest
might be present at childbirth in order to perform a quick baptism or
the last rites.[57] In fact, in early modern Europe, midwives in Catholic
territories were expected to baptize newborns who were at all frail,
to ensure that in case of death, the infant would receive a Christian
burial.[58] During the Reformation era, Protestant clerics ensured that
midwives received special instruction in emergency baptisms, to avoid
situations where a rebaptism might be necessary due to incorrect bap-
tismal procedure on the part of the midwife.[59]

For their part, the Mennonites' Anabaptist ancestors of the radical
Reformation found themselves in an opposite situation. Because they
opposed infant baptism as unscriptural, Anabaptist midwives were
accused of not baptizing newborn children while claiming that they
had. And Anabaptist midwives may in fact have done just that, as a
way of reducing the number of infant baptisms that occurred and, in
this way, spreading the movement. One example is Elsbeth Hersberger,
who was imprisoned for her Anabaptist beliefs several times in the
1530s and reportedly "influenced numerous parents not to have their
children baptized."[60] While research on this early period is minimal, it
has been suggested that there were a large number of midwives among
the Anabaptists.[61] Within this clandestine and subversive community,
the desire to use the services of midwives who shared their faith was

based on their need for assurance that the attending midwife would not baptize a sickly newborn child. Thus, the custom of calling out and appointing midwives within the ethno-religious fold had its origins early in the movement. At any rate, in this much earlier period, it is clear that midwives bore a significant burden in terms of the religious identity of the infant they helped to deliver, and as such, had a vocational role that carried a degree of spiritual authority that went well beyond the physical. Indeed, during the Middle Ages the activity of midwives came under the supervision of church authorities who used these "poor but honest" birth attendants – in addition to their role in baptisms – to access and report possible incidents of abortion or infanticide and determine paternity. The vocational linkage between midwife and undertaker certainly had its antecedents in earlier eras both for religious reasons and due to the fragility of life itself.

In her analysis of religion and homebirth, Pamela E. Klassen observes that in the nineteenth century both doctors and clerics ascribed more religious meaning to childbirth than became the case in the twentieth century.[62] It could be that Mennonite midwives of an earlier era who viewed their work as a 'calling' rather than a vocation integrated spirituality into their work more than the professionally trained doctor might have, especially a doctor who was 'English.' One woman recalled that the midwife who attended her, a woman trained in Russia, prayed throughout the entire birth process: "and once the baby was born, she knelt down beside the bed and thanked God for being with us and that the baby had come into the world, and that child and mother were alive."[63] That a certain common spiritual demeanor was required of both midwife and undertaker is suggested, though not stated explicitly, in the following description of Barbara Shuh, a turn-of-the-century midwife and cheesemaker in southwestern Ontario: "In her role as a mid-wife ministering at the birth of a child she rejoiced with the family. When the death of a loved one in the home was imminent, Barbara … without hesitation, joined the family in their walk through the valley of sorrow."[64] Shuh's role as community midwife, aside from the practical skill she brought to catching babies, clearly carried some religious significance as well, whether she was charming away a malady, assisting a woman in childbirth, or attending at a deathbed.

+++

The vocational identity of certain Mennonite women as both midwives and undertakers represents a fascinating confluence of life and death. It portrays the ways in which the vocational activity of women was multi-faceted and overlapping in an era before the compartmentalization and professionalization of occupations. The traditional Mennonite midwife held a position not unlike that of her Aboriginal counterpart who, in some locales, was referred to not as a midwife, but as the woman "who can do everything." In rural, isolated settings and particularly for definable immigrant or ethnic communities, midwives with abilities to catch babies, set bones, pull teeth, ease stomach pains, and prepare the dead fulfilled essential semi-public functions. To the extent that some elements in their array of healing skills had origins in particular geographic or ethnic customs from the 'old world,' the continued practice of such skills helped to maintain group identity and solidarity in new environments. The fact that some midwives included death rituals in their practices speaks not only to the nearness of death, lurking around the corners at childbirth, and to their own skill in handling things of the body but also to a pre-modern sense of the symbolic connectedness of birth and death that was implicit in their vocation.

NOTES

I would like to acknowledge research assistance from Conrad Stoesz, Agatha Klassen, and Bethany Leis.

1 Al Reimer, "Johann R. Reimer (1848–1918): Steinbach Pioneer," in *Preservings* 9 (1996): 41.

2 Wendy Mitchinson, *Giving Birth in Canada, 1900–1950* (Toronto: University of Toronto Press, 2002), Table 1, 175.

3 Jo Oppenheimer, "Childbirth in Ontario: The Transition from Home to Hospital in the Early Twentieth Century," in Katherine Arnup et al., eds., *Delivering Motherhood: Maternal Ideologies and Practices in the 19th and 20th Centuries* (London & New York: Routledge, 1990), 51.

4 'Baby-catching' is a colloquial term frequently applied to midwives past and present. It was and is widely used by midwives and others, and is not a Mennonite-specific term.

5 See for instance, Oppenheimer, "Childbirth in Ontario," and Suzanne Buckley, "Ladies or Midwives? Efforts to Reduce Infant and Maternal Mortality," in

Linda Kealey, ed., *A Not Unreasonable Claim: Women and Reform in Canada, 1880s–1920s*, 131–49 (Toronto: The Women's Press, 1979); C. Lesley Biggs, "The Case of the Missing Midwives: A History of Midwifery in Ontario from 1795–1900," in *Ontario History* 75 (March 1983): 21–36; J.T.H. Connor, "'Larger Fish to Catch Here than Midwives': Midwifery and the Medical Profession in Nineteenth-Century Ontario," and Dianne Dodd, "Helen Mac-Murchy: Popular Midwifery and Maternity Services for Canadian Pioneer Women." In Dianne Dodd and Deborah Gorham, eds., *Caring and Curing: Historical Perspectives on Women and Healing in Canada*, 103–34, 135–62 (Ottawa: University of Ottawa Press, 1994); Cecilia Benoit and Dena Carroll, "Canadian Midwifery: Blending Traditional and Modern Practices." In Christina Bates, Dianne Dodd, and Nicole Rousseau, eds., *On All Frontiers: Four Centuries of Canadian Nursing*, 27–41 (Ottawa: University of Ottawa Press, 2005).

6 See especially Wendy Mitchinson, *Giving Birth in Canada, 1900–1950*.

7 Cecilia Benoit, "Midwives & Healers: The Newfoundland Experience," in *Healthsharing* (Winter 1983): 22.

8 Judith Young and Nicole Rousseau, "Lay Nursing from the New France Era to the End of the Nineteenth Century (1608–1981)." In Christina Bates, Dianne Dodd, and Nicole Rousseau, eds., *On All Frontiers: Four Centuries of Canadian Nursing*, 18 (Ottawa: University of Ottawa Press, 2005).

9 See, for instance, Cecilia Benoit, "Midwives & Healers: The Newfoundland Experience," in *Healthsharing* (Winter 1983): 22–6; Cecilia Benoit, "Traditional Midwifery Practice: The Limits of Occupational Autonomy," in *Canadian Review of Sociology and Anthropology* 26 (1988): 633–49; Cecilia Benoit and Dena Carroll, "Aboriginal Midwifery in British Columbia: A Narrative Untold." In Peter H. Stephenson et al., eds., *A Persistent Spirit: Towards Understanding Aboriginal Health in British Columbia*, 223–48 (Victoria: Canadian Western Geographic Series no. 31, 1995); Katherine Martens and Heidi Harms, *In Her Own Voice: Childbirth Stories from Mennonite Women* (Winnipeg, MB: University of Manitoba Press, 1997).

10 Charlotte G. Borst, *Catching Babies: The Professionalization of Childbirth, 1870–1920* (Cambridge: Harvard University Press, 1995).

11 Wendy Mitchinson, *Giving Birth in Canada, 1900–1950*, 92.

12 John B. Toews, "Childbirth, Disease and Death Among the Mennonites in Nineteenth-Century Russia," in *Mennonite Quarterly Review* 60, 3 (July 1986): 462.

13 Ibid.

14 Susanna Epp's story is told in the following sources: Anna Ens, ed., *The House of Heinrich: The Story of Heinrich Epp (1811–1863) of Rosenort, Molotschna*

and His Descendants (Winnipeg: Epp Book Committee, 1980), 129; and "Agatha [Braun] Peters," in *Saskatchewan Mennonite Historian* 3, 3 (December 1998): 19.

15 Shirley Bergen, "Dr Katherina Born Thiessen: A Woman Who Made a Difference," in *Mennonite Historian* (September 1997): 8.

16 Irma Epp, Lillian Harms, and Lora Sawatsky, "Midwifery: A Ministry." In Leonard Neufeldt, ed., *Village of Unsettled Yearnings. Yarrow, British Columbia: Mennonite Promise*, 17–22 (Victoria, BC: TouchWood Editions, 2002).

17 Her story is told in Ruth Unrau, *Encircled: Stories of Mennonite Women* (Newton, KS: Faith and Life Press, 1986), 275–83.

18 See Sarah Dekker Thielman collection, Centre for Mennonite Brethren Studies, Winnipeg, Manitoba. Additional information about Sarah Dekker Thielman and other Mennonite midwives can be found in Marlene Epp, "Midwife-Healers in Canadian Mennonite Immigrant Communities: Women Who 'Made Things Right,'" in *Histoire Sociale/Social History* 80 (November 2007): 323–44, and in Marlene Epp, *Mennonite Women in Canada: A History* (Winnipeg: University of Manitoba Press, 2008).

19 "Introduction." In Hilary Marland, ed., *The Art of Midwifery: Early Modern Midwives in Europe*, 4 (London & New York: Routledge, 1993).

20 Reference to N. Leap and B. Hunter, *The Midwife's Tale: An Oral History from Handywoman to Professional Midwife* (London and New York: Routledge, 1993), in Hilary Marland and Anne Marie Rafferty, eds., *Midwives, Society and Childbirth: Debates and Controversies in the Modern Period*, 9 (London and New York: Routledge, 1997).

21 Royden K. Loewen, *Blumenort: A Mennonite Community in Transition, 1874–1982* (Steinbach, MB: The Blumenort Mennonite Historical Society, 1983), 219.

22 Regina Doerksen Neufeld, "Katharina Hiebert: Manitoban Pioneer Midwife," in *Mennonite Historical Bulletin* 61 (July 2000): 4.

23 Regina Doerksen Neufeld, "Katherina Hiebert (1855–1910): Midwife," in *Preservings* 10 (June 1997): 14.

24 Bergen, "Dr Katherina Born Thiessen."

25 Irma Epp, Lillian Harms, and Lora Sawatsky, "Midwifery: A Ministry." In Leonard Neufeldt, ed., *Village of Unsettled Yearnings. Yarrow, British Columbia: Mennonite Promise*, 20 (Victoria, BC: TouchWood Editions, 2002).

26 Lorraine Roth, *Willing Service: Stories of Ontario Mennonite Women* (Waterloo, ON: Mennonite Historical Society of Ontario, 1992), 28.

27 Ibid., 216–7.

28 See William Schroeder and Helmut Huebert, *Mennonite Historical Atlas* (Winnipeg: Springfield Publishers, 1996).

29 Charlotte G. Borst, *Catching Babies: The Professionalization of Childbirth, 1870–1920* (Cambridge: Harvard University Press, 1995), 5.

30 Hans Werner and Jenifer Waito, "'One of our own': Ethnicity Politics and the Medicalization of Childbirth in Manitoba," unpublished paper (2007) referenced with permission; published in *Manitoba History* 58 (June 2008).

31 Ben Fast, "Mennonite Pioneer Funeral Practices," in *Saskatchewan Mennonite Historian* 5, 1 (March 2000): 13.

32 N.N. Driedger, *The Leamington United Mennonite Church: Establishment and Development, 1925–1972* (Altona, MB: D.W. Friesen, 1973), 168–9; Astrid Koop, *The Mennonite Settlement on Pelee Island, Ontario: Memories of Life on "The Island," 1925–1950* (Leamington, ON: Essex-Kent Historical Association, 1999).

33 Hedy Lepp Dennis, *Memories of Reesor: The Mennonite Settlement in Northern Ontario, 1925–1948* (Leamington, ON: Essex-Kent Historical Association, 2001), 131–3.

34 Royden K. Loewen, *Family, Church, and Market: A Mennonite Community in the Old and the New Worlds, 1850–1930* (Toronto: University of Toronto Press, 1993), 47.

35 Loewen, *Blumenort*, 219.

36 Linda Buhler, "Mennonite Burial Customs," in *Preservings* 7 (December 1995): 51.

37 Esther Epp Harder, "Rites of Dying, Death, and Burial." In Leonard N. Neufeldt, ed., *Village of Unsettled Yearnings. Yarrow, British Columbia: Mennonite Promise*, 6 (Victoria, BC: TouchWood Editions, 2002).

38 Loewen, *Blumenort*, 219.

39 Jacob G. Guenter, "Life's End" (unpublished manuscript, Mennonite Heritage Village, Steinbach, MB). I am grateful to curator Roland Sawatzky for sharing this document with me.

40 Linda Buhler, "Mennonite Burial Customs: Part Three," in *Preservings* 10 (June 1997): 79.

41 Linda Buhler, "Mennonite Burial Customs," in *Preservings* 7 (December 1995): 51.

42 Ben Fast, "Mennonite Pioneer Funeral Practices," in *Saskatchewan Mennonite Historian* 5, 1 (March 2000): 13.

43 D. Plett, "Elisabeth Rempel Reimer: Matriarch of Steinbach," in *Preservings* 9 (December 1996): 5.

44 J.G. Guenter, ed., *Osler ... The Early Years and the One Room School #1238 (1905–1947)* (Osler, SK: Osler Historical Museum, 1999), 54.

45 Linda Buhler, "Mennonite Burial Customs: Part Two," in *Preservings* 8 (June 1996), part 2, 49.

46 Linda Buhler, "Mennonite Burial Customs," in *Preservings* 7 (December 1995): 51.

47 Peter C. Jupp, "Introduction." In Peter C. Jupp and Glennys Howarth, eds., *The Changing Face of Death: Historical Accounts of Death and Disposal*, 4 (London: Macmillan Press; and New York: St Martin's Press, 1997).

48 John B. Toews, "Childbirth, Disease and Death Among the Mennonites in Nineteenth-Century Russia,"in *Mennonite Quarterly Review* 60, 3 (July 1986): 462.

49 Olwen Hufton, *The Prospect Before Her: A History of Women in Western Europe, Volume One, 1500–1800* (London: Fontana Press, 1997), 179.

50 See figure 3 in Mitchinson, *Giving Birth in Canada*, 263.

51 Nanci Langford, "Childbirth on the Canadian Prairies, 1880–1930." In Catherine A. Cavanaugh and Randi R. Warne, eds., *Telling Tales: Essays in Western Women's History*, 150 (Vancouver: UBC Press, 2000).

52 Wendy Mitchinson, *Giving Birth in Canada, 1900–1950*, 261.

53 Ibid., 262.

54 Katherine Martens and Heidi Harms, *In Her Own Voice: Childbirth Stories from Mennonite Women* (Winnipeg, MB: University of Manitoba Press, 1997), viii.

55 Gelis, quoted in Brian Burtch, *Trials of Labour: The Re-emergence of Midwifery* (Montreal & Kingston: McGill-Queen's University Press, 1994), 55. Actual source is Jacques Gélis, *History of Childbirth: Fertility, Pregnancy and Birth in Early Modern Europe* (Cambridge, UK: Polity Press, 1991), 110.

56 David Harley, "Provincial midwives in England: Lancashire and Cheshire, 1660–1760." In Hilary Marland, ed., *The Art of Midwifery: Early Modern Midwives in Europe* (London & New York: Routledge, 1993), 34.

57 Alison Prentice et al., *Canadian Women: A History* (Toronto: Harcourt Brace Jovanovich, 1988), 48.

58 Olwen Hufton, *The Prospect Before Her: A History of Women in Western Europe, Volume One, 1500–1800* (London: Fontana Press, 1997), 188.

59 Merry E. Wiesner, "Nuns, Wives, and Mothers: Women and the Reformation in Germany." In Sherrin Marshall, ed., *Women in Reformation and Counter-Reformation Europe*, 24 (Bloomington and Indianapolis: Indiana University Press, 1989).

60 Guy F. Hershberger, "Hershberger (Hersberg, Hersberger, Herschberger, Hirschberger, Harshberger, Harshbarger)." In *Global Anabaptist Mennonite Encyclopedia Online*, 1956. Global Anabaptist Mennonite Encyclopedia Online. Retrieved 5 March 2007 at <http://www.gameo.org/encyclopedia/contents/h477 1ome.html>

61 William Klassen, "Midwives." In *Global Anabaptist Mennonite Encyclopedia Online*, 1989. Global Anabaptist Mennonite Encyclopedia Online. Retrieved 5 March 2007 at <http://www.gameo.org/encyclopedia/contents/m54me.html>

62 Pamela E. Klassen, *Blessed Events: Religion and Home Birth in America* (Princeton, NJ: Princeton University Press, 2001), 63.

63 Katherine Martens and Heidi Harms, *In Her Own Voice: Childbirth Stories from Mennonite Women* (Winnipeg, MB: University of Manitoba Press, 1997), 12.

64 "Excerpts from Diaries of Barbara (Bowman) Shuh, 1904–1920." In *Diaries of our Pennsylvania German Ancestors, 1846–1925*, 45 (Kitchener: The Pennsylvania German Folklore Society of Ontario, 2002).

65 Mitchinson, *Giving Birth in Canada*, 345, n 81.

3

+++++

On the Edge of Empire: The Working Life
of Myra (Grimsley) Bennett

LINDA KEALEY

In May 1921, thirty-two-year-old Myra Grimsley (later Bennett) arrived in a small isolated fishing outport in Newfoundland to take up a position as a nurse-midwife. She had trained in London as a nurse and later received the Central Midwives Board certificate that allowed her to also practise as a midwife. That certificate gave Bennett an advantage over her Canadian and American counterparts who had little access to formal midwifery instruction. These two different approaches to nursing and midwifery are reflected in the historiography as well. While English and Australian writers often group midwifery with nursing, with few exceptions, including Judith Young's essay in this book, historical writing about midwifery in North America tends to be distinct from discussions of nursing. Furthermore, nursing has been approached as a 'profession' attractive to the middle-class women that nursing reformers hoped would replace the working-class women who first took on the work. In established historiography midwifery, which persisted longer in remote rural areas of North America, has been most often treated as an outdated occupation that declined under the onslaught of organized medicine. More recently, scholars have recognized that there are varying experiences and patterns in midwifery that need to be explained.[1]

Cecilia Benoit's study *Midwives in Passage*, Janet McNaughton's doctoral thesis, and, more recently, Wendy Mitchinson's *Giving Birth in Canada* all suggest a more complicated picture. Benoit distinguishes between Newfoundland midwives who were informally trained ("granny midwives") and those who had some training resulting in a more respected professional role for midwives within clinics or the small cottage hospital system. McNaughton's study, completed around the same time as Benoit's, also attests to multiple models of midwifery and, like Benoit, she treats midwifery as a skilled occupation. Echoing Benoit and McNaughton, Mitchinson's work questions the emphasis on hostility between physicians and midwives and suggests that midwives operated in a variety of circumstances. Thus, the much-discussed 'decline of midwifery' occurs only partially and differently depending on location, a theme also noted by Judith Young and Marlene Epp in this book.[2] Bennett performed many health care roles in the rural outport of Daniel's Harbour, where access to medical treatment was very limited. Her career of over sixty years suggests the importance of and respect given to nurse-midwives in some rural communities even in the second half of the twentieth century. Unlike the granny midwives or those who worked in clinics or hospitals, Bennett operated her own clinic at home, sometimes as a formally recognized and remunerated health professional and sometimes informally, without pay or with pay in kind.

In some cases, midwifery has been discussed as an extension of women's domestic and community work, particularly in studies of informally trained women. When more closely examined, it is difficult to distinguish between those who were paid in some way and those who performed midwifery for reasons of mutual aid or as part of a 'calling.' As Epp's study in chapter 2 illustrates, rural Mennonite women performed an important community-based role as health care providers and most were not formally trained. Judith Young's research on nineteenth-century Toronto suggests a more market-driven context where older women and widows could make a living and gain respect as midwives who sometimes combined midwifery with nursing. Bennett (and probably other midwives) most likely did not see a contradiction between her profession and her role in the community. Nevertheless, her life history raises interesting questions about the relationship between paid and unpaid work, calling or vocation and profession. In this paper I examine Bennett's working life and her fragments of autobiography, including labour history, from several vantage points. Few scholars of nursing and midwifery have approached their subjects from the perspective of labour history.

Many more have turned to women's or gender history with some attention paid to the emergence of women's professions. A few have written about nursing within a framework critical of colonial relations and expectations.[3] In examining the working life of Bennett, this essay incorporates insights drawn from all three approaches – gender, labour, and colonial history.

In addition, I briefly look at Bennett's fragmentary autobiography as a type of life writing and what this might tell us about gender, class, and imperial relations. Bennett was a prodigious record keeper, saving daily diaries, correspondence, business records, medical casebooks, and her own writings about her experiences. These scripts suggest that she had a clear sense of her unusual life experiences and a consciousness that her story reflected larger themes in the history of Newfoundland, an outpost of the British Empire until confederation with Canada in 1949. In thinking about how to make sense of one woman's life, I turned for guidance to the publications of literary scholars who have worked in women's archives. As Carolyn Steedman has written, "Class and gender, and their articulations, are the bits and pieces from which psychological selfhood is made." She also notes that, "Specificity of place and politics has to be reckoned with in making an account of anybody's life, and their use of their own past."[4] Accordingly, I begin with a discussion of the context of place and politics before turning, in section II, to a more detailed examination of Bennett's life, emphasizing the transformation of a working-class woman into a trained professional. Her working life forms yet another important theme in section III. Section IV brings together these threads in a brief discussion of her fragmentary autobiography and what it tells us about class consciousness, gender identities, women's work, and power relations.

I. A Brief Context

In the early twentieth century Newfoundland was a British dominion and claimed a place within the empire. For hundreds of years West Country merchants had participated in the lucrative codfish trade that dominated the economy. Although the island was originally a way station for a seasonal fishing trade, it was gradually settled and the family fishery developed. At the time of the First World War, Newfoundland men supported the British Empire by enlisting, experiencing devastating losses on the battlefields of Europe, while at home local women's organizations mobilized to send bandages, socks, mittens, and other comforts to the troops. Many of these women became involved in the suffrage and child welfare movements.[5] The war underlined the importance of health issues to national survival; in England, the high percentage of men found unfit for military duty, combined with declining birth rates and climbing infant mortality, intensified concern about the future of the population, concerns echoed in Newfoundland. In the post-war period, health care and child welfare emerged as priority issues among the elite. Voluntary groups such as the Women's Patriotic Association (WPA) turned from rolling bandages to child welfare work after the war; in addition to raising funds for welfare work, the WPA also ran the child welfare services in the capital city of St John's, cost-sharing the nurses' salaries with government.[6] Lack of medical care for mothers in the city also led to the establishment of the Midwives Club in fall 1920; by 1924, some sixty midwives had undertaken training through the program. Founded by a nurse who worked for the Child Welfare Association, which in turn drew its membership from health professionals and wives of the St John's elite, the Club endeavoured to provide formal education to empirically trained midwives, mostly in St John's.[7] Problems remained, however, since there was no successful legislation mandating training and registration of midwives, a goal of the reformers, until 1936, despite several earlier attempts.[8] Also, nurse's training, available in St John's since 1903, did not provide obstetrical training for nurses thus necessitating travel elsewhere for instruction.

For the remote areas of the dominion, such as Labrador, the south coast and parts of the Northern Peninsula, however, there were even fewer trained nurses or doctors available. Midwives were trained by local women who did not have access to formal training themselves. In 1919, reports on the lack of medical care in isolated fishing outports reached the ears of Lady Harris, the wife of the governor-general; accompanying her husband, subsequent trips around the island confirmed her alarm. In response, in 1920, Lady Harris began to discuss the lack of medical facilities with members of the St John's elite, including clerics, doctors, businessmen, and eventually the prime minister, Sir Richard Squires. A committee was formed in May and the outport nursing scheme was conceived to provide trained nurses with midwifery certificates for the outports where doctors were not available.[9] The organization set up local committees in the outports to oversee the process and to assist in making the undertaking self-supporting. A clergyman or justice of the peace was to ensure that the nurse was not overworked and that the local committee carried out the details, including raising funds to support the nurse. The scheme was formally launched in fall 1920 when Lady Harris returned from England having engaged four nurses, one of whom was Bennett. As Harris noted, "we require a woman with a missionary spirit; and this is a spirit which it takes some years and a wider experience to develop."[10]

The arrival of four British-trained nurses in 1920–21 was not merely the result of each nurse's individual motivations nor of Lady Harris' philanthropic efforts. Although a sense of noblesse oblige likely accompanied the role of governor's wife, other aspects of the imperial framework were no doubt crucial. The spread of British power over much of the globe, including parts of Africa, Asia, North America, and elsewhere brought with it a demand for appropriate medical care, defined by British standards and personnel. In 1896 the wives of leading colonial officials established the Colonial Nursing Association (CNA) (later the Overseas Nursing Association) to meet these needs. The voluntary board of the CNA worked with the Colonial Office to provide "funds for and administer the provision of qualified nurses to British colonial communities world-wide."[11] While the impetus for these developments came from African colonies where Europeans experienced high death rates and objected to African caregivers, it was also the case that remote areas of Canada drew some of the CNA board's attention.[12]

Thirty years prior to Lady Harris' efforts to recruit nurses, Sir Wilfred Grenfell of the Royal National Mission to Deep Sea Fishermen had travelled to northern Newfoundland and coastal Labrador in response to reports of dire poverty and the lack of religious institutions and health care among the fishing population. Headquartered in St Anthony at the northern tip of the Northern Peninsula, the Grenfell Mission provided health care services as part of its 'civilizing' mission. By the 1930s it encompassed not only the hospital in St Anthony but also nursing stations, clinics, a craft industry, schools, and much more. Its medical personnel, both paid and volunteer, came from Great

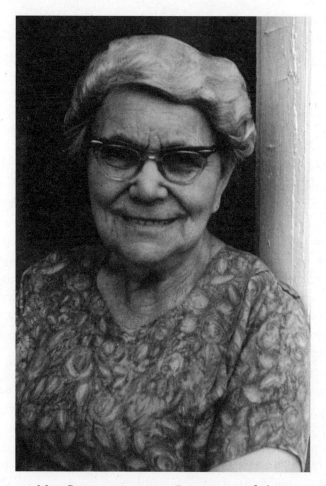

3.1 Myra Bennett, 1890–1990. Bennett, a certified midwife, moved from England to Newfoundland in 1921 and was called upon to perform a variety of medical and non-medical services.

Britain, the United States, and Canada and they were drawn into the work by a combination of appeals – to their religious sensibilities, to their desire for experience and adventure, and often by the convincing lectures of Grenfell himself, who spent his winters travelling around fundraising and recruiting. The Mission expected its workers to support its broad mandate of combining health care work with its religious and civilizing mission. Its female workers, nurses in particular, were to provide not only professional care but also to demonstrate the nurturant, feminine qualities that accompanied educated middle-class women from Anglo-Saxon, Christian backgrounds, standards that Bennett would probably have agreed with. The Grenfell Mission targeted English nurse-midwives for its remote posts where doctors visited rarely and where nurses often had to cope with medical emergencies normally referred to physicians.

Efforts to maintain nursing services in the outports faltered after the first two years; Lady Harris and one other member of the outport nursing committee left the island, some of the nurses' contracts ran out, and a number of the nurses married, including Bennett. No replacements were appointed and it appears as though funding dried up. The new governor, William Allardyce, and his wife came to the island in 1922 and Lady Elsie Allardyce soon became involved in the outport nursing movement. A revitalized committee organized a meeting in January 1924 to discuss how to make the scheme self-financing, an idea supported by Lady Allardyce and based on her acquaintance with practices in Scotland's Shetland and Orkney Islands. On these islands local committees looked after the welfare of nurses through the organization of home industries such as knitting and needlecraft, with the proceeds going to pay the salaries of the nurses. Lady Allardyce organized volunteers and samples were obtained from Scotland. This activity resulted in the creation of the Newfoundland Outport Nursing and Industrial Association (NONIA) in 1924 with several dozen communities participating. By the early 1930s only a handful of communities supported NONIA nurses and in 1934 the government took over responsibility for the remaining nurses.[13]

Indeed, 1934 signalled the beginning of a new era in Newfoundland. Driven into bankruptcy and faced with high levels of unemployment, poverty, and unrest, the island lost its status as a dominion within the empire and its government was replaced by a Commission of Government – six commissioners and a governor who were British appointees.[14] From 1934 until 1949, when Newfoundland joined Canada, the Commission embarked upon a number of ambitious reform projects, including the revamping of the health care system. During this time frame the government created a series of cottage hospitals in remote areas lacking health services. It also set up a district nursing service, commissioned a number of vessels to serve as travelling clinics, and experimented with food programs for target populations, especially children. A number of dietary studies conducted in the 1920s, '30s, and '40s alarmed health officials who worried about the consequences of poor diet. Lack of fresh milk, green vegetables, and fresh meat resulted in a number of problems, experts believed. Poor diet was blamed for tuberculosis, rickets, underweight and apathetic children, dental caries, and general malnourishment caused by a mono-tonous diet of salt meat, white flour, potatoes, and tea. Consequently, the government participated in the distribution of orange juice and cod liver oil to infants, children, and pregnant women as well as the dis-tribution of dried milk products to school children. Wartime prosper-ity, with the building of American military bases on the island and in Labrador, brought more income and the possibility for improved diets. Despite wartime improvements and confederation with Canada, authorities continued to pursue policies of supplementing foods for the vulnerable, fortifying flour and margarine with vitamins, and educat-ing through media campaigns well into the 1970s.[15]

II. Mobility Through the Professions

What attracted Bennett and women like her to nursing? What led her and other nurses to take the radical step of volunteering for duty in such remote places in the empire? How were they prepared or trained to work in isolated communities? Much ink has been spilled on the de-velopment of the 'women's professions' that attracted ambitious and relatively educated young women into nursing, teaching, and social work in the late nineteenth century. However, McPherson's study of twentieth-century nursing in Canada argues that nurses came from a variety of social-class backgrounds, including urban working-class women and daughters of farmers.[16] Bennett came from an East End London working-class background. Describing her father as working at several trades, Bennett's birth certificate listed him as a journeyman shoemaker, one of the trades compromised by mechanization.[17] She described her mother as a generous woman who consistently helped poor families living on the streets of London. Like most working-class children in the early twentieth century, Bennett left school at age four-teen to work, in her case in a dressmaker's shop. Her ambition was to become a teacher but her family could not afford it. While employed in

the garment trade she took Bible classes, attended temperance meetings, and participated in religious services.[18] According to notes Bennett
made in 1973, the superintendent of the Hoxton Market [Christian]
Mission approached her about taking nurse training with the promise
of financial support.[19] She found a place in a small hospital near
Manchester where she trained. Finishing her training in 1910, she took
a course in district nursing, which included maternity training, in 1913
in North London. When war broke out in 1914, nurses and midwives
assumed more maternity cases as doctors were needed in military hospitals. By 1915 Bennett had completed her midwifery training at the
British Hospital for Mothers and Babies in Woolwich. Certified by the
Central Midwives Board in December, she worked as a district nurse in
Woking for several years, earning praise from the medical men she
worked with: "I have always found her obliging, sympathetic, intelligent and keen in her work. Whilst she has been in Woking she has
gained the confidence of the medical men and a large section of the
population," wrote Dr George F. Vincent on 27 February 1919.[20] By
summer 1918 Bennett must have made a decision to explore nursing
posts overseas: an August medical certificate of good health testified
that she was fit for duties with the Overseas Nursing Association. While
awaiting an assignment overseas, she left the district nursing position
and accepted a post at an Anglican rescue home in Woking. The war
and the influenza epidemic left her exhausted so she decided to take a
less stressful position. From September 1919 to March 1921, Bennett
performed the role of matron-midwife and took advanced midwifery
training (instrumental and anaesthesia) in preparation for work abroad.
As Evelina Todd of the Winchester Diocesan Union for Preventive and
Rescue Work noted in her testimonial, "It is with great regret on my
part that she is leaving us, but she has felt the call to work where nurses
are greatly needed and the conditions hard."[21]

In reconstructing her life, Bennett emphasized her consciousness of
poverty, initially within her own family; as she once wrote, her own
home was "too poor for pleasures." As the only girl in a family of
brothers she "had no time for dreaming," she recalled. While her
family nominally belonged to the Church of England, they were not
churchgoers. Bennett, nevertheless, was attracted to the social outreach
activities of the Anglican mission. Perhaps prompted by earlier exposure to Bible classes and temperance meetings, she found a resonance

in the church for her own working-class moral code of helping others. As a young working-class woman with connections through the Church of England, Bennett was able to find satisfaction within the developing profession of nursing. Even in later life, she established a religious routine in her household with prayers on Sunday and a welcome for the itinerant minister who came to call. This melding of social conscience with the idea of a 'calling' and professional expertise perhaps best explains why Bennett, not really knowing what awaited her, set off for Newfoundland in April 1921. Equipped with a black bag of instruments, she no doubt felt a sense of purpose but perhaps also savoured the idea of adventure and exploring the margins of empire. The heavy casualties of the First World War made marriage a remote possibility in England. As an unmarried woman over thirty, maybe she sought more independence than could be found at home. Leaving home may have represented an opportunity to make oneself over again as well as an opportunity to bring medical skills and religious/moral values to those needing assistance.[22]

To some extent, the break with home combined with a professional designation allowed Bennett to reinvent her social-class position as well. Although born into a working-class London family, recordings of Bennett's voice late in her life reveal an upper middle-class English accent. In adapting to her new-found-land, Bennett may also have cherished her Englishness as key to her identity as a professional.[23] At the same time as nursing struggled to successfully establish itself as a respectable profession for middle-class women, it promised social mobility. Professional training emphasized not only technical skills in nursing but also a set of values based in middle-class respectability. Nurses were trained to fit into a clear hierarchy that demanded adherence to standards of female respectability. Bennett, who married into the community, found her skills in high demand but she also established herself as one of the few educated and cultured individuals in the community, writing letters for the illiterate, arranging visits for dignitaries, and organizing church events. These activities suggested a leadership role and middle-class values. In addition, Bennett was known for her precise standards and her imperious demeanour, which might be linked to the apprenticeship system in nursing. This relied on hierarchy in training, with senior nurses exerting authority over juniors. Discipline was also crucial in training nurses. Imitating military standards, nurses in training worked long hours and their lives were strictly regulated, with each day carefully planned to combine practical work with classroom learning. Dress codes, limited free time, and exacting standards prevailed. As McPherson has noted, "As ideological tools, discipline and subordination helped secure nursing's place within the social category of respectable femininity ... Rural and working class women had to acquire not only the specific skills of bedside attendance, but also 'character' as defined by bourgeois society."[24] For women from rural districts and working-class urban homes, nursing promised a valued set of skills but also the acquisition of a wider cultural experience and access to the middle class. In Bennett's case, nursing credentials were intertwined with class and ethnic background.

III. Work Life in Newfoundland

On 27 May 1921, six weeks after leaving England, Bennett arrived at her destination – Daniel's Harbour. She recalled that "dories were awaiting the arrival of the coastal steamer and the ice conditions had made its arrival so late, that normal stocks of food had become exhausted, and it was evident that the people had been on short rations. Goods were lowered into the waiting dories, rowed to shore, where boxes were broken open and tins distributed. Barrels of flour were being rolled away to the homes, men, women and children all working with a will to get the things handled and stowed away. Nobody wanted a nurse that day. Food came first."[25]

Daniel's Harbour was a small outport halfway up the Northern Peninsula with a population of a few hundred souls. Fishing was the major activity though, like many small communities, occupational pluralism best describes the economic activity. People made their livings from fishing, hunting, cutting wood, gardening, sealing, and fox farming. The coastal boat provided the main source of communication with other communities since there were no roads until the 1950s and 1960s, and it brought all the supplies and mail as well as passengers. Dependent on the weather, these vessels might not be able to stop when the seas were too rough or the ice too thick. From freeze-up in the late fall until spring break-up, communities like Daniel's Harbour were isolated and travel was limited to dog sled, snowshoes, or horse-drawn sleighs. Families bought supplies of salt meat, flour, tea, molasses, and other staples on credit to last them through the winter, and if the ice persisted for longer than usual in spring, families could be reduced to a diet of bread and tea.

The new nurse lodged with the local teacher and his family, in whose home she also set up a clinic. Within days, work commenced in earnest as patients began to arrive. One of Bennett's first patients came in suffering from a digestive problem and very bad teeth, both typical cases in Newfoundland at the time, given the diet and lack of dentists. From her ledger kept between May 1921 and April 1924, we know that about 20 per cent of her cases (789 total) involved dentistry. Fortunately, Bennett had brought with her a number of medical instruments, including several forceps useful for extractions. In addition, her inventory included syringes, catheters, kidney trays, breast pump, scissors, probes, knives, eyedroppers, and thermometers – all in a leather medical bag.[26]

Accidents and septic wounds were also common among patients, accounting for 14 per cent of her cases in the early 1920s. Maternity cases accounted for only 9 per cent of the cases she attended in the early 1920s. Occasionally she treated cases of scurvy and malnutrition. These cases often involved travel to neighbouring communities though a majority of her time was spent in Daniel's Harbour. From Bennett's records we also know that in 20 per cent of the cases no fee was charged. In an economy run by the truck system, cash was scarce and poverty meant some could not pay. For those who could pay, the usual charge was fifty cents for a tooth extraction or treating a septic wound and five to ten dollars for a confinement. Sometimes she was paid in produce or some other non-monetary item.

Children and childbirth were constant themes in Bennett's life, whether she was attending a birth, training local women to assist in births, or tending to her own family and those children and young adults she took in. Within eight months of her arrival in Daniel's Harbour, she met and married Angus Bennett, whose occupation was listed as "fisherman" on the marriage certificate. Perhaps aware of possible criticism for the age gap between them, Bennett shaved a few years off her age on the marriage certificate to disguise the fact that she was seven years older than Angus. The couple built their own house though it took some time to earn enough to buy the materials. Throughout the many years they lived in this home they made many additions to include a waiting area, surgery, and dispensary for the medical work. They had three children of their own and as well took in foster children and employed domestics. And sometimes young women were sent to Bennett for 'straightening out.' Since she might be called to a patient in a neighbouring community and her husband might be in the woods or out fishing, live-in domestics were key to bringing up a family. Much like midwife Martha Ballard in early nineteenth-century Maine, Bennett found that the reproduction of daily life, that is, accomplishing all the necessary domestic tasks to keep the family going, required helping hands.[27]

Trained to be a nurse-midwife, Bennett's experiences and case records help us to understand this part of her work life and the labour processes of her occupation. Taught to keep meticulous records, she brought with her the register or ledger supplied by the Central Midwives Board where she continued to write down information about the 343 maternity cases she attended in Newfoundland from 1921 to 1955. Record keeping, then, was part of the work process. She entered information about the mother – name, community, age, and previous pregnancies; particulars about the infant – sex, weight (in some cases), and name; and details about the actual delivery including the time of her arrival to the time of birth, the term of the pregnancy, presentation, and complications (if any) during or after labour. She also listed any interventions such as the use of forceps or the dispensing of drugs. If a student midwife or a doctor attended, she also wrote that down. The ledger is useful in telling us about the women who gave birth, the amount of time Bennett spent with her patients, and what services she provided. It cannot, however, give us a complete picture of Bennett's routines in childbirth cases. We do know that she rarely used forceps and lost only one mother and eleven babies, some of them stillbirths. Drugs – particularly ergot (to expel the afterbirth), morphine sulphate (painkiller), chloral hydrate (sedative), and chloroform (anaesthetic) – were administered in nearly two-thirds of the deliveries. The majority (two-thirds) of her deliveries took place in Daniel's Harbour. Thus, in one-third of her maternity cases, travel formed another aspect of her work, sometimes in dangerous weather. The rhythm of her work was unpredictable as well. Even when attending maternity cases in communities outside of Daniel's Harbour, she was sometimes called upon to look at other cases deemed to be urgent.[28]

From 1924 until 1936 Bennett carried on her medical work without official sanction or a salary. With the reorganization of health care under the Commission of Government and the creation of a district nursing service, Bennett was once again an employee of the state. As part of the health reform initiative to improve health care in rural areas, from the mid-thirties to the early 1960s, outport women were invited to St John's for midwifery training. Some nurse-midwives, including Bennett, were asked to train local women. Bennett chose five women from the local area to be trained and put them through a six-month course that involved lectures and assisting at deliveries. Bennett supervised exams at the end of the six-month period in summer 1936 and all five passed. Freda Guinchard, the daughter of the schoolteacher in Daniel's Harbour where Bennett first lived, continued to deliver babies until 1965. While Guinchard kept a little black book of her 556 cases, it recorded few details. However, she also filled out government forms reporting on each birth, records that still survive. Bennett's position as instructor of 'traditional' midwives underlines her leadership role and the value she placed on education. She often noted the lack of prenatal and postnatal care and campaigned against bottle-feeding as a regressive step.[29]

As the nurse for her area, Bennett handled general nursing activities such as surgical, pediatric, and dental cases. She visited schools and provided immunizations and also treated and reported incidents of communicable diseases, which often hit the school-age population. As well as filling in government forms, Bennett carried on correspondence with other health care professionals, particularly those located in St John's, St Anthony, Norris Point, and Port Saunders. In the latter two communities, cottage hospitals had been built, which meant that cases could be referred to the doctors – though in the case of Port Saunders, it was difficult to find and retain a doctor in such an isolated place. Despite his efforts to recruit in the United States and Canada, Dr LaSalle, who had worked there, reported to Bennett that he had no success, noting that the fee-based salary could not attract doctors, especially to such a large and isolated district. Acknowledging Bennett's efforts to support the hospital, Dr LaSalle recognized another aspect of her work life: the continuous struggle to draw attention to the health care needs of the area. In 1941 he wrote: "We all know that all your life there you worked towards the establishment of a Hospital. We can look back and see you rejoice when it actually went up and when you saw it in operation. And we can almost look into your soul and see the sadness there at the Hospital's disappearance after only such a short life,–and all for what? Nevertheless you have done good work there. We witnessed it ourselves, and Hospital or no Hospital, we know you will keep on keeping on."[30]

As early as 1929 Bennett had campaigned to get a replacement for her own volunteer labour by inquiring about how to get a NONIA nurse for her district. The requirements – a geographical description, a survey of the population, and the creation of a four- or five-person committee willing to raise hundreds of dollars – could not be met.[31] In addition to these activities, Bennett repeatedly lobbied the government for trained medical personnel from the 1940s to the 1970s, even writing to several ministers of health when she was in her seventies and eighties.[32]

A letter from Dr R.F. Dove of the Bonne Bay Hospital at Norris Point further illuminates aspects of Bennett's work: he offered to continue to assist her with medical problems noting, "especially I do appreciate the letters with important details of [patient] history that you send along. They have given me very valuable information which I could not have obtained otherwise." During the Second World War and in the immediate post-war period, Bennett also corresponded regularly with the superintendent of the nursing service, mixing the professional with the personal. The letters mentioned vacancies that could not be filled, the training of potential outport nurses, and the difficulties of recruitment along with personal messages. For example, the superintendent tried to comfort Bennett when she lost her first (and ultimately only) mother in spring 1946, a woman with eight children who died of heart failure delivering a stillborn ninth infant. This event, coupled with her son's tuberculosis, seems to have prompted Bennett to offer her resignation. The superintendent's reply included the comment, "We just have'nt [sic] got the nurses, and if you resign the end of March the people will just have to go without anyone." Bennett did not resign officially until 1953 though she continued to handle cases into old age.[33]

Finally, Bennett's work life also included helping her husband with his general merchandising business. She assisted in the shop and kept the books. At the end of 1946, for example, she had to give an account of banking transactions for income tax purposes. Here she revealed that the sums of money assumed to be profit from the business were actually repayments to her for loans she had advanced when the business had nearly failed. Rather than let him go bankrupt, she advanced him the money he needed from her savings.[34]

Bennett's work life was complex and multi-faceted. Although scholars most often use the term *occupational pluralism* to refer to the combination of subsistence activities undertaken by men in underdeveloped regions, the case can be made for applying the term to women's work as well. In Bennett's case, she engaged in a complex round of subsistence activities and medical work plus ran a business, raised a family, trained domestics, and entertained a constant stream of visitors and travellers. No one was turned away: local custom mandated open doors, cups of tea, and putting up travellers. No wonder there were frequent notations in her diary that conveyed her tiredness. On 5 April 1949 she wrote that her husband had brought ashore dozens of seals and that she "Did the washing in between pts [patients] & shop and am desperately tired tonight."[35] Confederation with Canada that year also meant the introduction of Canadian social welfare and health programs, including old age pensions, mothers' allowance, and other social benefits. Those who had some education or professional training found themselves helping the less educated fill out forms to obtain the benefit; Bennett's diary confirms that she too was called upon to fill out applications thus indicating her status as a local citizen of some note.

IV. A Fragmented Autobiography

Before Bennett died in 1990 at the age of one hundred, she wrote numerous fragments of autobiography as well as letters detailing parts of her life. As David Vincent noted over twenty-five years ago, "when an individual sets down a record of his life, he does more than provide an account of a series of actions. We are presented not with a collection of remembered facts but rather with a pattern of recollected experiences."[36] Bennett's fragmentary autobiography or life writing served several purposes: first, to provide her family with an account of her personal and professional life; and second, to fulfill what she seemed to see as a wider purpose in these accounts, as evidenced by her own words: "To attempt to record significant changes and improvements in the history of a country must of necessity be a stupendous task, but maybe a few notes on changes, especially those which have occurred during ones [sic] own life time, and in ones [sic] own district, may be of interest, or amusement to those who come after us, and who have never endured the trials and tribulations of their predecessors."[37] As Cynthia Huff has suggested of a nineteenth-century diarist, even though the diarist could not engage in the masculine occupation of soldier, "she could become part of the body politic by acting as its self-appointed chronicler," an observation that could be applied to Bennett.[38]

In her longest fragments, "Forty Years of Outport Life" (22 pages) and "Memoirs" (17 pages), Bennett provides a number of different types of 'stories' with five major tropes apparent: 1) her rendition of the quest, the epic journey from England to Newfoundland as well as her life's journey; 2) the heroic medical stories that feature sets of obstacles that need to be overcome and/or require improvisation; 3) trickster-type tales that persuade 'backward,' uneducated people to accept modern medical practices; 4) closely related to the trickster, pedagogical stories that demonstrate how she taught better health practices; and finally 5) stories of resilience, self-sufficiency, and generous giving associated with her vision of hearty Newfoundlanders. It is possible to see how these stories pull together the diverse threads of a life, helping to re-situate Bennett in terms of geography, class, and profession.

To take but one trope as an example, the pedagogical stories underline the lack of health knowledge among the people she served but they also simultaneously called up notions of colonialism, class difference, and professional expectations. Recreating the case of a malnourished baby brought in by its parents, Bennett comments on the parents' attempts to feed the child a combination of tea, molasses, and cocoa when the baby refused milk. Bennett also discovered that the sewn-up nipple on the bottle scraped the palate of the baby so that feeding was painful. Taking the baby with her to Daniel's Harbour, she gradually nursed the child back to health and commented that she hoped her actions would encourage others to seek help before it was too late. Another often-repeated story centred on her attempts to convince people that tuberculosis (TB) was infectious, despite the fact that some did not exhibit signs of the disease. Bennett complained that friends and family of patients helped spread the disease, especially in winter, by sitting in rooms tightly sealed against the weather. The stigma of TB also meant that some hid their symptoms. These stories convey the superiority of English middle-class professional expertise within a colonial setting, a theme echoed in the writings of nurses at the Grenfell Mission serving northern Newfoundland and coastal Labrador. Whether Bennett was conscious of creating such a narrative or not, its effect is to create distance between the nurse and her patients, between the middle-class professional and her petty commodity-producing clientele of fishermen, loggers, and their families.[39]

+++

Myra Bennett's story illuminates a number of themes: the potentially transformative nature of professional training in terms of class identification; the role of women's professions in creating new identities for educated women; the episodic nature of women's health care work as well as domestic labour; the fluidity between unpaid domestic and/or community work and remunerated professional health care work; and the attractions of life on the 'margins of empire' for some women who had ambitions, both philanthropic and personal. The emergence of nursing as a woman's profession opened up "new social territory" where women could examine the meaning of their lives.[40] For a nurse-midwife like Bennett, this new territory was physical as well intellectual. Having been raised in an English working-class family, she could see the benefits of travel to remote areas in need of her professional expertise: here an individual might find recognition and perhaps a new identity. Bennett's lifelong adventure in Newfoundland provided her with that recognition of her medical skills as well as of her leadership roles in the community. In exchanging her Cockney speech for an upper middle-class accent, Bennett reinforced her Englishness as well as her professional status. A close examination of her work patterns demonstrates a complex round of medical, domestic, accounting, shopkeeping, and community work, thus suggesting that some women's work can be described as occupational pluralism on a somewhat different scale than men's work. That work also demonstrated the easy

flow from domestic and community preoccupations to professional
ones and vice versa. Finally, Bennett's archive of written material
demonstrates the variety of narratives created by a single individual
seeking to explain and pass on her recollected experiences of a pur-
poseful life.

NOTES

1 On Australia, see for example, Glenda Strachan, "Present at the Birth: Midwives,
  'Handywomen' and Neighbours in Rural New South Wales, 1850–1900," in
  Labour History 81 (November 2001): 13–28; Madonna Grehan, "'From the
  sphere of Sarah Gampism': The professionalization of nursing and midwifery
  in the Colony of Victoria," in *Nursing Inquiry* 11, 3 (2004): 192–201; on the
  United States, see Katy Dawley, "Origins of Nurse-midwifery in the United States
  and its Expansion in the 1940s," in *Journal of Midwifery & Women's Health*,
  48, 2: 86–95. A revisionist account can be found in I.L. Bourgeault, C. Benoit,
  and R. Davis-Floyd, eds., *Reconceiving Midwifery* (Montreal & Kingston:
  McGill-Queens University Press, 2004). Kathryn McPherson, *Bedside Matters:
  The Transformation of Canadian Nursing, 1900–1990* (Don Mills: Oxford University Press, 1996), 1–3 makes the point that nursing is rarely considered as
  labour history; see also Judith Godden, "A 'Lamentable Failure'? The Founding of Nightingale Nursing in Australia, 1868–1884," in *Australian Historical
  Studies* 117 (October 2001): 276–291 who makes a point similar to McPher-
  son's on p. 279, that few studies of nursing utilize labour or gender history.
2 Cecilia Benoit, *Midwives in Passage: The Modernisation of Maternity Care* (St.
  John's: ISER Books, 1991); Janet McNaughton, "The Role of the Newfoundland
  Midwife in Traditional Healthcare, 1900–1970," PhD dissertation (St John's:
  Memorial University of Newfoundland, 1990 (1989)); Wendy Mitchinson, *Giv-
  ing Birth in Canada, 1900–1950* (Toronto: University of Toronto Press, 2002);
  Judith Young, "'Monthly' Nurses, 'Sick' Nurses, and Midwives: Working-Class
  Caregivers in Toronto, 1830–91," chapter 1 in this volume.
3 Dea Birkett, "The 'White Woman's Burden' in the 'White Man's Grave': The
  Introduction of British Nurses in Colonial West Africa." In N. Chaudhuri and
  M. Stroebel, eds., *Western Women and Imperialism: Complicity and Resistance*,
  179 (Bloomington: Indiana University Press, 1992).; see also Jill Perry, "Queen
  of Her Own Domain: Nursing for the Grenfell Mission, 1894–1938." In G. Burford and J. Symonds, eds., *Ties That Bind: An Anthology of Social Work and*

Social Welfare in Newfoundland and Labrador, 67–76 (St. John's: Jesperson Publishing, 1997).

4 Carolyn Steedman, *Landscape for a Good Woman* (New Brunswick, NJ: Rutgers, 1987), quotes from p. 7 and p. 6; Steedman ignores race/ethnicity in this statement. I thank Bonnie Hutchins for alerting me to some of this work including Helen M. Buss and Marlene Kadar, eds., *Working in Women's Archives: Researching Women's Private Literature and Archival Documents* (Waterloo, Ontario: Wilfrid Laurier University Press, 2001).

5 Margot Duley, *Where Once Our Mothers Stood We Stand: Women's Suffrage in Newfoundland, 1890–1925* (Charlottetown: gynergy books, 1993); Linda Kealey, ed., *Pursuing Equality: Historical Perspectives on Women in Newfoundland and Labrador* (St. John's: Institute for Social and Economic Research, Memorial University, 1999).

6 Margaret Gibbons, "The Child Welfare Association, 1919–1939," Honours dissertation (St John's: Department of History, Memorial University, 1996).

7 Evelyn Cave Hiscock, "Better Nursing in Newfoundland," in *The Newfoundland Quarterly* (Autumn 1924): 29–30.

8 McNaughton, "The Role of the Newfoundland Midwife," 78–85.

9 Lady Harris, "Outport Nursing," in *The Newfoundland Quarterly* 21, 1 (July 1921): 1.

10 Harris, "Outport Nursing," 4.

11 Birkett, "The 'White Woman's Burden,'" 177.

12 Ibid.

13 Edgar House, *The Way Out: The Story of NONIA, in Newfoundland, 1920–1990* (St. John's: Creative, 1990).

14 Three of the Commissioners were Newfoundlanders and the other three were English. See Peter Neary, *Newfoundland in the North Atlantic World, 1929–1949* (Montreal & Kingston: McGill-Queens University Press, 1988), chap. 3, 44–74.

15 Linda Kealey, "Historical Perspectives on Nutrition and Food Security in Newfoundland and Labrador." In C. Parrish and N. Turner, *Resetting the Kitchen Table: Food Security, Culture, Health and Resilience in Coastal Communities*, 177–90 (New York: Nova Science Publishers, 2008),

16 McPherson, *Bedside Matters*, 110–22.

17 Myra Bennett Collection (copy in the possession of the author), Miscellaneous Documents file, General Register Office, Somerset House, London. "Certified Copy of an Entry of Birth," Myra Maud Grimsley (dated 17 June 1959).

18 Myra Bennett Collection, Miscellaneous Documents file, "Memoirs."

19 Bennett Collection, Miscellaneous Documents file, "Questions for Mrs Bennett, 24 July 1973," "Memoirs."

20 Bennett Collection, Miscellaneous Documents file, testimonial letter, 27 February 1919, signed "Geo. F. Vincent, FRCSEd."

21 Bennett Collection, Miscellaneous Documents file, testimonial letter, 1 March 1921, signed "Evelina Todd."

22 Bennett Collection, Miscellaneous Documents file, "Questions for Mrs Bennett, 24 July 1973," "Memoirs."

23 See Mary-Ellen Kelm, "Part of a Large Company of White Folk," chapter 5 in this volume where she discusses Englishness as a unifying force in the face of the 'other,' in this case Aboriginal peoples.

24 McPherson, *Bedside Matters*, 33–4.

25 Bennett Collection, Miscellaneous Documents file, fragment.

26 Ledger, 29 May 1921 to 29 April 1924; see also Victoria Page Sparkes Belbin, "Midwifery and Rural Newfoundland Healthcare, 1920–1950: A Case Study of Myra Bennett, Nurse Midwife," Honours dissertation (St John's: Memorial University, 1996). As well as writing her dissertation on Bennett, Ms Belbin assisted with the copying and organizing of these files.

27 Laurel Thatcher Ulrich, *A Midwife's Tale: the Life of Martha Ballard, based on her diary, 1785 –1812* (New York: Random House, 1990).

28 Belbin, "Midwifery and Rural Newfoundland Healthcare," analyzed these cases and is the source of the information. See also "Register of Cases" in Bennett Collection. In total, Bennett recorded 595 births attended.

29 Government documents contain contradictory information on Bennett's re-employment date in the 1930s; on Guinchard see Provincial Archives of Newfoundland and Labrador, RC 98-004, Register of Midwives, 1937–1963.

30 Bennett Collection, Correspondence, Department of Public Health and Welfare File, 1938–1970, Dr LaSalle to Nurse Bennett, 20 January 1941.

31 Bennett Collection, Miscellaneous Documents file, W.F. Huthchinson to Myra M. Bennett, 11 April 1929.

32 Bennett Collection, Correspondence, Department of Public Health and Welfare, 1938–1970, Bennett to minister of health, 19 December 1969; Edward Roberts to Mrs M.M. Bennett, 2 January 1970; Miscellaneous Documents file, Bennett to Dr McGrath, minister of health, 10 March 1966.

33 Bennett Collection, Correspondence, Department of Public Health and Welfare, 1938–1970, Robert F. Dove to Mrs M.M. Bennett, 18 December 1942; Mary Green to Mrs M. Bennett, 5 March and 17 April 1946; 7 and 22 February 1947.

34 Bennett Collection, Miscellaneous Documents file, Bennett to "Dear Mr Roberts," 25 November 1946.

35 Bennett Collection, Book Number 9, Diary, January 1943 to December 1949.

36 David Vincent, *Bread, Knowledge and Freedom: A Study of Nineteenth Century Working Class Autobiography* (London: Europa Publications Ltd., 1981), 5.

37 Bennett Collection, Miscellaneous Documents file, "Memoirs," 13. Marlene Kadar defines life writing as a "genre of documents or fragments of documents written out of a life, or unabashedly out of a personal experience of the writer," quoted in Christl Verdun, ed., *Marian Engel's Notebooks: "Ah, mon cahier, ecoute"* (Waterloo: Wilfred Laurier Press, 1999), 5.

38 Cynthia Huff, "Textual Boundaries: Space in Nineteenth Century Women's Manuscript Diaries." In S.L. Bunkers and C. Huff, eds., *Inscribing the Daily: Critical Essays on Women's Diaries*, 136 (Amherst: University of Massachusetts Press, 1995).

39 Bennett Collection, Miscellaneous Documents file, "The Baby Who Wouldn't Drink Milk," and "Forty Years of Outport Life," 8; Perry, "Queen of Her Own Domain: Nursing for the Grenfell Mission, 1894–1938." In G. Burford and J. Symonds, eds., *Ties That Bind: An Anthology of Social Work and Social Welfare in Newfoundland and Labrador* (St. John's: Jesperson Publishing, 1997).

40 Jill Ker Conway, *When Memory Speaks: Exploring the Art of Autobiography* (New York: Vintage, 1999), 15.

Part Two

Writing Their Own Lives: Life Writing in Nursing History

4

+ + + + +

From the Streets of Toronto to the Northwest Rebellion:
Hannah Grier Coome's Call to Duty

ELIZABETH DOMM, RN

Hannah Grier Coome left to posterity a memoir of her life's work. For those engaged in the study of women's history this fact alone is interesting, given that the memoir was published in 1933 during an era when the history of women in Canada received very little attention. For those who study nursing history the text is of even more value. The book reveals the life of a deeply religious woman who shared a calling both to heal the ill and to help the disadvantaged. This essay explores the connection between spirituality and nursing to address the perspectives and motivations of a nineteenth-century Canadian pioneer nurse. Coome's work found her at the forefront of outreach nursing in Toronto and took her to the battlefield of the Northwest Rebellion. Yet, compared to her male counterparts, she has been ignored. In part, this is because historians of the Northwest Rebellion have focused most of their attention on the opposing interests of Louis Riel and the Métis, and John A. Macdonald and his expansionist policy. Because of the prominence of the politics of the rebellion, the actions of Coome and the other nurses on the battlefront have been neglected. Certainly, the desire to have a team of nurses at the site of the rebellion represented a Canadian response to a potential medical crisis. No doubt Florence Nightingale's Crimean example served as an important backdrop, but the call for trained nurses nonetheless emanated from the Canadian government. Coome's work in Toronto also begs attention since we are only just beginning to carefully delve into the history of nursing in nineteenth-century Canada. Influenced by developments in nursing in England and the United States, Coome and her Anglican Sisters were motivated to offer an increasing array of medical care and social services to their neighbours in Toronto. In order to understand how and why Coome carried out her work, and blended spirituality and nursing, it is first necessary to understand her background. Much of the information here was presented in her memoirs, which according to the preface, were written by "Many of the devoted men and women ... praying and laboring for this work years before it was brought into being ... for the younger members of our community and for future generations of sisters, associates, and friends."[1]

Sarah Hannah Roberta Grier was born on 28 October 1837, the third daughter and sixth of thirteen children, to Reverend John Grier and Eliza Lilias Grier of Kingston, Ontario. Her father was from County Antrim, Ireland, a trained Presbyterian minister who had attained a degree at Glasgow University, then was ordained in the Anglican Church of Canada. Reverend Grier later became the Rector at the Anglican Church in Belleville, Ontario. Eliza Grier's family had strong ties to the United Empire Loyalists. The Griers were a religious family and, as Grier would later recall, lived within a happy and busy home. She was raised in the Anglican faith, with the "Doctrine of the Real Presence," which was considered part of the traditional High Church Anglican ritual.[2] This religious upbringing would prove to be of critical importance to her life and career.

Grier met her future husband Charles Horace Coome in Belleville, Ontario, where he worked as an engineer for the Grand Trunk Railway. They married on 23 July 1859 and lived for some years in Kingston until Charles' engineering work took them to England and Wales. During her years abroad, Coome took an increasing interest in her religious life. She attended St John the Divine, Kennington church in London and she worked with and became close to the Sisters of St Mary at Wantage, whose mission house was in the "slums of Kennington."[3] She was also interested in the revival of the religious life in the Church of England. The Anglican Sisterhood in England met with controversy since it was seen as too Catholic. Nonetheless, the women involved were determined to commit to religion and good works within the context of a separate life and society for women.

While in Britain, Coome became pregnant, but miscarried, and as a result endured five years of "invalidism and suffering" which, if she had received proper attention at the time, would have been unnecessary.[4] This experience had a profound effect on Coome and she resolved that no woman should suffer as she had, if she could prevent it. As if that were not enough misfortune, only about one year after their return to America, her husband died of cancer.

Having moved to Chicago from overseas, Coome decided to stay in that city. She worked as the director of the Chicago School of Decorative Art and, at the same time, did much work for the altar guild of the Anglican Cathedral. She was concerned about those who were in need, and gave away most of her salary to help the less fortunate. Not long after, she chose to return to England and go into God's service, joining the Sisters of St Mary at Wantage. On her return trip she stopped in Toronto to see her mother and eldest sister Rose, who was the principal at The Bishop Strachan School. There, Coome was approached by Mrs Georgina Broughall, wife of Reverend Broughall of St Stephen's Parsonage in Toronto, to found an indigenous Canadian community of Anglican Sisters.

This was not the first time that an Anglican sisterhood for Canada had been imagined. In the early 1870s, Reverend William Stewart Darling of the Church of the Holy Trinity, Toronto had requested advice from Dr Littledale in England and received letters with suggestions. Dr Littledale was an "authority on the Religious Life and Communities in England."[5] While the first attempts failed, the idea did not altogether falter, and in Toronto, several Anglican Church communities set about collecting for the foundation of a Sisterhood.[6] At a meeting of the Anglican Church community in Toronto on 9 November 1881, a resolution was passed that "it was desirable to establish a Church of England Sisterhood in Toronto for the promotion of the Religious Life and Works of Charity and a building purchased should be vested in trustees and transferred to the Sisters as soon as they should be incorporated."[7] Very soon after that it was decided that Coome would be asked to found the first Anglican Church Sisterhood in Toronto. Georgina Broughall, as one of the key promoters of this Sisterhood, was asked to approach Coome. Broughall encouraged Coome to stay in Toronto and take up her work, arguing that as a native of Canada she knew its conditions. Reverend O.P. Ford, an Anglican minister at St Luke's Anglican Church in Toronto and elected warden of the church community promoting an Anglican Sisterhood, also encouraged Coome to start the foundation as a distinct vocation, not apart from a religious vocation. Nursing and religious work could be incorporated into one.

Coome seriously considered this request and asked for advice from her friends and advisors, including Canon Carter and Canon Brooke of St John the Divine, Kennington and other Anglican Church leaders. All agreed that the call to found an Anglican Community of Sisters in Canada was a distinct vocation and should be accepted; they suggested she should go to the United States rather than to England to take training, as the religious and social conditions there were similar to those in Canada. The training that was advised was similar to deaconess training. The education set out for deaconesses was meant to prepare women for various charitable works, including nursing and education of children, and a life of devotion. Coome agreed to be the foundress as soon as she could be professed after passing the novitiate. On 21 June 1882, she and "Miss Hare (later, the Novice Aimée"[8] left Toronto to do the novitiate at St Mary's Sisterhood at Peekskill, New York where she spent the next two years learning about religious life in the convent and taking nurse's training in the surgical wards in Trinity Hospital, New York. Even in her education, nursing and spirituality went hand in hand.

While Coome was in New York, Anglican Church community members in Toronto met several times and strengthened their resolve to support a Sisterhood that would do charitable works in the community, visit the sick, and spread the word of God. There were several "Sales of Work" by Anglican women, who raised the majority of the money to support the endowment. It was understood that unless the Sisters were experienced and had suitable finances, efforts would be futile to help the sick and the suffering, no matter how earnest the visiting church people were.[9] At one such organizational meeting, Dr O'Reilly, Inspector of Prisons and Public Charities for the Province of Ontario,[10] testified to the superiority of work done by women. He pointed to the number of cases treated by Roman Catholic Sisters in hospitals and in the community at this time, although Ontario's population was only one-fifth Roman Catholic. Reverend J.D. Cayley,

Rector of St George's Church, also spoke to the gathering and praised the efforts and work of women in helping the wounded and sick of the Crimean War, and in advancing the work of the church. Each meeting of the Toronto Anglican Church Community was asked to donate funds for the establishment of the Order of St John the Divine Anglican Sisterhood.[11] This concerted effort succeeded in providing an endowment for the Sisters so they would not have to be concerned with raising money for subsistence.

This venture to found a Canadian Sisterhood was unique, and undertaken with fervour by the High Church Anglicans in Toronto and surrounding parishes. Since the mid-1850s, the Church Missionary Society had sent Anglican missionaries to remote parts of Canada to work among Canada's indigenous people and bring the 'light of God's word to heathens' in these areas;[12] however, there were no Canadian Anglican Sisterhoods. Many of the Anglican missionaries who went to northwestern Canada were sent by the evangelical branch of the Anglican Church in England.

Coome made her profession of faith and became a Sister on 8 September 1884 in St Mary's Convent at the age of forty-seven, and then returned to Toronto to live with her sister at The Bishop Strachan School while waiting to begin as Mother Foundress of the Sisters of St. John the Divine. She stipulated that the Sisters were not to beg for their support, but money must be raised by the Anglican Church and freely given to endow the Sisters' work. In being firm about how she saw the Sisterhood unfolding, she showed herself to be a visionary, somewhat ahead of her time. In its efforts to meet her demands, the Anglican Church in Toronto guaranteed a house and an income for the Sisters. Soon, two small semi-detached houses on Robinson Street in Toronto were purchased; one had started out as a stable, and both had been used by workingmen in the parish of St Matthias. Work commenced to install sliding panels and archways to join the houses, and soon they were ready for occupation. It did not take long for Coome (now known as Mother Hannah), and the novice Aimée, and one other woman, a friend of Mother Hannah's from England, to move in. The conditions and décor were far from luxurious: the furnishings consisted of three beds; a few chairs and a table; a dishpan, coal scuttle, and shovel; some cups, saucers, and plates. In neighbourly fashion, someone brought food over, and Reverend Darling sent a frying pan, lamp, and two candles.

Within a short time, Mother Hannah completed a beautifully decorated altar for the first Eucharist in their new home. The women worked in the embroidery room and the first piece of beautiful needlework was given for the altar frontal at St Matthias Church.

The Sisters prepared food in the kitchen for themselves and for the sick and needy; they carried food to those in need when they went visiting from house to house. The Sisters were recognized in the St Matthias parish magazine for their good works in the community providing dinners twice a week for the poor at their house, a dispensary for the sick, a Bible class for boys, clothing for those in need, and visiting and feeding the hungry in the community. Indeed, Mother Hannah made it a practice that she or the Sisters visited all those who came to their attention as being in need, before any charity was offered, be it clothing, food, or nursing care. They worked both as nurses and as missionaries in an urban context, before the time of social service organizations, to help the sick and hungry.

A local advertisement claimed that the Sisters were in need of donations for their new house, and one parishioner of St Matthias (Mr Carter) went door to door asking for support for them. Apparently, Carter met with generosity and kindness, but also animosity and abuse, because the Sisters wore habits like Roman Catholic nuns. As in England, some Anglicans were affronted by Anglican Sisters wearing dark habits, and Mother Hannah was entreated to delay having the Sisters wear them until they were accepted in the neighbourhood, but she did not agree. The Sisters were noticed in their black habits and often mocked by a group of Protestants on their way to and from church. A group of Orangemen living in Toronto offered to give the Sisters a warm reception by burning their convent, but after the Sisters extended their help to many people in the community, they were not set upon; in fact, these same Orangemen donated to the Sisters. It was noted in Mother Hannah's memoirs that the Sisters were surprised by the volume of appeals for help from the sick, the aged, and the poor, and carrying food to them soon became a daily duty.[13] The Sisters also encouraged children to attend St Matthias Sunday School. When she was out late at night to minister to the sick and needy, Mother Hannah was recognized by her long habit and believed it helped to keep her safe. Her habit formed a protective shield. In some ways, wearing a habit allowed her to transgress the boundaries of respectable womanhood that she no doubt would have run up against in Victorian Toronto. Through her veiled body she could both work as a nurse and represent the Church at the same time, which was an advantage, given that Mother Hannah was often called out after dark to assist someone in need.

Called to Duty in the Northwest Rebellion

Early in 1885 in Canada's northwest (in an area that would become Saskatchewan), there was a rebellion of perhaps 250 Métis and First Nations people against the governing authority of the Dominion of Canada. The medical and nursing care at the time of the Northwest Rebellion involved many individuals from different areas; Mother Hannah was one of several that answered the call to duty. Doctors, stretcher-bearers, first aid–trained soldiers, nurses, and a few women came to care for the wounded and ill in less than ideal conditions in the Canadian prairies. They fulfilled their duty with courage, hard work, and resourcefulness.

When word of the provisional government of Louis Riel reached Ottawa, General Frederick Middleton from Eastern Canada was called upon to assemble an armed force to subdue the rebellion. In planning the military strategy, General Middleton sent close to 5,000 hastily re-cruited troops – drawn from retired battalions and the ranks of mini-mally trained soldiers – west on Canadian Pacific Railway trains. In some parts of Ontario, north of Lake Superior, the railroad tracks were not yet completed, so through that area some of the troops were sent in open wagons or marched between rail lines; some of these arrived in Winnipeg suffering from exhaustion and exposure to the cold.[14]

Medical care for the troops was needed. Dr Darby Bergin, Surgeon General of Canada, was asked to establish a medical corps to care for Dominion force casualties. Dr Bergin telegraphed companies ordering supplies of hospital cots, mattresses, instruments, and equipment to be delivered by railroad through Winnipeg to the battlefront. The public were asked to contribute dressings and bandages through church groups, Saint John Relief and Aid Society and the Red Cross Corps. He contacted and selected several physicians to go to the battlefront to care for casualties. Medical students from Toronto were recruited to give first aid and be stretcher-bearers. Some were given a week of training before they were sent west. Dr Bergin put out a public call for nurses to volunteer.

The Anglican Synod in Toronto volunteered nurses, and many individuals offered to go west in response to the call. General Middleton, General Laurie (in charge of the commissariat for the expedition), Deputy Surgeon General Dr Thomas Roddick of the Northwest Territories, and Dr James Bell, Surgeon Major in charge of base hospitals did not just want volunteers, they wanted trained nurses. This may have been due to the influence of Florence Nightingale's experience and writings following the Crimean War or insights gained during the American Civil War when trained nurses had been very effective in providing treatment and comfort to the sick and wounded. Nurses had shown they were able to improve health outcomes and reduce mortality not only for casualties but also for those with illnesses and infectious diseases in times of conflict and war. The idea and reality of trained nurses was fairly new but there were Nightingale training schools in New York City, at Bellevue Hospital, and in St Catharines, Ontario.[15]

Although many women volunteered, the telegraphed message clearly stated, "No volunteer nurses. If you can send an organized body under a trained head, they will be welcome."[16] This directive described Mother Hannah and the Sisters of St John the Divine: the Anglican Synod of Toronto asked Mother Hannah to volunteer. She consented to go to the front with one novice and two postulants of the Sisters of St John the Divine. In addition, three graduate nurses from Bellevue Hospital in New York City volunteered and were chosen. Mother Hannah agreed to take charge of the base hospital at Moose Jaw, with a budget of $200 from the Canadian government. It was noted at the closure of the Moose Jaw field hospital in July 1885 that Mother Hannah returned $50 from the original budget.[17]

Mother Hannah left the Mother House in Toronto to the care of six dedicated women, as she set out for Moose Jaw with the nurses from Toronto in mid April 1885, crossing the Great Lakes by boat then continuing by train. The journey took six weeks from the time they accepted this call to duty until their arrival on 30 May 1885 in Moose Jaw. Travel was arduous, and Mother Hannah's memoirs record that while crossing Lake Superior she cut off her long dark hair and dropped it overboard. She felt that this was an example to the small contingent of women that she was travelling with of her practical nature, for if the care of her hair was proving difficult now, what would happen when they reached what they thought of as the wilderness?[18]

After the battle between General Middleton's forces and the Métis at Fish Creek in April 1885, the injured from each side were taken behind battle lines and given first aid in tents as the weather alternated between heavy rain, wind, hail, and snow. Doctors and first aid–trained soldiers tended the wounded from the Dominion force, and Métis women tended the wounded Métis soldiers. Most of the injuries were from gunshots, but there were also compound fractures and amputated limbs. Arm and shoulder wounds were most common.[19]

A few of the injured died at Fish Creek, but a week later, when it was deemed safe to travel, others who were sick or wounded were taken on a forty-two-mile, two-day journey to Saskatoon. To make the journey as comfortable as possible for those travelling, canvasses and cowhides were slung on the sides of wooden wagons, with canvas awnings covering the wagons, offering a measure of protection from the elements. Nevertheless, the jolting travel in wagons was reported to be extremely difficult, causing the wounded much pain and discomfort.[20]

Thirty wounded men arrived in Saskatoon after the Battle of Fish Creek and were billeted first in a school or in some of the twenty private homes of the community. Soon, the largest houses on the banks of the South Saskatchewan River were commandeered to house the wounded. Women from Saskatoon were asked to help the doctors and provide what care they could for the wounded and those with illnesses such as rheumatism, scalds, infected wounds, and syphilis.[21]

A robust response team is necessary to give immediate medical and surgical care to the wounded and sick, close to battles and in field hospitals. The small pool of doctors and stretcher-bearers couldn't be in both places, at the battlefront and caring for wounded in the commandeered houses in Saskatoon. Dr Roddick and Dr Campbell worked in the base hospital in the houses on 11th Street starting on 3 May. Four days later, Dr Roddick summoned a trained nurse from Winnipeg, the closest major hospital, to care for the wounded in Saskatoon. On 12 May 1885 Nurse L. Miller arrived and immediately set to work organizing the care of the wounded.[22] Nurse Miller was a graduate nurse from the Montreal General Hospital and was working as head nurse in the Winnipeg General Hospital.

On 12 May 1885 the Battle of Batoche ended with the defeat of the provisional government. Louis Riel and Gabriel Dumont surrendered, but approximately eighty men of the Dominion force were wounded. Reverend Father Moulin, a Catholic priest, was wounded and trapped in the upper story of a church; however, he was rescued by the ardent efforts of stretcher-bearers. On 14 May, twenty-seven wounded men were moved to the base hospital in Saskatoon, which was reported to be quite crowded with eighty wounded and ill persons being cared for by two doctors, Nurse Miller, and four dressers. In the doctors' medical report, it was noted that the soldiers' health had been adversely affected by clothing inadequate for weather conditions, and lack of water to drink or wash in (most of the enlisted men had not bathed for almost two months).[23]

By contrast, the base hospital in the houses in Saskatoon run by Nurse Miller provided a clean, orderly haven. The only recorded defect with the accommodations was the inferior quality of the cots, which were discarded. The mattresses from the cots were put on wooden pallets.[24] On 23 May 1885 Surgeon Major Douglas reported: "Two nurses, an assistant and a helper, arrived today by trail and were at once put on duty under the superintendence of nurse Miller. The latter had hitherto been most indefatigable in her attendance of the wounded. In fact, much of the success which attended the treatment of our wounded at Saskatoon was undoubtedly due to the skill, kindness and untiring devotion of nurse Miller. Nurses Elking [sic] and Hamilton are likewise deserving of praise for their unremitting attention to duty."[25]

Nurses Elkin and Parsons and Miss Hamilton, an assistant, arrived from Winnipeg after travelling three days by train to Troy (now Qu'Appelle, Saskatchewan) then over land in a horse-drawn democrat. Nurse Parsons reported that it was the nurses' duty to assist with medical treatment of the wounded, carry out physicians' orders, and monitor patients' progress, with little time for anything else.[26] She noted the wounded in the Saskatoon hospital were from both the army and the opposing force; the nurses were not asked to go to the battlefront. Nurses did not wear uniforms but plain print dresses, covered with a small tea apron, and a Red Cross band on one arm for identification. Clean old linen, blankets, sheets, and clean nightshirts for wounded in hospitals were received from women from Winnipeg.

When nurses were off-duty, they made and rolled bandages from the clean linen or slept in tents on cots by the river. Surgeon Major Dr James Bell reported, "much of the success of the treatment of the wounded at Saskatoon was due to the skill[,] kindness and untiring devotion of the nurses."[27]

Near the end of May it was decided that some of the convalescing wounded and ill were well enough to travel to a base hospital in Moose Jaw. They were transported on the steamer *Northcote* to the elbow in the South Saskatchewan River, then loaded into nine wagons and taken overland to Moose Jaw on 26 May 1885. The wounded soldiers cared for each other on the trip. Surgeon Major Douglas reported the trip overland was hard for the wounded: "I would suggest that no serious cases of wounds be sent by this route, the journey overland in unsuitable vehicles being too trying."[28] Dr Roddick and Mrs Bellamy, wife of one of Moose Jaw's residents, organized volunteers to feed and care for the arriving wounded until Mother Hannah and the nurses arrived in Moose Jaw. The purveyor general requisitioned the Moose Hotel, a building in Moose Jaw that could accommodate about thirty patients with medical attendants and nurses.

The Moose Hotel was chosen as the site of the second field hospital, as it was claimed to have the finest accommodation for travellers west of the Manitoba border. Mother Hannah described the interior walls as covered by tar paper with slats holding it in place, and decorated with white "no smoking" signs. It was a long, narrow two-storeyed building, with the ground floor partitioned into an office to be used as an apothecary, a large room for ten beds, a large kitchen, and storerooms. There were ten small rooms suitable for two beds each in the upper storey. Privies and cesspools were outside the back door. Water was kept in barrels hauled to the back door of the building, and wastes were hauled away through the same door. The Sisters and nurses were allocated a building adjoining the hospital for their residence.

Mother Hannah and her nurses arrived in Moose Jaw on the next to last day of May, accompanied by Dr Carniff. Dr Douglas was delighted by the arrival of new helpers in the field: "Their arrival was most opportune as some of the men were much in need of skilled nursing."[29] The women were met at the train station by Dr Roddick and General Laurie, escorted to the Moose Hotel, and ceremoniously given the keys. It was noted in Mother Hannah's memoirs: "There was

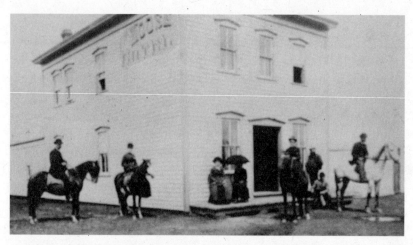

4.1 Moose Hotel, built in 1883, Moose Jaw, Saskatchewan.

no organization, and no facilities, so the Hospital had to be made out of nothing."[30] Apparently, Mother Hannah had no trouble getting started. Dr Douglas wrote: "The Lady Superior at once took charge, so that in a short time, things were put into good shape."[31] By the evening of their arrival, Mother Hannah, the novice and two postulants, and three nurses from New York had arranged the field hospital for the wounded. Mother Hannah reported the only nuisance that continually plagued the field hospital were gophers running in and out at will.[32]

The nurses cared for the sick and wounded twenty-four hours a day in the field hospital.

It soon became apparent to Mother Hannah that the crowded quarters for the sick and wounded in the Moose Hotel were not the best for healing or convalescence. She did not like to keep the wounded soldiers indoors all the time, in the stale air and environment of the sick. She felt those that were able to get up or be moved would benefit from fresh air, sunlight, cleanliness, and good food. Initially, all food was prepared on a kitchen stove in the house, and the sick and wounded either ate in the kitchen or were fed in bed. The odours from the kitchen (from cook stove fuel and cooking) and close habitation could be quite overwhelming. Mother Hannah believed that if a person was to heal properly, it was necessary to put a body in an optimal environment for healing – which included good sanitation and fresh air, as Florence Nightingale had written about in her *Notes on Nursing*.[33]

Mother Hannah and Dr Roddick made rounds and visited each patient every day, and Dr Roddick and General Laurie made every effort to procure what was needed to run the field hospital. At Mother Hannah's request, a recreation tent, cook shop, and marquee with blue and white striped canvas for convalescents were erected outside, on a grassy area adjoining the hospital. She arranged for dining tables to be set up under the trees and the marquee, and some cots with mattresses and pillows were placed outside for the wounded to lounge upon during the day. Donations were received from women in Toronto that pleased the convalescents: magazines, books, newspapers, chess and cribbage boards, cards, pipes, and tobacco. Ladies from Portage la Prairie sent donations of fruit, cakes, and fresh eggs, which enhanced and gave variety to the food served to the men. Mother Hannah believed many of the men were not so ill that they should be confined to bed after their bandages were changed. The wounded were encouraged to spend their time outside during the fine days of June, getting fresh air and exercise and assisting their bodies to recover.

It was recorded in Mother Hannah's memoirs that members of a remnant band of Sitting Bull's Sioux from Montana were camped close to the field hospital on the other side of the Moose Jaw Creek. Several members of the band came to the field hospital for treatment of various ills, and some of the women were employed to clean the hospital. Mother Hannah wrote that Black Bull, Sitting Bull's brother, was the leader of the band.[34] He drew a fine picture of a buffalo for Mother Hannah in return for care that members of his band received at the hospital.

The Wounded Transferred to Winnipeg and the Nurses Return to Eastern Canada

Early in July, Mother Hannah and the nurses accompanied the only remaining wounded man from Moose Jaw to the Winnipeg General Hospital. Prior to their departure, they were invited to dine with General Laurie, which was unusual, given the strict gender and military hierarchies maintained. General Laurie later accompanied the women to the train station along a road lined by cheering men who had gathered to express their gratitude for the care they had received from the nurses, and to send them off in style. After turning over care of the last patient to those at the Winnipeg General Hospital, the nurses returned to Toronto. Mother Hannah's memoirs record that she looked back fondly on the time spent in the west, and was frequently stopped by people who said they remembered her from the Moose Jaw field hospital. It was reported that she once met a man in Toronto with a grizzled beard, still suffering from the effects of his injuries, who reminded her that she had cared for him in the field hospital: "Remember me? I was the one in the cot by the door to the kitchen."[35] Before Mother Hannah left Moose Jaw in 1885, the Canadian government awarded her a medal for her work in the field hospital.

The last twenty wounded men from Saskatoon were moved to the Winnipeg General Hospital on 3 July 1885 on a barge named *Sir John A. Macdonald* towed by the steamer *Alberta*. By the standards of the day, the barge was quite luxurious: it had cabins for two doctors, four nurses, three dressers, and a female servant. Another barge with "two milk cows, fresh meat, vegetables and comforts for the wounded" followed. The wounded men were transferred 1,100 miles by barge and steamers and claimed the water trip was "more comfortable than the short overland trip from the hospital to the barge."[36]

The history of medical and nursing care during the Northwest Rebellion provides insight into the challenges and responses of the people at this time. Acknowledgement of the presence of nursing Sisters in the rebellion of 1885 is especially necessary since the rebellion has often been portrayed as a male endeavour. The military and doctors who were recruited had a guaranteed place in the history of the uprising, but women's participation has for too long been neglected. The nurses were all female and the call was for "trained" volunteer nurses, when recognition of the difference to survival of wounded that trained nurses made in military disputes was only just beginning. Nurses Miller, Elkin, Parsons, Hamilton, and Mother Hannah and her nurses, were highly praised for bringing order and care to the wounded in the hastily assembled field hospitals, and Mother Hannah's memoirs state that their service went a long way in removing the animosity and prejudice against female nurses and these Sisters.[37] In fact, the positive outcomes for many of the wounded were attributed to the skilled care they received from these nurses. Mother Hannah used organizational and nursing skills acquired while training for her vocation to help the wounded and suffering. Nurses treated both First Nations people and

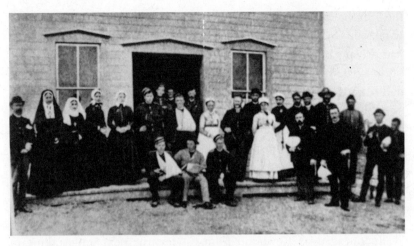

4.2 June 1885. Dr Roddick, on the far left side, next to Mother Hannah, the novice, and the two postulants in front of the field hospital at Moose Jaw. Three nurses from the Bellevue Hospital in New York are to the right of the entrance.

the Dominion forces wounded within a framework of ethical care. Although the conditions were primitive, the doctors and nurses called to duty in Saskatoon and Moose Jaw fulfilled their commitment to provide medical aid and succor to their fellows injured in battle.

Mother Hannah Back in Toronto

Prior to leaving for duty in the Northwest Rebellion, the Sisters of St John the Divine "had no thought of taking up Hospital work," however, upon her return, Mother Hannah saw the need for a hospital to provide nursing care to the sick, and consented to begin this work.[38] While the Sisters were away, a large frame house adjoining the Mother House on Robinson Street was leased and renovated by the clergy and people of the parish of St Matthias and the Toronto Anglican community. The house was intended as a clinic where the nurses would receive patients for surgical and medical care.[39] The profound impact of Mother Hannah's early experience of losing a baby made her determined that this would be a surgical hospital for the treatment of women. She recognized that maintaining a hospital must be one of the chief works of the Sisterhood. Their new house became the first surgical hospital for women in Toronto, and was used by leading surgeons. The hospital had private and public rooms for women, and a tiny room at the end of the upstairs hall that was used as an operating room. Mother Hannah trained the Sisters herself in the nursing care of women patients, and "the Hospital was blessedly free from poisoned cases, though the antiseptic and hygienic arrangements were of the simplest."[40] Acquiring and equipping the hospital coalesced with the movement for skilled nursing care and the growth of calls for the professionalization of nursing. The hospital was at once filled and busy. The labour involved in managing the hospital stretched the endurance of the six Anglican Sisters, with nursing becoming "the chief feature of their work."[41]

Encouraged by Reverend John Cayley, the next undertaking in 1886 by the Sisters of St John the Divine was a "Home for the Aged"[42] in a small double house in St George's Parish. Few in number, the Sisters were already working very hard, but they were constantly urged to found an Anglican home for elderly men and women. There were no professed Sisters to take up the work away from the Mother House, but two novices were sent from the Order, and with the help of an aged cook and laundress, set up and operated the home.

✦✦✦

This chapter is the story of a dedicated woman who was ahead of her time. In a country still in its infancy, Mother Hannah Grier Coome was a visionary. She was able to see and accomplish what was needed for fellow humans in suboptimal conditions, with few resources, and during a time when women were not recognized as powerful or voting members of society. An intelligent, skilled, and kind woman, she lived a life of devotion. Following two years of religious training that included in-hospital training as a nurse, Mother Hannah responded to the call to found the first order of Anglican Sisters in Toronto. Her dedication to religious life and charitable works was evident in her service to people in the Toronto community, to men in the Moose Jaw field hospital, to women in need of surgery, and to elderly in need of a home. Mother Hannah and the Sisters participated in mission work; provided meals, essentials, and in-home visits amongst the poor and needy; nursed the sick and suffering; organized and ran a field hospital in the North West Rebellion; set up the first surgical hospital for women (which was considered to provide exemplary care) with a convalescent home for those recovering from surgery and illness; and established a church home for the aged – at a time when these social supports, common today, did not exist.

NOTES

I would like to thank Dr Tricia Marck, Associate Professor, University of Alberta, and Dr Myra Rutherdale, Assistant Professor, York University, for their support and encouragement in the preparation of this paper. Thank you also to the reviewers for their comments.

1 Hannah G. Coome, *A Memoir of the Life and Work of Hannah Grier Coome, Mother-Foundress of the Sisterhood of St John the Divine* (Toronto: Oxford University Press, 1933), Preface.

2 Ibid., chap. 1.

3 Ibid., 20

4 Ibid., 20, It was noted early in the book that Coome resolved to start a Women's Surgical Hospital if she ever had the opportunity, which came years later in Toronto.

5 Ibid., 8.

6 Ibid., 28.

7 Ibid., 27.

8 Ibid., 53

9 Ibid., 29.

10 Charles Pelham Mulvany and G. Mercer Adam, *History of Toronto and county of York, Ontario* (Toronto: C.B. Robinson, 1885), 122.

11 Coome, *A Memoir*, 29.

12 Myra Rutherdale, *Women and the White Man's God: Gender and Race in the Canadian Mission Field* (Vancouver: UBC Press, 2002).

13 Coome, *A Memoir*, 86.

14 Marguerite E. Robinson, *Saskatchewan Registered Nurses Association: The First Fifty Years.* (Regina, SK: Saskatchewan Registered Nurses Association, n.d.), 9.

15 M. Patricia Donahue, *Nursing the Finest Art: An Illustrated History*, 2nd ed. (St. Louis: Mosby Year Book, 1996), 289.

16 Sessional Papers. *Fourth Session of the Fifth Parliament of the Dominion of Canada*, 5, 6 (Appendix 5), Report of the Surgeon Major, Dr J. Bell, 10 May 1886, 358–9.

17 Sessional Papers, Dr J. Bell, 359.

18 Coome, *A Memoir*, 91.

19 Leith Knight, "Historically Speaking" in *Moose Jaw Times Herald* 17 December 1969: 18.

20 Sessional Papers, *Fourth Session of the Fifth Parliament of the Dominion of Canada*, 5, 6 (Appendix 1), Report of the Brigade Surgeon, Dr George Orton, 21 May 1885, 381–4.

21 Sessional Papers. *Fourth Session of the Fifth Parliament of the Dominion of Canada*, 5, 6 (Appendix 5), Report of the Surgeon Major, Dr Douglas, 13 May 1886, 368–9.

22 Robinson, *Saskatchewan Registered Nurses Association*, 10.

23 Sessional Papers, Dr G. Orton, 383.

24 Sessional Papers, Dr Douglas, 368.

25 Ibid., 368.

26 John M. Gibbon and Mary S. Mathewson, *Three Centuries of Canadian Nursing (Illustrated)* (Toronto: MacMillan, 1947), 200–2.

27 Sessional Papers, Dr J. Bell, 358.

28 Sessional Papers, Dr Douglas, 368.

29 Ibid., 370.

30 Coome, *A Memoir*, 92.

31 Sessional Papers, Dr Douglas, 370.

32 Coome, *A Memoir*, 93.

33 Florence Nightingale, *Notes on Nursing: What It Is and What It Is Not* (New York: Dover, 1969; original work published 1859), 133.

34 Coome, *A Memoir*, 93–4.

35 Ibid., 94.

36 Robinson, *Saskatchewan Registered Nurses Association*, 11.

37 Coome, *A Memoir*, 94.

38 Ibid., 91.

39 Ibid., 96.

40 Ibid., 97.

41 Ibid., 102.

42 Ibid., 103.

5

+++++

Part of a Large Company of White Folk: Making 'Whiteness,' Marking Gender in the Letters of Nurse Margaret Butcher

MARY-ELLEN KELM[1]

For decades, those committed to anti-racist struggle demanded that the construct of 'race' be thoroughly interrogated. In the waning decades of the twentieth century, scholars began to answer that call.[2] Study of the making of alterity demonstrated the complex frameworks of biology and culture, gender and class, place and space that were required to construct categories like 'the Indian' or 'the Chinese.'[3] Scholars, demonstrating that race is always constructed, challenged the claims of whiteness to normalcy, to naturalness, to an unchanging and almost imperceptible presence.[4] Scholars in labour history placed whiteness into the history of class formation and class struggle.[5] Recognizing the imbrication of whiteness and sexuality fundamentally deepened our understanding of the production of masculinity and femininity.[6] Emerging definitions of whiteness stressed three features: "Whiteness is a location of structured advantage, or race privilege. Second, it is a 'standpoint,' a place from which white people look at ourselves, at others, and at society. Third, 'whiteness' refers to a set of cultural practices that are usually unmarked and unnamed."[7] Rather than being an immutable but ill-defined presence, whiteness was revealed to be contingent on the same organizing regimes that produced alterity. Wary as scholars were not to re-inscribe its privileged position, they have forced whiteness to the table of race studies.[8]

Constructions of whiteness were particularly important in colonial situations where the right to rule rested on a shifting yet crucial foundation of difference between colonizers and colonized.[9] In settler colonies, including the dominions of the British Empire, tensions associated with becoming indigenous to the land without 'going Native' haunted the subjectivities of settlers, their governments, and those who observed them.[10] Complex definitions of citizenship, inheritance, and belonging emerged whenever settlers entered the colonial scene.[11] Constructing the 'other' meant that the Western white self had to be articulated as well. This was not always a straightforward task.[12]

In British Columbia, as elsewhere, making race was central to structuring society. The continuing presence of First Nations as well as significant Asian populations made British Columbia a multicultural society, even as it avowed itself to be principally, and fundamentally, British.[13] But a clear sense of the various racial divides was not something that emerged without anxiety. Nor was it a 'natural' or accidental process for whiteness to emerge as the marker of dominance. Backwoods masculine culture, relationships formed between European men and Aboriginal women, even the discourses of missionary writers, all offered – admittedly tentative – alternatives to a society of firmly entrenched racial hierarchy in nineteenth-century British Columbia.[14] The spatial segregation that became evident by the next century grew upon and contributed to a more pervasive cultural sense of 'knowing one's place.'[15] Constructing whiteness was part of that process, and it *was* a process. As Adele Perry makes clear: "Whiteness was constructed, problematic, and fragile ... at once powerful and precarious."[16] Because it was so precarious, it needed to be asserted and re-asserted throughout British Columbia's history.

Using the letters of Margaret Butcher, an early twentieth-century nurse and midwife in Kitamaat, BC, we can see this process in action. Butcher arrived at the Haisla Village of Kitamaat in 1916. She had been hired by the Methodist Women's Missionary Society to be the sewing instructor at the Elizabeth Long Memorial Home, a residential school first opened in 1896. But it was her experience as a nurse and midwife that brought her into sustained contact not only with the Aboriginal children in the school but also with the Haisla Villagers and the non-Native settlers of the Kitamaat Valley.[17] In her letters home, Butcher spent considerable effort describing settler society, making note of its whiteness, its coherence, and its superiority. These missives were intended to be shared by family and friends of the mission who could pass them around, and perhaps also offer financial support. The intended audience would read about the conditions in the 'heathen lands' but would also be exposed to the new self being created by Butcher. The repeated and self-conscious construction of whiteness in these letters seems to contradict the definition above that whiteness is unmarked and invisible. Yet this rupture reveals a great deal: as Ruth Frankenberg argues, "In times and places when whiteness and white domination are being built or reconfigured, they are highly visible, named and asserted."[18] The construction of whiteness, then, in Butcher's letters reveals not only the internal definitions of whiteness but also the anxieties that its assertion was supposed to lay to rest.

The world that Butcher entered on the north coast was a dynamic one. The Haisla had only recently consolidated settlement around Kitamaat, partly in accordance with the meager reserve allocation of Indian Reserve Commissioner Peter O'Reilly, and partly because the population had been greatly reduced by disease.[19] By the 1910s, the Haisla were taking out logging licenses and hiring on in the salmon canning and the pulp and paper industries.[20] Meanwhile the promise of a railway terminus attracted European, Canadian, and American settlers to the Kitamaat Valley. Though these hopes proved false, some settlers stayed to join a very small population of former mission personnel who had taken up residence in the Kitamaat Valley.[21]

Butcher's white world was a small and disparate community made up of the all-female school staff, isolated missionaries, mobile workers, and hard-pressed settlers. The 'fine company of white folk' to which Butcher referred found themselves far flung along a thousand-kilometre coastline. Butcher's was a transient and tumultuous world where well-loved missionaries went off to war, where loggers died at their work, where women found themselves abandoned on newly hewn pre-emptions, where families tried to build a life on the land but failed. Yet it was this population whose presence justified the dispossession of First Nations from the land. This was the community that was supposed to demonstrate the superiority of European culture. Justifying her work at the residential school, based as it was on the idea that Aboriginal people needed to be transformed as much as possible into white people, meant that Butcher also had to transform for her readers the settler society of the North Pacific Coast into a coherent white community deserving of its privileged status in the colonial hierarchies of race.[22]

This community had certain key features. While Butcher downplayed class, ethnicity troubled the category 'white.' On one hand,

Butcher was proud of the diversity of whiteness and settlers from many European backgrounds were included in her definition of white. On the other, 'Englishness' was highlighted and became a point of commonality for the white community Butcher encountered. But this was not an Englishness that was necessarily tied to birth or citizenship; rather, it was a portable concept that could be bestowed or denied. Gender, however, needed to be carefully managed. In Butcher's eyes, her fellow workers and settler women were masters of domesticity, eradicating dirt and primitiveness wherever they were found. For Butcher, 'doing gender right' was more difficult. As Myra Rutherdale has noted, among Anglican missionaries, the exigencies of the field challenged gendered norms of behaviour. In describing her activities, Butcher revealed the variety of tasks, the range of experiences to which she was exposed. In her writing, she sought to appear competent but not beyond needing male assistance and protection. White men, too, walked a fine line. Adaptability was a key feature of white masculinity, as Butcher described it, and among the settlers only men were ever described as 'belonging' to this new and strange land. But belonging too much could be transgressive. White men who married into Haisla society placed themselves outside whiteness, in Butcher's words, "belonging nowhere." As in so many other colonial contexts, white man's sexuality provided the contaminating opportunity, the contact that breached cultural difference. Butcher's white world excluded such men, as, she argued, did the rest of the white community of the North Coast. Whiteness, thus, claimed the power to include and exclude. Constructing a homogenous whiteness necessitated downplaying some divisive elements, like class, while reserving the markers of belonging for those whose conduct preserved the cultural divide between colonized and colonizer.[23]

Englishness

Feeling a sense of belonging and finding the familiar filled Butcher's letters as she depicted the white community on the North Pacific Coast. Everywhere Butcher looked, 'Englishness,' both real and fictive, surrounded her. Indeed, Butcher's understanding of Englishness conforms to Paul Gilroy's proposition that Englishness as an identity and a descriptor could not be confined by ethnicity or geography but that it was complex and contested, shaped by the British Empire as much as by the metropole.[24] For Butcher, Englishness did not segment the white community; rather, it unified it. She came to gloss over internal differentiation within whiteness. Butcher's early recognition of class, for instance ("I was greeted by quite a bunch of White men – settlers of varying degrees of roughness") was soon replaced by the assertion that "One has to get away from the habit of judging by clothes out in these regions."[25] Ethnicity was similarly elided. Although she sometimes identified individuals by their country of origin, collectively, they were a "large company of white folk."[26] When what mattered was the "mustering of white faces" for church and companionship, ethnicity only advertised the diversity, the broad ascendancy, of whiteness. Butcher's use of Englishness, then, spoke less of nationality than of belonging.

Though other ethnicities were submerged in the category 'white,' Butcher delighted in finding Englishness all around her. In the mission, she was one among a group of "old country women ... [who] ke[pt] the Home running."[27] In the Valley, she was among fellow Englishmen whom she fit into her own extended kin network. Her particular favourite was Charlie Moore, who was not only English but a Londoner as well. Butcher wrote: "When I first saw him there seemed something familiar in his bearing and his speech was very pleasant to my ear. At last I said, 'Are you from London?' and sure enough he is. It was not the Englishman that pleased me but the City man – the Londoner."[28] Butcher's English neighbours in the Valley became part of her extended and international network of family and friends. She and Charlie Moore, for instance, speculated that they were related by marriage, sharing a 'cousin Flo,' and later discovered that Moore knew acquaintances of Butcher's sister Nell.[29]

Just as whiteness was not a natural descriptor for any particular group of people, Englishness was not merely a natural signifier for those born in England. Declaring someone or something 'English' was Butcher's way of claiming that person or place as familiar, valuable, as belonging to her white world. Canadians she liked were returned into the English fold. Butcher's encounter with the down-at-heel Canadian Mrs Pearson is typical. Visiting Vancouver in 1918, Butcher stayed with Mrs Pearson, whose family had recently lost its fortune through some form of financial mismanagement. Pearson proved herself to

Butcher, however, by praising England and the English saying that she "loved the beauty of the country, the homes, the ancient landmarks and remark[ing] 'Canada seemed so crude, so hoydenish, so unfinished ... and I think how wonderfully adaptable the English are to fit in our country so well.'" Butcher reported that she was astounded to hear this from a Canadian and, promptly claiming Pearson as English, reported she replied that, "the English strain must be strong in her even though her father was born in Canada."[30] Similarly, Butcher made fictive kin, and hence fictive Englishmen, of the settlers she admired. She wrote of George Anderson: "Mr Anderson won my heart by a certain likeness to Uncle Harry [of Worthing]. Some trick of manner when he starts a yarn & just the same happy way of telling appropriate yarns. I dubbed him Uncle & he calls me niece."[31] Englishness, more than a product of birth, was a portable concept to be bestowed to enhance the sense of belonging that being white created.

The land, too, was claimed as English. Like so many other travel writers and missionary correspondents, Butcher was struck by the need to depict the land as both exotic and familiar, dramatic and yet readily exploitable.[32] Even the remarkable landscape of the Kitamaat Valley was re-visioned in this way. The land along the river was, to Butcher, very "Englishy" with trees she recognized, though their Canadian names escaped her. She distinguished among the pre-emptions she visited: "That home [was] the first pre-emption work that has appealed to me. I like the class of land because it is Englishy."[33] When the more dramatic mountain vistas did not fit the common view of the English countryside, Butcher made mental connections to more fabricated scenes from her English life. The towering mountains around Douglas Channel thus became like "the pasteboard hills around Earl's Court Exhibition."[34] Butcher often compared the climate to that of England, commenting how the cold in England was more biting but concluding, in the end, that the climate of the North Pacific Coast was "very Englishy only more so."[35]

Hospitality and Entertaining Englishness

Claiming the land and climate as English figuratively tamed the North Coast in Butcher's writing. The rugged coast, however, tested settlers' abilities to form community and here, too, Butcher's depiction of whiteness was mobilized to overcome the challenges of this foreign land. The extent to which the white community was built on travel between isolated sites made hospitality a key feature of whiteness in Butcher's letters. In celebrating community, at gatherings in Kitamaat and elsewhere, settlers travelled some distance to share the material culture of whiteness, most often, but not always, associated with things English. When Butcher travelled, the white community granted her accommodation and care that permitted her to move about alone, guarding her respectability as a white woman. By accommodating women such as Butcher, the white community created a space for independent women who were so necessary for the community's replication both literally and figuratively. It also claimed for itself characteristics of hospitality, camaraderie, and chivalry.

The white community of the North Pacific Coast was geographically dispersed. Along the intricate coastline of the Pacific, cannery managers and their wives joined the missionaries scattered in places like Kitamaat, Hartley Bay, Port Simpson, and Rivers Inlet to form the core of white settlement. With few white people in any one place, building a sense of community required travel. Kitamaat provided a kind of hub where missionaries and other workers from farther-flung places retreated to visit and celebrate Christmas and other holidays. Visits from other white folk, offering her relief from the isolation of mission work, punctuated Butcher's letters. In the world Butcher described, vessels were announced excitedly, greeted and visitors were always asked in for tea. Early in her letters, she tried to convey the importance of these visits to her readers. Describing the inspector of Indian agencies who was there on government business as a "good talker, easy, anecdotal and humorous and … a fine refreshing companion," she concluded: "this does not read as of any importance but I can assure you that it was a mighty event in our routine lives."[36] The arrival of vessels brought the mail, news from the outside world, particularly of the war, fresh food, and companionship. When, just before Christmas 1917, the vessel *Charles Todd* called in at Kitamaat, Butcher gleefully wrote of a meal of cold chicken, celery, and tea which "took [their] fancies." The captain also told exciting stories of submarines that brought home, for Butcher, the war's impact. Still it was companionship more than information that Butcher longed for. And after such an evening, "next day [they] were all lively as crickets on account of the complete change of thought [that] the touch with the outside world had brought."[37]

Englishness marked the trappings of community celebrations with Valley residents as well. Butcher consistently described her Christmases in Kitamaat as time when "all the white people" assembled.[38] Christmas dinner of 1916 was composed mainly of country foods and though Butcher boasted that her English cousins would envy such a spread of venison and the like, for her, Charlie Moore's "real English plum pudding" made from his mother's recipe was the highlight. As Butcher concluded her description of her first Christmas at Kitamaat, "Canadian mince pie is good but not quite up to the English."[39] English goods were the star attraction of the next year's Christmas as well, when mission supporters sent both holly and mistletoe to garnish the table – "so very English." St Patrick's Day too warranted festivities as one of the settler women sacrificed her green petticoat to decorate the gathered number, including horses and dogs, in green ribbon.[40] A century later one scholar would refer to St Patrick's Day as a "high holy day" of whiteness; here in the Kitamaat Valley, St Patrick's Day was indeed a special day, emptied of any Irish content – certainly any Republican content – celebrating only whiteness.[41]

The camaraderie of the white community extended beyond the Kitamaat Valley to the whole of the coast. In 1918, when Butcher travelled to Vancouver to a meeting of the Women's Missionary Society, she enjoyed the hospitality of other workers in the field. Upon arriving in Prince Rupert, for instance, she called upon Fanny Kergin, a former teacher at the Crosby Girls' Home in Port Simpson. Butcher described the scene: "She is a delightful woman. We had not met before but that I was from Kitamaat was sufficient introduction. The freemasonry between Workers is very pleasant."[42] Further down the coast, Butcher arrived at the cannery site, Butedale, at nearly three in the morning. Here again, the white community proved hospitable as the bookkeeper of the company store met Butcher at the dock and brought her home, where a room awaited her. The next day, his wife took Butcher on a hike to the falls above the town that generated the hydroelectric power to the cannery. The cannery foreman's wife, "another white woman" in Butcher's words, took her in for dinner until the SS *Chilcotin* left that evening. On her return trip, Butcher arrived at the dock, in the late evening, and was told that she was expected up at that manager's house. Though the manager and his family were away, Butcher was told, a "white woman was in his house." Butcher climbed the steep hill to the house, knocked on the door for some time and was about to turn away when "the door was opened by a man who had just finished washing himself. Behind him stood a comely bright-faced woman drying her face and neck. They gazed in astonishment which did not decrease when I begged a night's lodging. However, they soon got over it and accepted me on my own credentials, relieved me of wraps, seated me in a warm room for awhile, then shewed [sic] me a good bathroom and a bedroom, so I was in a comfortable bed by 10:30."[43] Such intimacy among strangers seems remarkable. In the presence of Aboriginal and Asian workers, whiteness provided a common bond and allowed familiarity in situations where it would have otherwise been improper. In contrast to the immediate intimacy that was possible among white people was the need for absolute separation from those who transgressed the boundary between colonizer and colonized. Later in Butcher's travels, she hoped to obtain passage aboard a launch but its owner, a Mr Hanson, refused saying that "he would not like her sleeping with Mr Cordello and his Indian wife aboard."[44] Within the white community, belonging ensured safety for white women, a safety that permitted women like Butcher to have mobility and independence. Safety, however, was not just physical. The white community sought to keep women such as Butcher safe from the taint of hybridity as well, and in so doing it protected both Butcher's respectability and claimed its own. Casting out, keeping separate – these were also functions of community-creation, as essential as establishing belonging and companionship.

Doing Gender Right: The Family of Women

Whiteness laid the groundwork for respectability, but maintaining gendered norms ensured it. Butcher wrote as well of camaraderie and congeniality as characteristics of the white women with whom she worked. Although being a white woman might have opened the doors of other white people in communities along the coast, not getting along in an isolated community could be exceedingly uncomfortable. Belonging was crucial: Butcher was warned before her arrival in Kitamaat "to lay especial emphasis upon 'fitting in.'" In her letters, Butcher depicted her life with her fellow workers as one of domestic contentment. On one hand, it is slightly ironic that domesticity was the paradigm she chose. Mission work was one of the few respectable ways in which middle-class women of Europe and North America could escape a life confined to the private sphere. Early in her letters, Butcher admitted that she chose mission work precisely to avoid domestic responsibilities and observed the quirk of fate that, instead of a husband and children of her own, she was looking after over thirty children belonging to others. And her work in the residential school centred on transferring appropriate gendered skills to Aboriginal children. So the world of the residential school was a *very* domestic one. Butcher remarked when her sister Nell took on war work: "Now we are all in some measure Public women, even if only in a small way. Of course, there is nothing very Public about me at present excepting my letters ..." In this context, then, it is perhaps not surprising that Butcher cast her relationships with the other women in the school in familial terms.[45]

In Butcher's institutional family, Matron Ida Clarke was mother. Butcher called her, "our backbone, our stay, our prop, our sure confidence."[46] Throughout Butcher's letters, Clarke sustained staff with her wise advice, intervened with troublesome parents and Haisla Villagers, and ensured that the teachers took time off, ate well, and rested.[47] She continued that, appropriately for a mother-like institutional head, Clarke "never asserted herself as Matron, nor ma[de] any show of discipline, yet [kept] everything running smoothly and on time."[48] Butcher wrote that when Clarke was away, the teachers were "like children keeping house without Mother."[49]

Butcher portrayed the other workers as giddy schoolgirls with whom she got along amiably. Her first Christmas, she wrote, was full of "abundance of good feeling, kind heartedness, frolic, nonsense, bearing of one another's burdens ..."[50] Later, she carried on that "there is no end of kindness shewn [sic] to me by these ladies."[51] When a new teacher was on her way to the school, Butcher expressed regret at the change to their little domestic scene: "It would be nice if we could go on just as we are for we are so happy together but the work is a little strenuous." Months later, when still more personnel changes were afoot, she remarked: "We are a congenial bunch now that one dreads the thought of change. Imagine being shut up with uncongenial folk – it would be dreadful."[52] Despite all the talk of congeniality, however, Butcher had to work at getting along, at least on some level. She did

this by describing herself as a kind of younger sibling to the more experienced teachers in the school. Until a new worker joined that staff in
1917, Butcher was the Home's newest addition and so she positioned
herself in the 'family' as its youngest child, despite turning forty-six
during her first year at the Home. Above her in her sibling hierarchy
was the formidable Miss Scotun, a veteran mission worker who could
do almost anything.[53] Scotun did not, it appears, suffer fools gladly. In
a rare description of conflict among the workers, Butcher relayed the
following exchange between Scotun and herself:

> One evening I settled in front of the fire. "My feet are so cold,
> I'm going to warm them before going any further."
>   Miss Scotun replied: "Well they may be cold when you wear
> stockings like that. Why don't you put on some good woolen ones?"
>   Another time, I said: "I've got a chilblain; it isn't comfort-
> able." The same lady replied: "You deserve to have them wearing
> flimsy stockings and pretty slippers."
>   I said, "Please ma'am I have woolen combinations that reach
> below my knee and I always wear walking shoes unless it is my
> rest day and I don't like thick stockings [as] they fill my shoes
> & keep my feet cold."
>   "Well, then wear larger shoes."
>   "Please ma'am my shoes are so big for me that it is hard to
> keep them on."
>   Well, when it got frosty I put on woolen stockings and went
> in triumph for her approval.
>   "Call those winter stockings! They are only fit for summer
> wear. Get some good '2&1' like mine."
>   Today we went into the woods so I wore my heavy boots and
> just now, sitting by the fire, took them off. We had no light &
> presently Miss Scotun moved & stumbled over them.
>   "Don't trouble, " I said, "they are only my boots."
>   "Are they good boots or only flimsy slippers?" She threw
> at me, going out of the room so when she returned I made her
> examine them and she pronounced them "respectable."[54]

Rather than depicting Scotun's irascibility, Butcher concluded for her
readers that this exchange proved that she "was being well looked

after." Portraying herself as someone who required looking after was the cost, it seems, of fitting in to the family of women.

Domesticity was also the gauge by which Butcher measured the women settlers in the Valley. While at the school, Butcher had to laboriously teach her Aboriginal students the domestic arts. In contrast white women, it seemed, made homes in the wilderness without any visible labour. Butcher was absolutely impressed by the standards of feminine care that settler women took with their homes. Butcher praised both the Anderson ranch and the Moore homestead, finding both welcoming and comfortable. But her favourite example of bush domesticity was the home of Mrs Mitchell. The Mitchells lived in the boathouse of a scow. It had no more than three compartments: kitchen, sitting room, and bedroom. Nevertheless, Butcher was very impressed by Exilda Mitchell's ability to turn the mere rudiments of habitation into a home, saying that it was "as compact neat and dainty as few, save Mrs Mitchell, could make it."[55] Butcher saved her most fulsome description for Mitchell's housekeeping abilities at camp. Butcher spent her summer holidays in 1917 at the logging camp of Mitchell and Hallett. Amid detailed descriptions of timber cruising and falling, Butcher related the domestic arrangements of the camp. She was awed by Mitchell's abilities to construct a comfortable and tasteful abode at an industrial site and indeed, the appointments of the ladies' tent were remarkable: "A little to the right, facing the camp, far enough away to be out of the run of the men, is the Ladies Tent. Mrs Mitchell has it very comfortably fitted up, with a large double spring bed, dressing table and chest of drawers (combined), large corner-hanging wardrobe. A small cook stove with oven, washstand made from a box, a double flap table and a small table holding the phonograph [complete the furnishings]. Photos, pictures and flags are pinned to the tent wall. The floor is covered with cork carpet. A rocker, three chairs, white draperies etc. all go to make for comfort and ease."[56]

Moreover, creating such a space also had the effect of taming the men who worked at camp. Butcher defended them from imagined aspersions: "Loggers are proverbially a 'tough lot,' if so, this Camp must be an exception for the men are well conducted and orderly. Some come to our tent every evening and laugh and chat whilst the Gramophone plays."[57] Entering the ladies' tent and listening to music, it seemed, smoothed the rough edges, domesticating but not emasculating these capable and hardy men.[58] In writing about the domestic feats of white women, however, Butcher tellingly left one thing out. Unlike her work in the school teaching Native children how to make a home and unlike the work of the men logging, Butcher is absolutely silent on the labour that white women must have performed in order to keep their homes as neat, clean, and orderly as Butcher maintained they were. Anne McClintock argues that the women's work in the home was necessarily invisible in order "to disavow and conceal within the middle-class formation the economic value of women's work."[59] Labour in the home, according to McClintock, evoked a dangerous blurring of public and private. Perhaps Butcher tried in her writing to maintain the fictitious boundary between work and home for white settler women. That her work was to teach Aboriginal girls how to make a home only underscored how primitive and backwards Aboriginal people were, in her eyes, not only because they had to be taught but because in so doing they forced the rupturing of the line between public and private. If as McClintock argues the domestic servant became "figured by images of disorder, contagion, disease, conflict, rage and guilt," then the world of Aboriginal girls taught to be servants must have been one of dangerous isolation in which they were expected to breach the bounds of respectability even as they conformed to the lessons of residential schooling.[60] Butcher's erasure of settler women's labour preserved the divide between public and private for white women, but Butcher's own work in the school, making domestic work public, potentially put her in a precarious position.

Humour and the Rhetoric of Containment

Butcher occupied a liminal position. Running the Elizabeth Long Memorial Home as part of an all-woman staff forced Butcher and her colleagues to perform duties that were not normally considered part of women's sphere. This was true for all women in newly settled districts of various colonies.[61] Maintaining respectability was difficult under such circumstances and constructing lines of race and class were important indicators of the maturation of settler colonies.[62] Displaying the markers of class, of whiteness, for instance, was a key component of the configuration of the domestic space.[63] Women missionaries were doubly burdened: while they themselves were often acting out of their gendered sphere, they were simultaneously teaching the importance of that sphere to Aboriginal women and children and were themselves subject to scrutiny.[64] Butcher's letters offered women back home in England a glimpse of a woman who, by virtue of her occupation and her location, was partially unfettered from domestic constraints, yet her passport to such a realm was guaranteed only by her respectability. So when describing her work and her adventures, Butcher was careful to limit the impact of these descriptions on her readers. She did this principally through humour.

Mission life required special skills. Soon after her arrival, Butcher praised Miss Scotun for being "clever at carpenting [sic], plumbing and gardening."[65] She seemed proud that the female staff of the school were "a company of women ... mak[ing] the best 'do'... fixing washers, mending pipes, carpentering, whitewashing etc."[66] Yet when Butcher undertook difficult tasks, her descriptions emphasized the comic nature of women undertaking such things as fixing stove pipes – and as she related it: in the end, a man must always come to the rescue. She relayed her experience of cleaning stovepipes with a team of her students like this:

> Do you savvy that there are sixteen joints in my bedroom and six in [the] sewing room and one between the ceiling and floor? Well I wandered and ran up and down those stairs getting them right and presently Louisa separated the joint between the ceiling and floor which I had been most careful to keep fixed also she mixed all the pipes in the cleaning although they were all laid in order when taken down. Do you think that joint between ceiling and floor would fix? No such thing! I went downstairs, fixed a chair on the stove, shoved the pipe up high into my room rested the bottom of the pipe on the chair, went upstairs again to fix it and presently down went the pipe and a scream came from the girl below who was balancing it ... There were eight joints to fix as we lifted two lengths at once. There were two elbows to the whole structure. Well those pipes joined in one place and fell apart in another. They wobbled and creaked. The step ladder I used was very rickety and gave me jumps ... I was in despair of ever getting them up when Mr. Allen's [the missionary in Kita-

maat Village] voice sounded below. I called him up. He came and with very little trouble compared with mine, the thing was fixed, the fire lighted, the two rooms freed from soot.[67]

In a similar story, bursting water pipes were set to right by Mr Moore, who "soon put all our pipes and taps in order." Visits to the Anderson ranch also presented Butcher with labour for which she felt particularly unprepared. Milking a cow, for instance, required "some pluck," while churning butter was worthy of detailed description.[68] As Butcher got more accustomed to an isolated mission life, she soon delegated more 'manly' tasks to settler men and carried on with the equally difficult, but more feminine, tasks of fumigation and food preservation. When a new furnace was purchased, neither Butcher nor the students participated in its installation. Charlie Moore alone handled that task. ("Mr Moore fitted up the precious thing single-handed. It was a colossal task but that is the way of things up here.") But Butcher and the girls were not idle. While Moore was doing his job, they fumigated the school after an attack of whooping cough and then salted the meat for the winter's supply. No longer finding such work humorous, Butcher dealt with it succinctly in her letters, neither minimizing nor highlighting. In her words: "We did strenuous work but the tale is soon told."[69] Domestic labour was again made invisible.

Outside of the school, the rules of gender were more difficult to live by. Butcher clearly enjoyed adventures in the bush. Yet as an urban English woman from the middle classes, the picture of modernity, she was quite unprepared for them. After her first experience riding a horse bareback on her way to the Anderson ranch, Butcher exclaimed: "Is it possible that [this] woman was born in 1870? Surely there is some mistake."[70] Her experiences in Kitamaat seemed to move her out of the modern, but perhaps more important, her adventures moved her beyond the domestic both physically and, sometimes, socially. As she wrote about her forays out of the white world of the mission community, Butcher deployed self-deprecating humour to contain the gender disruption that her writing necessarily captured.[71]

Butcher clearly loved the landscape of the North Pacific Coast. Though she often tried to make the landscape fit English ideals, she just as often conceded that this was a foreign country in which the Haisla, not English ladies, belonged. Early in her stay, she took the girls from the residential school for a walk in the woods and encountered the feeling of foreignness: "The children look so pretty in the woods. Their dark skin and hair and bright dresses seem to belong to the woods. They slip along through dense undergrowth and are out of sight in no time and we poor white women are left far behind."[72] Nevertheless, hikes in the woods were a regular feature of Butcher's time on the coast. And while she wanted to convey the difficulty of the terrain, she did not do so with a view to proving her competence, as did male writers of her day. For her the beauty and ruggedness of the place demanded physical skills that she apparently lacked.[73] And so, guided often by settler men, she made her way through the woods, ill equipped and often falling in rather dramatic ways. On a trip to see the falls above Kitamaat, all the missionaries struggled to keep up to the lithe Charlie Moore. The missionary Mr Allan, for instance, joked that, "If they went backwards they might arrive sooner since their heels wanted to go first," but it was Butcher who fell dramatically, reporting that: "I stepped on an insecure log and slipped down, hanging to the path by my arms, brush below me." At the end of the expedition, she concluded: "Ah me, I was tired! However the beauty of the Falls, the grand woods, the lovely patches of flowers here and there more than compensated for the weary and bruised limbs and tattered garments with which we returned home. I was the only torn one – one stocking was ripped and two tears in my skirt."[74] Butcher never described herself as anything but completely ungainly on any of these ventures. On an early spring jaunt, she travelled by "leaping, scrambling, sitting down and sliding," and even a trip to the Village in February occasioned this slapstick scene involving Butcher and Matron Clarke: "Miss Clarke got me down the steps allright but a few yards further on I slipped over. She tried to save me but fell on top. She got to her feet and held my hand to pull me up but I only got to my knees, sat down, twirled around and slid down the path backwards for a yard or two."[75] Eventually, she became accustomed to feeling foolish and perhaps the people around her came to expect a certain clumsiness. Logging boss Frank Hallett was close at hand when Butcher slipped on a snow-covered plank while embarking a launch to return to the mission after one winter visit to the Anderson ranch.[76] Similarly, on her return visit to Butedale, she was helped to the wharf by two men who, she related, "constantly assur[ed] me that I could not fall into the water," while they hauled her onto the wharf like a "bundle of hay." All the while she was "occupied with [her] ludicrous position," writing that it was "not at all dignified to be hauled up by one's arms, legs waving in air to find a foothold, but it all comes naturally after a time."[77] Unlike urban men writing in the same time, Butcher did not gain physical strength or skill from her time in the wilderness; rather, reliance on men and looking ungraceful became the norm.[78]

Why did Butcher write so often of her ungainly behaviour? We have a hint that she feared that readers, and her fellow mission workers, might find her outings unseemly. Not only did she have to travel beyond the realm of the domestic in order to enjoy the landscape, she needed to do so in the company of men. All of them, admittedly, were married men, but early in her letters, she wrote that she worried whether her time spent walking with Charlie Moore would "scandalize the Ladies."[79] Similarly, she took time to discuss her riding apparel when she reported having to ride a horse astride in order to attend a birth in the Valley. She even recorded Matron's admonition that she wear her bloomers for the trip. Here again, the picture was humorous even as it was meant to show her modesty. She wrote: "Oh my dears, my dears! Can you imagine me essaying a three mile ride along a flooded track! I have recently made myself a full serge skirt; quite three yards around the bottom and was wearing it but even a three yard skirt will not cover a woman's legs when she straddles on horse back! Mag – in close fitting wool cap, warm coat, serge skirt just over the knees – (I hope it was) – a bit of stocking showing, gaiters, fastened on galoshed feet. Got the picture? Not quite – my clothes were stuffed into two white flour sacks which were tied together and slung across the saddle in front of me."[80]

The picture of an inelegant, slightly incompetent Margaret Butcher was clearly intended to forestall any conclusion that she was slipping the bonds of appropriate behaviour. Just as she willingly submitted to the scolding of Miss Scotun and to being the younger sibling in the family of women so, too, did she wish to appear the child in her outings with men and on the land. Ridiculous and unthreatening then, we see Butcher's repeated 'falling' as a pre-emptive defense against being perceived as 'fallen.' The anxiety revealed by the constant containment of textual references to expanded opportunities for women underscore the importance of strongly differentiated gender roles in the white

community. The tension between the demands on women in an isolated community and the importance of 'doing gender right' in the
missionary-imperialist context was another key component of whiteness on the North Pacific Coast.

White Men: Adaptability and Belonging

Butcher's depiction of white men contrasted her portrayal of her own
limited adaptation to the North Coast. More than any other characters in Butcher's letters, white men appeared as able, competent, and
kind. This image of mission and settler men was, of course, the per-
fect partner to Butcher's portrayal of herself as clumsy and childlike,
in need of protection. And the image of white man as strong, protective, and able to adapt to a rugged environment dominated colonial
discourse of the time, whether as the 'frontier' thesis or as muscular
Christianity among turn-of-the-century missionaries. Butcher used
these tropes to express her approval of the majority of the white men
of the Kitamaat Valley and in so doing further diminished whatever
residual unease readers of her letters may have had about her behaviour among them.

Among the men, Charlie Moore was Butcher's favourite. She connected with him immediately as a fellow Londoner – "the city man,"
she called him. Yet, it was Moore's uncanny ability to transform himself from an urbanite to a homesteader that most impressed Butcher.
It was Moore who, along with Mr Allen, saved the day of the crash-
ing stovepipes and who, later, installed the new furnace in the school.
It was Moore who put the school's plumbing in order. Moore built the
new dispensary for the government nurse Miss Alton.[81] More than
that, Moore was Butcher's guide to the wilderness she loved but feared.
His presence and his competence made the dangerous landscape safe.
When on an early hike, Butcher wanted to take pictures of the swirling
rapids of the Kitamaat River, Moore used his own body as tripod and
guardrail. As Butcher described it: "Mr Moore helped me to the edge
of the canyon, hewed down a small tree that obstructed the view, sat
down that I might rest the camera on his head, put his axe against a
tree to form a rail in front of me and I proceed [ed] to take a sight in
the view finder. The tail of my eye caught a boil of water just below us,

far below. Of course it made me squeamish but nothing mattered so much as the photo 'til I raised my head – then I didn't like it but we sat down for a few moments and the sickness passed right away."[82]

Butcher longed for Moore's manly life and when he told her about his trapping adventures one February, she pined, "one could picture the delight of sleeping out in the pure clean air."[83] But Moore was more than a manly man living rough in the bush and saving women from falling to their deaths in swirling waters – he had also mastered a few domestic arts as well. Moore's mince pie, based on his mother's recipe, was a pure English treat offering Butcher a taste of home during her first Christmas at Kitamaat.[84] Moore delivered his wife's baby alone in a blizzard and then, when Butcher arrived to help, became "a second nurse" being principally responsible for cooking and washing. And Moore fit into the Valley, almost naturally. After a walk in the woods, Butcher wrote that, Moore "moves so easily through the woods – he seems to 'belong' as do the Indian children." Moore, then, was both English and almost indigenous – claiming to be a part of the land not by birth but through competence. His belonging was earned. Moore so impressed Butcher that she anticipated someday "writ[ing] a panegyric on Mr Moore."[85] Moore was clearly her epitome of the white man.

But he was not entirely alone. Bob Mitchell was a Harvard man who had ended up in the Valley, running a logging camp. Getting to know him, Butcher learned not to assume class based on occupation or clothing alone in the Valley. Declaring that she had previously found him to be a 'stick,' when Butcher spent her vacation at his logging camp in the summer of 1917, she reported that "his speech was good … and his judgment [was] … calm; his camp, well-conducted, there was no drinking, no Sunday working."[86] Here again. Mitchell's ability to adapt his Harvard education to a life in the bush while keeping his morals largely intact (Butcher commented that the missionaries did not always speak well of Mitchell and he had only recently brought in a non-Native woman to be his wife) earned him a position in Butcher's category of white men whom she was "delighted to know." Similarly, the younger missionary William Allen, though inexperienced compared to these other men, showed himself to be generous with his labour and concern for the mission women's safety and comfort.[87]

Belonging Nowhere: The Taint of Hybridity

In contrast to all of these men stood George Robinson. Robinson had come to Kitamaat in 1884, joining the famous Methodist missionary Thomas Crosby in outreach to the Haisla. For several years, George Robinson worked as a lay missionary and he was credited with introducing the Haisla to brass instruments, a particularly masculine expression of Christian conversion.[88] In the 1890s he started a trading post that he was still running when Butcher arrived in 1916.[89] He had married into the Haisla at a time when some Christian workers believed that such marriages would show the universalism of the church.[90] He had married into a high-ranking family, to a woman who would be called a 'princess' by a later ethnologist.[91] So Robinson was a prominent member of Kitamaat society. And he was a major thorn in Butcher's side as she tried to describe white men in ways that would make clear their dominance, their inherent difference from and superiority to Native men.

Butcher first introduced George Robinson by saying that he was an "Englishman." In this case, however, it did not prove to be the basis for a common bond linking him to Butcher. Butcher commented that, "one surmises that he came of good stock and had fair education."[92] How far he had fallen, in Butcher's mind. Butcher described Robinson as living a "retired, secluded life, belonging nowhere."[93] He was not Indian so he could not be involved in Village life, Butcher believed, but his marriage cast him out of white society as well. Butcher had little hope for the Robinson children, though they were beautiful and, she argued, with Robinson's wealth they could be well educated. Instead they were "being brought up as Indians." Even their "heritage of beauty" was a drawback, according to Butcher, as the stain of hybridity contaminated all that was good in them.[94] Unlike Moore, who through competence could 'belong' to the land, Robinson forfeited his right to belong when he traded English-ness for cross-race marriage. Like "Mr Cordello and his Indian wife," crossing the boundary between white and Native was itself contaminating and, in order that whiteness remained pure, those men who crossed that line could no longer belong in Butcher's white world.

Indeed, any inter-relationship between the white world as Butcher saw it and the Indian was, it seemed to Butcher, inevitably doomed.

Another half-breed man, Henry McIvor, was the subject of one of Butcher's sadder tales. It seemed that McIvor was the offspring of a white man and a Native wife. The father had been dead for some time and the mother had married a Haisla man of the Kitamaat Village. Henry had "lived white, made a good name for himself, married a dainty little white woman, who had one boy and two girls." However, McIvor's essential Indian-ness emerged when he moved his family back to his mother's village in order to take up logging. Butcher anticipated tragedy: "We were aghast when we found so neat a little woman living amongst the Indians, but could not dream of the finale." The finale came when Henry McIvor was found dead on his newly purchased gas launch and the woman, and her children, were left alone among the Indians who, according to Butcher, cared little for her plight.[95] Significantly to Butcher, in telling this tale, the tragedy began with the first white man's intermarriage. The son McIvor, as a 'fabricated European,' was doomed. His 'dainty little white' wife was not to blame, but it was she who bore the burden of being duped by the deceptive sameness of the hybrid. Butcher asserted that mission staff could not interfere to save the woman, lost now among Indians, but had to wait until the Haisla cast the woman out. Unlike the white community whose chivalry protected women, for Butcher, First Nations and their offspring could not be counted on to save even their own. The immutable difference between Indian and white was proven by the tragedies that ensued from its breaching.

An Absent Presence: Health and Whiteness

There is a remarkable absence in Butcher's narrative. Although the ill health of the Haisla community and the residential school students was a constant theme in Butcher's letters and she saw tragedy as the consequence of hybridity, she hardly mentioned the health of the white community. When Frank Hallett was evacuated following an industrial accident in the woods, Butcher reported this only obliquely in a story about the difficulties of communication. A mis-spelled wire seemed to indicate that halibut not Hallett required evacuation. Later, Butcher discussed Hallett's long stay in hospital in Vancouver only to praise her sister's attention to this acquaintance from the Kitamaat

Valley. Similarly, Lizzie Moore's difficult confinement, to which Butcher travelled on horseback in high water, warranted mention only to show the varied skills of Charlie Moore. But tragedy stalked the white community of the Kitamaat Valley. Shortly after the arrival of a woman known only as Mrs Deighton, her husband dropped dead of a heart attack while working on his pre-emption. Within a year of the birth of her second child, Butcher's good friend Lizzie Moore came to live at the school so that Butcher and other staff could care for her as she slowly and painfully died from abdominal cancer. At the end of Butcher's narrative, both Deighton and Moore were living in the Elizabeth Long Memorial Home and a pall of sadness is clearly evident in Butcher's letters. For most of the three years she was at Kitamaat, Butcher used the prevalence of tuberculosis among the Haisla to highlight their need for missionary intervention into the intimate contours of their lives. This dichotomy that situated ill health with indigenity in opposition to whiteness implied a healthiness for the latter that was, of course, unattainable. For this reason, although Butcher's nursing eyes must have perceived illness and tragedy within the non-Native as well as the Native community on the North Coast, the structure of her narrative and the purpose of her letters may have caused her to downplay experiences of sickness, injury, and death when crafting whiteness in the Kitamaat Valley.

+++

The missionaries of the North Pacific Coast in the nineteenth century, men like William Duncan and Thomas Crosby, set themselves in opposition to settler society and the provincial government that represented it. These missionaries feared the drunk and disorderly society of men that grew up around the fur trade, mining, and other resource-based industries. Crosby, in particular, advocated on behalf of First Nations, supporting them in protests over the allocation of reserve land, hoping that Aboriginal people would be provided with assistance, time, and distance from the baleful effects of contact as they learned to take their proper place within the Family of Man.

Margaret Butcher's view of Aboriginal people was very much rooted in a more twentieth-century conception of race. Though committed to assimilation through her work at the residential school, the Elizabeth Long Memorial Home, Butcher doubted that Aboriginal people would ever be equal to their white counterparts. Her task was to impart to her students the skills needed to make them useful to white people rather than join with them as inheritors of this province. And indeed, white settlers were, according to Butcher, the rightful heirs to the land. Butcher's letters elevate the settler society of the Kitamaat Valley, proving it to be a community worthy of the efforts made on its behalf. Correspondingly, Butcher constructed a different Family of Man than that of her nineteenth-century counterparts: hers was based on immutability, on the stability of race based in biology rather than culture.

In Butcher's writing, whiteness was ascendant and but not necessarily unchanging. Culture, like Englishness, could be bestowed upon individuals or even landscapes so that their value would be made plain. In this respect, we see culture cut loose from nationality, since all that was English need not be born in England; rather Englishness was a marker for a whiteness that could be, when necessary, ethnically diverse. Race rooted in biology, however, made reproduction the mainspring of society and gender exceedingly important. In Butcher's white world, the boundaries between races and the borders around gender were meant to be impregnable. While the categories of "White Man, White Woman, Woman of Color, Man of Color" were all present in Butcher's letters, so were those who disrupted this taxonomy.[96] For some the disorder could be contained. For Butcher, like other independent women in the mission field, life demanded more than frailty, so she used humour to contain the rupture that writing about her life made in the categories of race. For others, like white men who married Aboriginal women, the consequences were figurative, if not literal: banishment from the terrain of whiteness. Butcher's letters, then, reveal that rather than a stable identity, whiteness was, in Ruth Frankenberg's words, "more about the power to include and exclude."[97] The strategic and contingent nature of whiteness is laid bare.

What is the importance of any of this? Margaret Butcher was a little-known nurse working in a residential school long since closed. Few people saw her letters; just a handful of family and friends circulated them – but they were preserved. Today they reveal a great deal about community identity formation, about the construction of race. First, we see how a very ordinary woman constructed whiteness, self-consciously and with great care. This proves that, at least for Butcher, the need for such construction was apparent. There was nothing natural about the ascendance of the white community on the North Coast and those involved in its settlement knew that. Second, as Michael Marker argues, educators of Native children asserted and negotiated cultural identity for themselves as well as trying to shape that of the pupils. Recognizing this is an important step in ending the disavowal of whiteness as cultural work. Dissecting Butcher's self-conscious depiction of whiteness therefore picks apart the insidious nature/culture divide that posits white perspectives as 'natural' and Native views as 'cultural,' a strategic inversion of the historic nature/culture divide currently used to dismiss Aboriginal views of history.[98] Ascribing ordinariness to whiteness both perpetuates the exoticization of Aboriginality and erases the power relations inherent in the history of peoples becoming white. As our activist contemporaries tell us, historicizing whiteness is a crucial step in unlearning racism.

NOTES

Special thanks to Dan Watt for the Herculean task of transcribing the hand-written letters of Margaret Butcher and for subsequent research. Colin McLean fielded a number of last-minute questions on material in various Vancouver archives. His labour is much appreciated.

1 BCARS, MS-0362 Margaret Butcher, "Letters" are the base text for this chapter. The letters have now been published as Mary-Ellen Kelm, ed., *The Letters of Margaret Butcher: Missionary-Imperialism on the North Pacific Coast* (Calgary: University of Calgary Press, 2006).

2 Anti-racist workshops of the 1990s asserted that racial hierarchy *produced* racism in individuals (the 'we are all racists' argument) who could then unlearn their racism. By arguing that all members of such societies were racist, these workshops avoided essentializing race and, to a degree, diffused an 'us versus them' mentality that racism itself thrives on. If racism itself produces race, then it becomes the work of everyone in racist society to examine their own racialization. Ruth Frankenberg links the growth of the study of whiteness to the anti-racist movement in Ruth Frankenberg, *White Women, Race Matters: The Social Construction of Whiteness.* (Minneapolis: University of Minnesota Press, 1993): 1 and Ruth Frankenberg, "Local Whiteness, Localizing Whiteness." In Ruth Frankenberg, ed., *Displacing Whiteness: Essays in Social and Cultural Criticism*, 17 and 33 cf 24 (Durham and London: Duke University Press, 1997).

3 See on the Chinese, Kay Anderson "Cultural Hegemony and the Race – Definition Process in Chinatown, Vancouver: 1880–1980," in *Environment and Planning D: Society and Space* 7 (1988): 127–49 and in *Vancouver's Chinatown*
(Vancouver: UBC Press, 1991). On the construction of the 'Indian,' see Robert
F. Berkhofer Jr., *The White Man's Indian* (New York: Knopf, 1978); Brian W.
Dippie, *The Vanishing American: White Attitudes and U.S. Indian Policy.* (Mid-
dleton, CT: Wesleyan University Press, 1982); Daniel Francis, *The Imaginary In-
dian: The Image of the Indian in Canadian Culture* (Vancouver: Arsenal Pulp
Press, 1992); Reginald Horsman, "Scientific Racism and the American Indian in
the Mid-Nineteenth Century," in *American Quarterly* 27 (May 1975): 52–168;
Horsman, *Race and Manifest Destiny: The Origins of American Racial Anglo-
Saxonism* (Cambridge: Harvard University Press, 1981); Ronald Takaki, "The
Tempest in the Wilderness: The Racialization of Savagery," in *Journal of American History* 79, 3 (December 1992): 892–912; John Lutz, "Making 'Indians'
in British Columbia: Power, Race and the Importance of Place." In Richard
White and John M. Findlay, eds., *Power and Place in the North American West*,
61–84 (Seattle and London: University of Washington Press, 1999); Peter Jackson and Jan Penrose, eds., *Constructions of Race, Place and Nation* (London:
University College London, 1993).
4 Mike Hill, "Introduction: Vipers in Shangri-la: Whiteness, Writing and Other
Ordinary Terrors." In Mike Hill, ed., *Whiteness: A Critical Reader*, 2 (New
York: New York University Press, 1997).
5 See the special issue of *International Labor and Working Class History* no. 60
(spring 2001) for a series of articles debating the validity of the concept and the
usefulness of the scholarship. See particularly, James R. Barrett, "Whiteness Studies: Anything Here for Historians of the Working Class?" in *International Labor
and Working-Class History* 60 (Fall 2001): 33–42; Victoria C. Hattam, "Whiteness: Theorizing Race, Eliding Ethnicity," In *International Labor and Working
Class History* 60 (Fall 2001): 61–8; David Roediger, *Wages of Whiteness: Race
and the Making of the American Working Class* (New York: Verso, 1990) and
Colored White: Transcending the Racial Past (New York: Verso, 2002); Noel Ig-
natiev, *How the Irish Became White* (New York: Routledge, 1995).
6 Ruth Frankenberg, *White Women, Race Matters: The Social Construction of
Whiteness* (Minneapolis: University of Minnesota Press, 1993); Vron Ware, *Beyond the Pale: White Women, Racism and History* (London: Verso, 1992).
7 Frankenberg, *White Women, Race Matters*, 1.
8 Barbara J. Fields, "Whiteness, Racism and Identity," in *International Labor and
Working Class History* 60 (2001): 48–56.

9 Frankenberg, *White Women, Race Matters*, 16. The literature on this is vast. Key texts include: Catherine Hall, *Civilising Subjects* (Chicago: University of Chicago Press); Ann Laura Stoler, *Carnal Knowledge and Imperial Power* (Berkeley: University of California Press, 2002). Frederick Cooper and Ann Laura Stoler, "Introduction." In *Tensions of Empire: Colonial Cultures in a Bourgeois World*, 3 (Berkeley: University of California Press, 1997).

10 Cooper and Stoler, "Introduction," 26; Adele Perry, *On the Edge of Empire: Gender, Race and the Making of British Columbia, 1849–1871* (Toronto: University of Toronto Press, 1991); Mary Louse Pratt, *Imperial Eyes: Travel Writing and Transculturation* (London and New York: Routledge, 1991); Ann Laura Stoler, *Carnal Knowledge and Imperial Power: Race and the Intimate in Colonial Rule* (Berkeley: University of California Press, 2002).

11 Angela Woollacott, "'All This Is Empire, I Told Myself': Australian Women's Voyages 'Home' and the Articulation of Whiteness," in *American Historical Review* 102, 4 (October 1997): 1003–29.

12 Frankenberg, *White Women, Race Matters*, 16.

13 The diverse nature of British Columbia's population has been the subject of a great deal of scholarship over the years. W. Peter Ward, *White Canada Forever: Popular Attitudes and Public Policy Toward Orientals in British Columbia* (Montreal & Kingston: McGill-Queen's University Press, 1973) and Patricia E. Roy, *A White Man's Province: British Columbia Politicians and Chinese and Japanese Immigrants 1858–1914* (Vancouver: UBC Press, 1989) are two early classics. In the 1980s there were a series of debates over which social category was most significant, see W. Peter Ward, "Class and Race in the Social Structure of British Columbia, 1870–1939," in *BC Studies* 45 (Spring 1980): 17–36. Rennie Warburton, "Race and Class in British Columbia: A Comment," In *BC Studies* 49 (1981): 79–85, followed by W. Peter Ward, "Race and Class in British Columbia: A Reply," In *BC Studies* 50 (1981): 52. Geographers have productively probed the spatiality of racism and of population distribution. See, for example, Dan Clayton, "Geographies of the Lower Skeena," in *BC Studies* 94 (1992): 29–58. Kay Anderson, *Vancouver's Chinatown: Racial Discourse in Canada, 1875–1990* (Montreal & Kingston: McGill-Queen's University Press, 1991). Cole Harris with Robert Galois, "A Population Geography of British Columbia in 1881." In *The Resettlement of British Columbia: Essays on Colonialism and Geographical Change*, 137–60 (Vancouver: UBC Press, 1997). Syntheses of the province also grapple with the diversity of its demographics and the British-ness of its avowed culture. See Jean Barman, *The West Beyond the*

West, paperback ed. (Toronto: University of Toronto Press, 1996) and Hugh Johnston, *The Pacific Province: the History of British Columbia* (Vancouver & Toronto: Douglas and McIntyre Press, 1996). For Britishness in British Columbia, see particularly Jean Barman, *Growing Up British in British Columbia* (Vancouver: UBC Press, 1984). .

14 For the social impact of fur trade marriages and the gradual displacement of fur trade society, see Sylvia Van Kirk, *Many Tender Ties: Women in Fur Trade Society in Western Canada, 1670–1870* (Winnipeg: Watson and Dwyer, 1980). Sylvia Van Kirk, "Tracing the Fortunes of Five Founding Families of Victoria," In *BC Studies* 115/116 (1997–8): 148–79; Erica Smith, "'Gentlemen, This is No Ordinary Trial': Sexual Narratives in the Trial of the Reverend Robert Corbett, Red River, 1863." In Jennifer S.H. Brown and Elizabeth Vibert, eds., *Reading Beyond Words: Contexts for Native History*, 1st ed. (Peterborough, ON: Broadview Press, 1996). Brent Christophers argues in *Positioning the Missionary* that the precepts of Augustinian Christianity sought not to make distinctions based on race but rather on the distinction between civility and savagery. Brent Christophers, *Positioning the Missionary: John Booth Good and the Confluence of Cultures in Nineteenth Century British Columbia* (Vancouver: UBC Press, 1998), 21. This corresponds to the early nineteenth century notion among evangelical Christian missionaries of the 'family of man'; see Hall, *Civilising Subjects*, 140–71. On the energy expended on making British Columbia white in the colonial period, see Adele Perry, *On the Edge of Empire: Gender, Race, and the Making of British Columbia, 1849–1871* (Toronto: University of Toronto Press, 2001).

15 For a superb discussion of the inter-relationships between cultural placement and spatial segregation, see Steven Hoelscher, "Making Place, Making Race: Performances of Whiteness in the Jim Crow South," in *Annals of the Association of American Geographers* 93, 3 (2003): 657–86.

16 Perry, *On the Edge of Empire*, 197.

17 J.R. Miller, *Shingwauk's Vision: A History of Native Residential Schools* (Toronto: University of Toronto Press, 1996), 152–58;Vancouver School of Theology, United Church of Canada Archives, Isobel McFadden, "Living by the Bells: A Narrative of Five Schools in British Columbia, 1874–1970." Unpublished manuscript written for the Committee on Education for Mission and Stewardship of the United Church of Canada. Rosemary Gagan, *A Sensitive Independence: Canadian Methodist Women Missionaries in Canada and the Orient, 1881–1925* (Montreal & Kingston: McGill-Queen's University Press, 1992), 198. BCARS, MS-0362 Margaret Butcher, "Letters" – page references in text are

to the original letters. The letters have now been published as Mary-Ellen Kelm, ed., *The Letter[[Letters?]] of Margaret Butcher: Missionary-Imperialism on the North Pacific Coast.* (Calgary: University of Calgary Press, 2006).

18 Frankenberg, "Local Whiteness, Localizing Whiteness," 5.

19 Cole Harris, *Making Native Space: Colonialism, Resistance, and Reserves in British Columbia*, (Vancouver: UBC Press, 2002), 176, 182–7; Robert Boyd, *The Coming of the Spirit of Pestilence: Introduced Infectious Diseases and Population Decline among Northwest Coast Indians, 1774–1874*, (Seattle: University of Washington Press, 1999), 227.

20 John Charles Pritchard, "Economic Development and the Disintegration of Traditional Culture among the Haisla," unpublished PhD dissertation (Vancouver: UBC, 1977).

21 Elizabeth Anderson Varley, *Kitamaat, My Valley* (Terrace: Northern Times Press, 1981).

22 Kim Greenwell, "Picturing 'Civilization': Missionary Narratives and the Margins of Mimicry," in *BC Studies* 135 (Autumn 2002): 3–54.

23 Paul Gilroy, *The Black Atlantic: Modernity and Double Consciousness*, (London & New York: Verso, 1993), 11.

24 Ibid.

25 Butcher, "Letters," 11, 56.

26 Ibid., 55, 65.

27 Ibid., 47.

28 Ibid., 12.

29 Ibid., 12, 90.

30 Ibid., 107.

31 Ibid., 13.

32 Myra Rutherdale, *Women and the White Man's God: Gender and Race in the Canadian Mission Field* (Vancouver: UBC Press, 2002), 74–9; Sara Mills, *Discourses of Difference: An Analysis of Women's Travel Writing and Colonialism* (London & New York: Routledge, 1991), 22, 75, 79; See for contrast the eroticized image of the land in male travel writing, Anne McClintock, *Imperial Leather: Race, Gender and Sexuality in the Colonial Contest* (New York, London: Routledge, 1995), 25.

33 Butcher, "Letters," 11–12.

34 Ibid., 105.

35 Ibid., 93, 26, 31, 90, 91.

36 Ibid., 43.

37 Ibid., 80.

38 Ibid., 28.

39 Ibid.

40 Ibid., 86, 101.

41 John Hartigan Jr., "Locating White Detroit." In Frankenberg, ed., *Displacing Whiteness*, 188.

42 Ibid., 109.

43 Ibid., 109, 103, 106.

44 Ibid., 110.

45 Ibid., 17.

46 Ibid., 43.

47 Ibid., 12, 13, 14, 25.

48 Ibid., 13.

49 Butcher, "Letters," 20; Barbara N. Ramusack, "Cultural Missionaries, Maternal Imperialists, Feminist Allies: British Women Activists in India." In Nupur Chaudhuri and Margaret Stroebel, eds., *Western Women and Imperialism: Complicity and Resistance*, 120 (Bloomington: Indiana University Press, 1992); Mariana Valverde, *The Age of Light, Soap and Water: Moral Reform in English Canada, 1885–1925* (Toronto: McClelland & Stewart, 1991), 17, 30.

50 Butcher, "Letters," 30.

51 Ibid., 92.

52 Ibid., 70.

53 Ibid., 30.

54 Ibid., 23.

55 Ibid., 101.

56 Ibid., 57.

57 Ibid., 59.

58 For a similar discussion of transplanting European domesticity to the field, see Rutherdale, *Women and the White Man's God*, 88–92.

59 McClintock, *Imperial Leather*, 164.

60 Miller, *Shingwauk's Vision*, 150.

61 Elizabeth Jane Errington, *Wives and Mothers, School Mistresses and Scullery Maids: Working Women in Upper Canada 1790–1840* (Montreal & Kingston: McGill-Queens University Press, 1995).

62 Sylvia Van Kirk, "Tracing the Fortunes of Five Founding Families of Victoria," *BC Studies* 115/116 (1997–98): 148–79; Erica Smith, "'Gentlemen, This is No Ordinary Trial': Sexual Narratives in the Trial of the Reverend Robert Corbett,

Red River, 1863," in Jennifer S.H. Brown and Elizabeth Vibert, eds., *Reading Beyond Words: Contexts for Native History*. 1st ed. (Peterborough, ON: Broadview Press, 1996).

63 Rutherdale, *Women and the White Man's God*, 90–1; Andrew Porter, "'Cultural Imperialism' and Protestant Missionary Enterprise, 1780–1914," in *Journal of Imperial and Commonwealth History* 25, 3 (September 1997): 385; Mary Taylor Huber and Nancy C. Lutkehaus, "Introduction," in *Gendered Missions: Women and Men in Missionary Discourse and Practice* (Ann Arbor: University of Michigan Press, 1999), 2.

64 Rutherdale, *Women and the White Man's God*, 90–1; Gagan, *A Sensitive Independence*; Kwok Pui-lan, "The Image of the White Lady: Gender and Race in Christian Mission," in *Concilium* 6 (1991): 19–27.

65 Butcher, "Letters," 30.

66 Ibid., 31.

67 Ibid., 34-35.

68 Ibid., 31, 13, 45.

69 Ibid., 117.

70 Ibid., 45.

71 Mills, *Discourses of Differences*, 102–3, 95.

72 Butcher, "Letters," 48.

73 This was a not uncommon preoccupation; Blake writes that women travellers often found themselves asking: "Will I manage; How will I look?" Susan Blake, "A Woman's Trek: What Difference Does Gender Make?" In *Western Women and Imperialism*, 19.

74 Butcher, "Letters," 53.

75 Ibid., 98.

76 Ibid., 102.

77 Ibid., 103–6.

78 See for contrast Cliff Kopas, *No Path But My Own* (Madiera Park, BC: Harbour publishing, 1996) tells the story of one man's victory of over weakness by in the course of a pack horse trip through the Rockies.

79 Butcher, "Letters," 12.

80 Ibid., 72.

81 Ibid., 35, 117, 31, 70.

82 Ibid., 53.

83 Ibid., 31.

84 Ibid., 28.

85 Ibid., 73, 53, 65.

86 Ibid., 56.

87 Ibid., 56, 26, 35.

88 Susan Neylan with Melissa Meyer, "'Here Comes the Band!': Cultural Collaboration, Connective Traditions, and Aboriginal Brass Bands on British Columbia's North Coast, 1875–1964," in *BC Studies* 152 (Winter 2006–07): 67–96.

89 Vancouver School of Theology, United Church Archives, Church History Files, G.H. Raley to Rev. J.C. Goodfellow, 25 February 1938, Alex Mogee, 1 February 1930; Elizabeth Varley, *Kitamaat, My Valley*, 15.

90 Varley, *Kitamaat, My Valley*, 15.

91 Ivan A. Lopatin, *The Social Life & Religion of the Indians of Kitimat, British Columbia*, social science series, #26 (Los Angeles: University of Southern California, 1945).

92 Butcher, "Letters," 32.

93 Butcher, "Letters," 14.

94 Ibid., 55, 32–3.

95 Ibid., 95.

96 Frankenberg, "Locating Whiteness," 11–13.

97 Ibid.

98 Michael Marker, "'That History Is More a Part of the Present than It Ever Was in the Past': Toward an Ethnohistory of Native Education," in *History of Education Review* 28, 1 (1999): 24.

6

+++++

Nursing in the North and Writing for the South:
The Work and Travels of Amy Wilson

MYRA RUTHERDALE

During the 1950s and 1960s it became increasingly popular for new-comers to northern Canada to write their autobiographies, or partic-ipate in the preparation of their biographies. Often these newcomers were part of a professional class who moved to the North to work as doctors, teachers, nurses, missionaries, RCMP officers, and federal government bureaucrats. Sometimes they were simply travellers, pass-ing through the region and believing that even a short stint in the North somehow conferred upon them the status of an expert on mat-ters northern. Alluding to just this tendency, Ernie Lyall, author of *An Arctic Man: Sixty-five Years in Canada's North*, sought to set the record straight in his autobiography. He had seen too many of these 'northern experts': "There's a saying up here that goes something like this – if you come up here from the south and you stop over at some place in the north for an hour, you can write an article for a news-paper; if you stay overnight you can write a big article for a magazine; and if you stay for three days, you're an expert and you can write a whole book."[1] At the outset of his autobiography Lyall attempted to establish himself as an authority on the North, in opposition to what he called "those three-day experts."[2] His sixty-five years were in many ways extensive and impressive.

Despite Lyall's cynicism, thousands of southern readers were at-tracted to the genre of northern life writing during the 1960s and 1970s.[3] Canadian publishers, notably McClelland & Stewart and

Ryerson Press, particularly welcomed northern adventure writing.[4] The authors of these tales usually cast the North as the central protagonist in romantic terms and in language that deliberately contrasted it to the south. Nordicity was conflated with hardy individualism, especially masculinity. Historically, northern life writing was the domain of men. Explorers, gold miners, and sojourners eagerly prepared their journals for publication. Historians of the North, who until recently were most often male, turned to those tales when constructing their narratives of northern history.[5]

Women's northern travel writing and life writing was less common, or at least more rarely included in northern historiography.[6] Scholars of women's travel writing have since offered reasons for this neglect. In her analysis of this genre, Sara Mills argues that texts by British women written during the age of high imperialism were frequently the site of "discursive conflicts." Not only did women transcend boundaries by travelling and writing about their adventures – and therefore step well beyond the private sphere – but they also occasionally offered opinions on the politics of empire, which was perceived to be out of place for women. Mills recognizes that women travel writers were "caught in a double-bind." Their narratives had to be structured with the right balance, noting that if they relied too heavily on the "discourses of femininity" their work was dismissed as "trivial," whereas if their texts leaned too much toward the "adventure hero type narratives" they were seen as inauthentic, or mannish.[7] Karen R. Lawrence agrees that women's travel narratives had to strike just the right note. Too often travel narratives – and the women travellers themselves – were portrayed as akin to eccentric, "mildly batty," strange birds.[8] Not all women writers were so easily dismissed and it is the invention of the travelling self that concerns Lawrence. She is especially conscious of the fact that the travel genre could allow for varying identities to be forged: "Travel can accommodate the ambivalent impulses of Florence Nightingale's radical individualism and her service as handmaiden to the British Empire."[9] Lawrence is particularly curious about how women mediated between what she describes as "black and white and female and male on the imperial frontier." One narrative strategy that she highlights is the "fraternal mode."

Appropriating masculinity, or the fraternal mode, seemed for many women writers to be a useful strategy, although it functioned to highlight the 'mannish' woman. However, as Renée Hulan reminds us, northern literature is all about masculinity: "Heroic, rugged individuals, usually male, people the literature set in the north, and they usually share common characteristics."[10] Generally, these characters are on a quest, and are at the same time enjoying the freedom from "social connection, responsibility and moral reason."[11] Hulan agrees with Lawrence that women on the other hand either had to adopt a "passive role or take on the same 'masculine' characteristics."[12]

After the Second World War, women's autobiographies and biographies began to attract southern readers. Their stories of transcending gender norms by travelling and often working for a living in Arctic environs were appealing to southerners who could read about, and at the same time experience, adventure vicariously. Their lives stood in stark contrast to other middle-class Canadian women in the 1950s and 1960s who were living lives shaped by new suburban realities.[13] One such text is *No Man Stands Alone*, an autobiographical account written by Amy V. Wilson. The purpose of this essay is to assess Wilson's text and determine what this richly detailed and textured example of writing from the region and era can tell us about nursing and northern health care, Native/newcomer relations, gender dynamics in northern Canada, and the act of memorializing a life in autobiographical form. The first important question is: given the range of historical experience and social contingencies, how much value can we place on the observations of one person alone? And furthermore, given the propensity for northern tales to be overwhelmingly masculine, how did Wilson approach the task of writing her life?

Amy Wilson: Making a Northern Nurse

Amy Wilson was born in southern Alberta in 1905. Like thousands of others in the first decade of the twentieth century, her parents were drawn to the Canadian prairies from the United States – in this case, Missouri – by the promise of agricultural success. Amy was one of seven children and her mother died when she was three. She remembered her childhood as happy if not materially wealthy.[14] Her sister, Lucy Sutherland, recalled in hindsight that Amy was "a girl who favoured outdoor activity. She loved to hunt and fish, skate and play baseball."[15]

Upon completing high school, Wilson began a three-year nurse training program at the Calgary General Hospital. Sutherland, also a graduate nurse, claimed that Wilson always felt attracted to nursing: "Her objective from the time of childhood was to become a nurse and to care for the unfortunate and underprivileged."[16] Although this may have been the case, it is likely, too, that both were drawn from rural Alberta to Calgary to pursue nursing because there were few other options. According to Kathryn McPherson, rural prairie women were often made redundant by the inheritance practices of farm families, who tended to bequeath the family fortune to the first-born son. McPherson makes it clear that nursing was a viable white-collar profession for women who wanted to pursue a career: "Nursing promised board and room for three years, during which time women from the countryside could familiarize themselves with urban life, make contacts in the urban job market, and acquire highly portable skills and certification."[17] The Wilson sisters were two out of hundreds of young women who moved from rural prairie communities to urban training hospitals in the decades before the Second World War. Like others of their generation, they sought to change their fortunes and take advantage of new opportunities, largely unavailable to women in their mother's era.

But, finding employment after the three years of nurse training was not always easy. After taking her Florence Nightingale pledge, Wilson realized, as she put it, "I was a full-fledged nurse, and it was in the middle of a full-fledged depression."[18] However, she was not daunted, and took up her first hospital posting in a mining community. After this, she was hired by the Department of Public Health as a district nurse, and was posted first to the Peace River country, and then to Lesser Slave Lake in northern Alberta. Again, her employment choices represented certain patterns to be found among graduating nurses in Western Canada. Public health nursing in rural areas was not the most desired kind of work; nonetheless, it provided a wide range of experience and vested those who practised rural medicine with a sense of mission and accomplishment. Based on her reading of Canadian Nurse (CN), Kathryn McPherson found that rural public health nurses in Western Canada started to see themselves as quasi-missionaries: "Testimonials published in the CN suggested that graduate nurses who were working in isolated rural districts resolved the contradictions inherent in their position as single working women by justifying their presence in rural communities in terms of uplifting downtrodden and needy citizens." Those who needed salvation included newcomers to Canada, bachelor men, economically deprived farm families, and Aboriginals. With so many struggling souls, the Canadian trained nurse could reinvent herself as a beacon of hope or, as McPherson puts it, a missionary "of the Canadian state."[19]

In fact, it is through Wilson's work with the Canadian federal government that we come to know her as a nurse. From the late nineteenth century, the Department of Indian Affairs (DIA) – often in partnership with either the Catholic or Anglican churches – helped to fund reserve hospitals in Western Canada. But Maureen Lux, in her acclaimed *Medicine That Walks*, hastens to remind us that the care provided to Natives was on an ad hoc basis and that the government as late as 1946 proclaimed that "neither law nor treaty imposes an obligation on the government to establish a health service for the Indians and Eskimos."[20] The government's parsimony is reinforced in Laurie Meijer Drees's study of the Blood and Blackfoot reserve hospitals during the period from 1890 to 1930. Drees, however, is determined to correct the assumption that the federal government refused to take responsibility for Native health care prior to 1940. She finds instead that such medical treatment as there was, was firmly imbued with the ideas of social purity and moral reform. In agreement with McPherson, Drees claims "social reformers in this era targeted the poor and the rural for reform, and Indian peoples were included in their agenda through the Department of Indian Affairs."[21] So although the government denied full responsibility for Aboriginal health care, they simultaneously – with the help of Anglican and Catholic churches – operated a parsimonious program with a skeletal staff on reserves and in Aboriginal communities across Canada. However, in 1945 the DIA's health work came to a halt with the creation of the Department of National Health and Welfare. Hereafter, Aboriginal health would be placed under the jurisdiction of the Indian and Northern Health Services Branch, which very quickly began to advertise nurse's positions in northern and Aboriginal communities.

For several years, CN regularly featured job announcements calling for nurses. All categories of nurses were encouraged to apply for this "interesting, challenging, satisfying work." The advertisements featured nurses in their uniforms and in northern outdoor clothing:

"Nursing With Indian and Northern Health Services – Opportunities For Registered Hospital Nurses, Public Health Nurses, and Nursing Assistants or Practical Nurses for Hospital Positions and Public Health Positions in Outpost Nursing Stations, Centres and Field Positions in the Provinces, Eastern Arctic and North-West Territories."[22] Amy Wilson no doubt saw a job advertisement similar to this. In 1949, she applied for the position of "Alaska Highway Nurse," through the Department of National Health and Welfare.[23] She was interviewed by the regional superintendent of Indian and Northern Health Services and, as she claimed, "the position meant being field nurse for the 3,000 Indians in the Yukon Territory and Northern British Columbia, an area covering roughly 200,000 square miles. Such a challenge! And I couldn't resist it."[24]

Wilson was clearly professionally prepared for her appointment as the Alaska Highway nurse.[25] After all, she had worked as a hospital nurse in a mining community and recalled an affinity for public health nursing in northern Alberta: "I enjoyed the work in this area; first aid, home nursing classes, immunizing the children, attending maternity cases, trying to be counsellor and friend as well as nurse to these people whom I understood and respected."[26] She felt she understood the local population because of her experience growing up in southern Alberta, which shaped her attitude toward new challenges. As she herself commented, "gloom was never part of [my] personality," and she, not unlike her parents, was excited by "the thought of new territory and new adventures."[27]

Wilson's career with the Indian Health Services Branch lasted six years and would certainly take her to territory that was new for her. She travelled extensively throughout British Columbia and the Yukon. Some of these "new adventures" were recorded in *No Man Stands Alone*, published retrospectively in 1965. Perhaps the most adventurous part of Wilson's sojourn was in coming to terms with herself as one of the new – to borrow McPherson's phrase – missionaries of the state.

Encounters with Aboriginal Medicine

It should have come as no surprise to Wilson in her position as Alaska Highway nurse to see just how much Aboriginal people in her jurisdiction relied on their own medicine. While growing up in rural

Alberta, she would have been familiar with midwives, or at the very least home-based curatives. In her study of seventy-eight rural home-steading women in Saskatchewan and Alberta, Nanci Langford demonstrates just how much women depended on each other for midwifery support and health care: "they assisted each other at child-birth because they were the only ones available to do so."[28] But she also recognized that it was rather uncommon for Native women to assist at the birth of non-Native children, at least in the southern communities. The one exception highlighted in Langford's study was a case in northern Alberta where the midwife Nokum Julie helped the white settler Mary Lawrence in her delivery. Lawrence was relieved by the technique of kneeling rather than lying down: "I was so convinced of the logic of this natural method over that to which white women are enforced that I abided by it henceforth."[29]

As for Aboriginal midwifery and medicine, recent scholarship reinforces the ways in which Aboriginal people from British Columbia, Alberta, and the Plains were, as Maureen Lux demonstrates, adamant in their "refusal to forsake their own medicine."[30] A pluralistic system had emerged by the 1920s, but in some communities, especially in the provincial norths, as Langford acknowledges, there was still more reliance on Native midwifery and medicine than Western medicine well into the 1940s.[31]

In her autobiography, Wilson described Aboriginal medicine makers she encountered in her northern travels. In fact, she sought to learn from them, and to forge relationships with Aboriginal women in particular. She described how one "medicine woman" in northern Alberta's community of Lesser Slave Lake became "quite a good friend."[32] According to Wilson this woman, who unfortunately remains name-less, had spent the better part of fifty years working as a midwife in her community and had garnered respect because of her birthing accomplishments. Wilson claimed that when she moved to Lesser Slave Lake the midwife did not treat her as competition, but rather that "when a newcomer, and a white one at that, came in, she felt no resentment."[33] In the shadow of colonization there was indeed room for resentment, but instead she and Wilson appeared to enjoy each other. Importantly, too, we can see that Wilson identified herself as a white woman. She was conscious that she was the outsider, or the 'other,' in this encounter.

Wilson's description of a visit to the medicine woman's cabin provides insight into the common interest shared by these two women:
"One day when I called at her cabin, she pulled a cardboard box from
under her bed and showed me the collection of 'medicine' that it contained. One that particularly interested me she called 'Iskwao Muskike'
or Woman Medicine. This, she said, was her best medicine, and she
explained its use in these terms: 'Only for woman who is going to have
baby. If egg break and baby come too soon, lots of blood come. If not
can stop, woman die. This medicine stop him.'"[34] Wilson spent many
hours with her new friend learning about the various "herbs and
roots" that she used in her day-to-day encounters with ill patients. Wilson was not critical of the cures offered but, rather, interested and
curious to learn about the natural remedies.

In her journey through the North Wilson would meet other midwives and attend many births.[35] She was usually invited to births only
if midwives were concerned that there was some jeopardy. In one such
case, in Minto, Yukon, Wilson reported on what she saw as a typical
pattern of delivery for most Aboriginal women: "When an Indian
woman goes into labor her favorite midwife comes to help her. Quite
often it is her mother or mother-in-law. If there are no complications
no one else is called. If it is a difficult birth all the old women come.
The patient is sometimes standing, or on her knees, leaning over a pole
put across the tent. She is pummeled and squeezed. Often a blanket is
tied around her as tightly as two women can pull it. They think this
will force the baby's birth. Nothing particularly clean is used, yet it
is surprising how few die."[36] Typical of her generation and training,
Wilson passed judgment on the cleanliness of the environment, but she
obviously recognized the success of the birthing practice itself, measured in the numbers of babies who survived. She also commented on
the practicality and success of the muskeg moss diapers. In this particular instance Wilson noted that the moss had been gathered,
washed, and dried by the mother before the baby's birth and as she
concluded: "One seldom sees a baby with sore buttocks if muskeg
moss has been used as a diaper."[37]

Wilson's response, however, may not have been typical. Scholars who
have studied the impact of Western medicine in northern communities
suggest that newcomers were far more intrusive and disruptive. For
example, in Patricia Jasen's study on Inuit women's birthing practices,

she claimed "a traditional sense of community and self-sufficiency has
been eroded by a process of colonization that introduced health risks,
and by a civilizing mission that undermined old knowledge."[38] There
is no question about the devastation caused by colonization, and the
impact it had not only on childbirth but also on the health of northern Aboriginals. Certainly, the intrusive nature of the Alaska Highway
cannot be underestimated. Interviews with Native elders and northern
newcomers forced anthropologist Julie Cruikshank to conclude that
the health conditions of Native inhabitants rapidly deteriorated with
exposure to construction workers and other re-settlers: "Among the
most immediate and horrifying results of the coming of the highway
were the epidemics brought to settlements along the route. Any discussion of genealogies or old family photographs leads to commentary
on people who 'died in '42' or people who became ill during or after
the construction. A doctor described how families remained at the Teslin
post in the winter of 1942–43, hoping for jobs. During that winter
they were overwhelmed with measles, dysentery, jaundice, whooping
cough, mumps, tonsillitis, and meningitis. Only the Indian population
was affected."[39] Nurses like Wilson were hired to provide health care
to ameliorate these conditions, but they were also meant to introduce
new technologies and practices. Individually they, like Wilson, may
have shown appreciation for Aboriginal medicine, but at the same time
they were part of a larger medical mission with specific cultural aims.[40]
Given the prospect for a rivalry between medical traditions, Wilson's
views seem somewhat enlightened.

It was not only in the context of childbirth that Wilson recognized
the value of Aboriginal health care. As she travelled up and down the
Alaska Highway she regularly met patients who had been treated successfully by Aboriginal healers. Sometimes the healers were unwilling
to share information about their remedies.

This was the case with a Southern Tutchone, Kluane First Nation
woman named Old Lucy who Wilson met in Snag, Yukon, northwest
of Whitehorse on the Alaska border. Wilson was called to a community
close to Snag, and learned there of Lucy. Her curiosity led her to pay
a visit. Arriving in Snag, she noted that many of the children were just
recovering from the measles and observed that, despite this, no one
looked extremely ill. She heard Lucy treated them: "Thinking she must
have some specific medicine for measles, I made a special trip to the

ramshackle log cabin that was her home. There she sat on a log by the cabin door. Snow-white hair, much matted by scratching, hung down to her shoulders. When I asked her what kind of medicine she used, she grinned toothlessly and pretended she could not understand English."[41] Lucy managed to cure her people, and at the same time temper the ill effects of the measles by using a traditional remedy that she was unwilling to share with Wilson. Wilson went away unsatisfied in her quest but, nonetheless, undoubtedly reassured that the people in Snag were well cared for. Lucy's reluctance is of course understandable, too, since many northern newcomers tended to be suspicious rather than appreciative of Aboriginal healing practices.[42] What is striking about this account is that Lucy is named, whereas the woman who helped Wilson in Lesser Slave Lake is not. And while she fetishized Lucy's personal hygiene, Wilson expressed an appreciation for natural remedies and tended not only to seek them out but also to highlight them in her book.

In contrast to most of the missionaries who served the North before the Second World War and even some post-war northern nurses, Wilson held a substantial appreciation for Aboriginal medicine.[43] She did not dismiss the remedies and cures that she witnessed. In fact, Wilson yearned to learn more about them. She did not, like many missionaries before her, suggest that alternatives be found for Native midwives, nor did she think that Native medicine should be eradicated. In this way her text, and her opinions, seem unique. Wilson's text is a practical guide to some of the Aboriginal uses of local plant life. For example, Wilson noted how fireweed both camouflaged burned forests and provided the basis of a valuable salve: "The Indians dry the roots and pound [sic] it into powder. When mixed with water, it makes a pasty salve, and on more than one occasion I have come across patients with sores and varicose ulcers in different stages of healing using the soothing salve of the fireweed root."[44] Sometimes however, Wilson was skeptical of the value of Aboriginal medicine. When she first encountered the use of bulrush seeds for reducing swelling, she remained a non-believer until she tried it: "After a few moments I found out that the woman had made a good rubefacient ointment. My arm was red and hot."[45] Explicit in these descriptions is an acknowledgement of the success of traditional cures.

As the Alaska Highway nurse, Wilson not only would learn much about local medicine but also would often rely on Aboriginals to assure that her program was successful. At the same time, Wilson did not pretend that everyone accepted or welcomed her or her associates, or "white man's medicine." There were those who greeted this northern nurse, and her paraphernalia, with a certain degree of suspicion. The X-ray van, sent from the Charles Camsell Hospital in Edmonton to X-ray the lungs of all Aboriginal people and newcomers along the Highway, aroused just such doubt. As Wilson herself pointed out, "there were those few who were openly opposed to X-rays. These were usually elderly Indians who distrusted the white man's medicine."[46] But clearly not all illnesses could be cured by indigenous medicine. The most severe disease outbreak that Wilson had to contend with was a diphtheria epidemic.

In mid-December 1949, Wilson learned that some illness had gripped the Tsattine community of Mosquito Flats on Halfway River, about sixty miles northeast of Hudson's Hope. A man from Mosquito Flats travelled to the Hudson's Hope ham radio office to plea for help. Four members of his community had choked to death. This sounded to Wilson like diphtheria, but she could not be sure until she saw the patients. She moved quickly and gathered as many dosages of antitoxin and other medical supplies as she could pack for her flight. Wilson recalled in her memoir how, as she was packing, she suddenly realized the position she'd be in as a medical professional in the midst of a potential disaster: "The last item to be packed into my medical bag was a tracheotomy tube borrowed from the Fort St John Hospital. Inclusion of this little tube suddenly made me realize how very much on my own I would be. Certainly no one but a surgeon should insert it into a windpipe of a choking patient, but if it were necessary in an effort to save a life, it would be done."[47] In the end, Wilson did not have to use the tube, but she did face a crisis. She arrived at the village of Mosquito Flats just as it was being visited by diphtheria, and worked day and night to vaccinate children and adults.

Once the disease was under control, she spent the rest of the winter administering vaccinations, not just to the Tsattine but also to other Aboriginals along the Highway. First, however, she had to convince the community elders that the antitoxin was necessary. In at least one case she claimed to have the support of an old chief who himself was badly scarred from smallpox. He remembered how many of his people

died during the smallpox outbreak of his childhood. Wilson appealed
to him to encourage the others to line up for the vaccine to avoid another "white man sickness," as he labelled it.[48] "And tell them he did,"
Wilson asserted, "No parents refused the injections, either for themselves or for their children."[49]

A Northern Brotherhood

After the diphtheria epidemic of 1949, Wilson and her nursing partner Aileen Bond, who followed her to Mosquito Flats, were called to
Victoria to receive official government recognition for their work and
dedication during the diphtheria outbreak. In describing the written
citation of the awards Wilson deflected the personal attention being
bestowed upon her and focused instead on the brotherhood of the
North: "The writing on both read: "For Distinguished Service." We
felt proud but very humble, for we knew that equally deserving of
those honors were the men who, with no thought of self, had provided
us with transportation and shelter – who had fully lived up to the true
interpretation of "Men of the North." We never stood alone."[50]

Wilson saw herself as part of a northern fraternity standing in service with the Royal Canadian Mounted Police, the Royal Canadian Air
Force as well as bush pilots and ham radio operators.

Not only were Wilson and Bond commended by the government of
British Columbia but they also became minor celebrities south of the
border. *Time* magazine featured a short article about their battle against
diphtheria with a photograph of Wilson holding her nurse's kit in one
hand and snowshoes in the other. The article juxtaposed modernity and
barbarity: "In the windowless, filthy hovels, modern nursing techniques
were impossible."[51] Despite this impossibility, of course, the modern
scientific nurses would prevail. The journalist was given plenty of opportunity to provide this contrast. For example, Nurse Bond herself did
much to construct a sharp contrast between cultures: "It was not the eas-
iest thing to look professional in Arctic regalia, crawling into a tepee
on hands and knees and having to squat on the saliva-spattered ground
while the smoke from the bonfire blinded one. Our favorite expression
soon became *klootna-kloon* [too much smoke] ... and it was flattering

to enter the wigwams and be greeted with *chai-wootcha* [good woman]."⁵² The *Time* journalist went on to assure his readers that no matter what the nurses looked like, in the end they "won the battle."⁵³

Another article, this one in the style of a Ripley's Believe It or Not cartoon, appeared in several American newspapers. The top of the newspaper piece proclaimed "IT HAPPENED IN CANADA." Beneath these emboldened letters was the phrase, "An Intrepid Nurse." The article then went on to describe how Wilson heroically travelled "by every sort of northern conveyance" to administer the antitoxin that in the end successfully brought "the epidemic under control." The piece included a likeness of Wilson, which portrayed her as much more masculine than feminine. She was bundled up in heavy winter clothing holding a nurse's kit; in the background is a quintessential log cabin. At the bottom of the article is some information meant to stoke the imagination of American readers: "Hard to realize it in this age of jets, but it is possible to travel all the way from the Rockies to the Atlantic by water or even to turn north to reach the Pacific or Arctic." Wilson appeared as the embodiment of a robust, almost masculine Canadian who heroically risked life and limb to come to the aid of suffering northern Tsattine. Northern-ness here was linked to the canoe, the log cabin, and the strong, hardy, manly looking Canadian woman.

In her autobiography Wilson did little to dispel the conflation between nordicity and masculinity. More than anything, Wilson identified with what she called the "true brotherhood of the north." She did not see herself as either domesticated or feminine. The title of the book itself indicates that Wilson saw herself as part of a fraternity.

Dispensing medication and providing health care were important parts of Wilson's daily activities, but in her autobiography she also shaped an identity for herself and her readers as an adventurous northern traveller. She chose to see her time in the North as an adventure, as a sojourn, and as a time for personal and professional growth. Professionally, the challenges were far greater for a nurse in the North. Wilson often found that she had to carry out tasks that she would not have been responsible for in the south. She diagnosed illnesses, supervised the care and control of epidemics, and even extracted teeth. She felt fulfilled in this work and, upon returning from a leave in the south, she stated: "My leave seemed almost too long and often there was a tug at my heart. The Yukon called, and I longed to be back where I felt needed."⁵⁴

THE WORK AND TRAVELS OF AMY WILSON

As much as *No Man Stands Alone* can be read as a narrative on the morbidity and mortality of Aboriginals along the Alaska Highway, it should also be placed within the context of the genre of northern travel writing. Wilson's book is not a conventional travelogue by any means; rather, it may better be understood as a tale of adventure and a construction of nordicity. But interestingly, the North she portrays is not a feminized or even feminine North. Oddly enough, Wilson writes about a North that is better suited to hardy men.

Wilson's *No Man Stands Alone* seems to fit nicely within the "fraternal mode." While she wrote about her work relationship with other women, she identified more closely with the male camaraderie of the North. In the prologue to the book, the publishers commented on how Wilson had once been told that, "the Yukon is a wonderful country for men and dogs but it kills women and horses."[55] The North was constructed as a place best suited to male newcomers, a place where women would be uncomfortable and even in danger because of their delicate natures.

Wilson, however, revelled in the adventure of travel. She wrote extensively about her journeys up and down the Highway and into the backwoods. She travelled by car and by dog sled. She described moments when she wondered if she would survive. For example, at one point she crossed an ice bridge by dog sled. Her guide asked if she would rather walk across or stay on the sled and as she claimed she could neither walk across the bridge nor crawl. She chose to hang on to the sled: "The team sprang to its little feet. They clawed their way up the short slippery approach. I was in a cold sweat. For the first time on the whole trip I was thoroughly scared. The sled veered, then straightened out as the little lead dog unhesitatingly led them across on the dead run." Wilson survived to write about many more close calls. She described various modes of transportation, from her car, which she drove over treacherous roads, to snowshoeing and riding horseback. But she also drew colourful portraits about the people she met along the way. Her interest was in both Natives and newcomers. She was particularly eager to listen to the stories offered by male prospectors and traders. She often heard their tales of trapping and travelling along the Liard and Mackenzie Rivers, or listened to their concerns about the decline in fur markets. "It was new and exciting to listen to these men of the North," Wilson commented. "This was their country and they loved it."[56]

Wilson saw no inherent problem in describing the North as the country of the prospector and trader. It did not occur to her that these men were newcomers to the land that had been occupied for many generations by the Natives of the North. Nor do we see in this description a recognition that although the North was portrayed as a land for hardy white men, it had been lived upon by Aboriginal women for generations. The men of the North liked to talk about how they were the men of the North, especially to women who ventured into "their country." And Wilson liked to retell their tales. But for whom? We have some evidence of how reviewers responded to her book as part of the emerging genre of northern life writing for southern audiences. Three reviews appeared shortly after its publication (though there may have been others): all were written by women and each depicted Wilson's autobiographical account as a northern adventure. One reviewer commented that this book was about more than just nursing: "Nursing is only one facet of such a career for there is arduous travelling on horseback, or snowshoes, in aircraft or alone by car."[57] Another reviewer commented on how Wilson and her associates had "risked their lives travelling over almost impassable roads and flying through snowstorms to answer emergency calls."[58] The review for the journal *North* observed that Wilson portrayed the northern landscape in romantic yet realistic terms: "Through Nurse Wilson's eyes we see the beauty of nature from majestic mountains to tiny roadside flowers, but we also see its harshness."[59] Reviewers praised Wilson for her ability to depict a landscape that was an ideal space for a fraternal culture. They saw the book as a northern narrative about nursing, but within a travel writing genre. They commented on how Wilson had accommodated to life in the North, a life most southern women would have balked at.[60]

The book itself started out at a print run of 5,000; in the first few weeks 1,000 copies sold. The publisher, Gray Campbell of Sidney, British Columbia, professed to be thrilled by these numbers and pleased that the book was published simultaneously in England. As far as he was concerned this was the first book of its kind to do so well: "It is the first time a Canadian author writing a story of this type has had her first book accepted for such distribution right off the bat."[61]

The book was launched from Wilson's home in Calgary in September 1965; unfortunately, Wilson died only one month later. She was in her late fifties by that point, and apparently in the process of writing another book. After her one-year sojourn in the Yukon, she moved to British Columbia where she nursed in Merritt, Lillooet, and Williams Lake. At the time of her death, the *Williams Lake Tribune* noted that, "The many Cariboo friends of Amy Wilson, both Indian and white were shocked last week to hear of her sudden death."[62]

+++

Wilson's *No Man Stands Alone* offers a unique perspective. Because of her sensitive portrayal of Native medicine it does not fit squarely within the colonial literature by white women who preceded Wilson to the North. And since Wilson was working as a nurse and not simply travelling for the sake of travel, it does not fit perfectly into the category of leisurely middle-class women's travel narratives. However, it does share some of the characteristics of this genre – particularly the idea that women had to appropriate a fraternal mode of expression in their writing. The existence of a fraternal culture of newcomers in post–Second World War northern Canada can hardly be doubted. It is this culture that is given voice by Wilson who, ironically, went to the North to do the work that had for so long been considered the epitome of femininity: nursing and caring for others. At the same time, Wilson's work and her experiences provide unique perspectives. The most striking and significant aspects of Wilson's autobiography are her open-minded attitude toward indigenous medicine and her willingness to sacrifice what many saw as southern comfort for both her professional objectives as well as for her desire to live and travel in the North. Her experiences as a nurse and later as a writer also serve to confront stereotypical views about women's positions in Canada following the baby boom and the post-war surge to the suburbs. Some women clearly made different choices.

NOTES

1 Ernie Lyall, *An Arctic Man: Sixty-five Years in Canada's North* (Edmonton: Hurtig, 1979), 13

2 Lyall, *An Arctic Man*, 14.

3 On the history of southern representations of the north, see Sherill E. Grace, *Canada and the Idea of North* (Montreal & Kingston: McGill-Queen's University Press, 2001).

4 Mena Orford, *Journey North* (Toronto: McClelland & Stewart, 1957); Pierre Berton, *The Mysterious North* (Toronto: McClelland & Stewart, 1956); Margery Hinds, *School-House in the Arctic* (London: Wyman & Sons, 1958); Archibald Lang Fleming, *Archibald the Arctic* (New York: Appleton-Century-Crofts, 1956); Robert John Renison, *One Day At A Time: The Autobiography of Robert John Renison* (Toronto: Kirkwood House, 1957). Some later examples of this northern life writing genre include Betty Lee, *Lutiapik: The Story of a Young Woman's Year of Isolation and Service in the Arctic* (Toronto: McClelland & Stewart, 1975); Sheila Burnford, *One Woman's Arctic* (Toronto: McClelland & Stewart, 1973).

5 This has recently started to change with close attention being paid to the lives of northern women. On newcomers, see, for example, Charlene Porsild, *Gamblers and Dreamers: Women, Men, and Community in the Klondike* (Vancouver: UBC Press, 1998); Barbara Kelcey, *Alone In Silence: European Women in the Canadian North Before 1940* (Montreal & Kingston: McGill-Queen's University Press, 2001); Myra Rutherdale, *Women and the White Man's God: Gender and Race in the Canadian Mission Field* (Vancouver: UBC Press, 2002). On Aboriginal women, see Julie Cruikshank, with Angela Sidney, Kitty Smith, and Annie Ned, *Life Lived Like a Story: Life Stories of Three Yukon Elders* (Vancouver: UBC Press, 1990); Nancy Wachowich, in collaboration with Apphia Agalakti Awa, Rhoda Kaukjak Katsak, and Sandra Pikujak Katsak, *Saqiyuq Stories from the Lives of Three Inuit Women* (Montreal & Kingston: McGill-Queen's University Press, 2001).

6 There are fewer northern narratives about women's experiences in the early twentieth century, but there are nonetheless some very useful texts, including S.A. Archer, ed., *A Heroine of the North: Memoirs of Charlotte Selina Bompas (1830–1917)* (London: Macmillan, 1929); David Richeson, ed., *The New North: An Account of a Woman's 1908 Journey through Canada to the Arctic by Agnes Deans Cameron* (Saskatoon: Western Producer Prairie Books, 1986); Laura Beatrice Berton, *I Married the Klondike* (Toronto: McClelland & Stewart, 1954).

7 Sara Mills, *Discourses of Difference: An Analysis of Women's Travel Writing and Colonialism* (London: Routledge, 1991), 118.

8 Karen R. Lawrence, *Penelope Voyages: Women and Travel in the British Literary Tradition* (Ithaca: Cornell University Press), 105.

9 Ibid., 21.

10 Renée Hulan, *Northern Experience and the Myths of Canadian Culture* (Montreal & Kingston: McGill-Queen's University Press, 2002), 99.

11 Ibid., 100.

12 Ibid., 134.

13 For a detailed account of women's suburban lives in southern Canada, see Veronica Strong-Boag, "'Their Side of the Story': Women's Voices from Ontario Suburbs, 1945–1960." In Joy Parr, ed., *A Diversity of Women. Ontario 1945–1980*, 46–74 (Toronto: University of Toronto Press, 1995). See also Valerie Korinek, *Roughing It in Suburbia: Reading Chatelaine Magazine in the Fifties and Sixties* (Toronto: University of Toronto Press, 2000).

14 Amy Wilson, *No Man Stands Alone* (Sydney: Gray's Publishing, 1965), 19.

15 Glenbow Museum and Archives, Joy Duncan Frontier Nursing Project, M4745, File 61, Wilson, Amy.

16 Ibid.

17 Kathryn McPherson, "'The Country Is a Stern Nurse': Rural Women, Urban Hospitals and the Creation of a Western Canadian Nursing Work Force, 1920–1940," in *Prairie Forum* 20, 2 (Fall 1995): 177.

18 Wilson, *No Man Stands Alone*, 22.

19 McPherson, "'The Country Is a Stern Nurse,'" 195.

20 Quoted in Maureen Lux, *Medicine That Walks: Disease, Medicine and Canadian Plains Native People, 1880–1940* (Toronto: University of Toronto Press, 2001) 138, from Brooke Claxton, minister of health and welfare. CHC, Sessional Papers, Joint Committee of the Senate and House of Commons Appointed to Consider the Indian Act, Minutes of Proceedings and Evidence, no. 1, 28–30 May 1946, 65.

21 Laurie Meijer Drees, "Reserve Hospitals and Medical Officers: Health Care and Indian Peoples in Southern Alberta, 1890s to 1930," in *Prairie Forum* 21 (1996): 155.

22 Alice K. Smith, "Nursing with Indian and Northern Health Services," in *Canadian Nurse* 54, 2 (February 1958), 167.

23 For the history of the Alaska Highway, see Ken Coates, *North to Alaska* (Toronto: McClelland & Stewart, 1991); Ken Coates and W.R. Morrison, *The Alaska Highway in World War II: The U.S. Army of Occupation in Canada's*

Northwest (Norman: Oklahoma University Press, 1992). For a very useful history of Native/newcomer relations in the Yukon, see Ken Coates, *Best Left As Indians: Native-White Relations in the Yukon Territory, 1840–1973* (Montreal & Kingston: McGill-Queen's University Press, 1991).

24 Wilson, *No Man Stands Alone*, 26.

25 On the history of nursing in Canada, the most comprehensive study is Kathryn McPherson, *Bedside Matters: The Transformation of Canadian Nursing, 1900–1990* (Toronto: Oxford University Press, 1996).

26 Wilson, *No Man Stands Alone*, 23.

27 Ibid., 24.

28 Nanci Langford, "Childbirth on the Canadian Prairies, 1880–1930," in Catherine A. Cavanaugh and Randi R. Warne, *Telling Tales: Essays in Western Women's History*, 170 (Vancouver: UBC Press, 2000).

29 Quoted in Langford, "Childbirth on the Canadian Prairies, 1880–1930," from M. Lawrence, Memoirs "Keewatin," Glenbow Archives, Accession no. M3481, 163.

30 Maureen Lux, *Medicine That Walks*, 225. See also Mary-Ellen Kelm, *Colonizing Bodies: Aboriginal Health and Healing in British Columbia, 1900–1950* (Vancouver: UBC Press, 1998).

31 Langford makes the case that Native midwifery was common in the North and that it was not so unusual for a white woman to have a Native midwife: "In the culture in which Lawrence had lived in the North this was not unusual; but for the settlers included in this study it was atypical," 156.

32 Wilson, *No Man Stands Alone*, 24.

33 Ibid.

34 Ibid.

35 There is a large and rich literature on the history of midwifery in Canada. For southern experiences, see C. Lesley Briggs, "'The Case of the Missing Midwives': A History of Midwifery in Ontario from 1795–1900," and Helene Laforce, "The Different Stages of the Elimination of Midwives in Quebec." In Katherine Arnup, Andrée Levesque, and Ruth Roach Pierson, eds., *Delivering Motherhood: Maternal Ideologies and Practices in the 19th and 20th Centuries*, 20–50 (London: Routledge, 1990). For a discussion on contemporary debates on midwifery, see Brian Burtch, *Trials of Labour: The Re-emergence of Midwifery* (Montreal & Kingston: McGill-Queen's University Press, 1994). For the Arctic, see John D. O'Neil and Penny Gilbert, eds., *Childbirth in the Canadian North: Epidemiological, Clinical, and Cultural Perspectives* (Winnipeg: Northern Health Research Unit, University of Manitoba, 1990).

36 Wilson, *No Man Stands Alone*, 48.

37 Ibid., 49.

38 Patricia Jasen, "Race, Culture, and the Colonization of Childbirth in Northern Canada." In Veronica Strong-Boag et al., eds., *Rethinking Canada: The Promise of Women's History*, 363 (Toronto: Oxford University Press, 2002).

39 Julie Cruikshank, "The Gravel Magnet: Some Social Impacts of the Alaska Highway on Yukon Indians." In Kenneth S. Coates, ed., *The Alaska Highway: Papers of the 40th Anniversary Symposium*, 182 (Vancouver: UBC Press, 1985).

40 John D. O'Neil, "The Politics of Health in the Fourth World: A Northern Canadian Example." In Kenneth S. Coates and William R. Morrison, eds., *Interpreting Canada's North: Selected Readings*, 279–99 (Toronto: Copp Clark, 1989). See also J. Karen Scott with Joan E. Kieser, *Northern Nurses: True Nursing Adventures from Canada's North* (Oakville: Kokum, 2002).

41 Wilson, *No Man Stands Alone*, 78.

42 The legacy of disease and ill health that followed contact has been well documented by historians. Two recent studies that are especially strong on the relationship between disease and colonization are Maureen K. Lux, *Medicine That Walks: Disease, Medicine and Canadian Plains Native People, 1880–1940* (Toronto: University of Toronto Press, 2001) and Mary-Ellen Kelm, *Colonizing Bodies: Aboriginal Health and Healing in British Columbia, 1900–50* (Vancouver: UBC Press, 1998). For the Arctic, see Pat Sandiford Brygier, *A Long Way From Home: The Tuberculosis Epidemic Among the Inuit* (Montreal & Kingston: McGill-Queen's University Press, 1994).

43 Myra Rutherdale, *Women and the White Man's God: Gender and Race in the Canadian Mission Field* (Vancouver: UBC Press, 2002). See also Winifred Marsh, ed., *Echoes from a Frozen Land: Donald B. Marsh* (Edmonton: Hurtig, 1987), 117–18.

44 Wilson, *No Man Stands Alone*, 64.

45 Ibid., 120.

46 Ibid., 86.

47 Ibid., 3.

48 Ibid., 61.

49 Ibid.

50 Ibid., 45.

51 "Choking Death," *Time*, 6 February 1950.

52 Ibid.

53 Ibid.

54 Ibid., 97.

55 Ibid., prologue.

56 Ibid., 39.

57 Malvina Bolus, "Review of *No Man Stands Alone*," *Beaver*, Spring 1966,

58 Helen Dawe, "Review of *No Man Stands Alone*," *British Columbia Library Quarterly* 29, 2 (October 1966): 27.

59 Sue Park, "Review of *No Man Stands Alone*," *North* 13, 3 (September–October 1966): 43.

60 Ibid.

61 Glenbow Museum and Archives, Joy Duncan Frontier Nursing Project, M4745, File 61, Wilson, Amy. Ian Smith, "Publisher Excited by Nursing Story," *Colonist*, 19 August 1965: 23.

62 "Death Claims Cariboo Nurse," *Williams Lake Tribune*, 20 October 1965, 14.

Part Three

Regulating Nurse Training and Professional Boundaries

7

+ + + + +

Training Aboriginal Nurses: The Indian Health Services in Northwestern Canada, 1939–75

LAURIE MEIJER DREES

Mr Harkness (Conservative – MP, Calgary): A considerable number of doctors, nurses, cleaners, helpers, ward aides and housemaids are covered by this item [Indians and Eskimos health services – operations and maintenance]. Could the minister state how many Indians are employed in these positions?

Mr Martin (Liberal – Minister of Health and Welfare): I cannot give the exact number, but we are endeavouring in the main to employ Indians in certain kinds of posts. Obviously there are posts where that cannot be done. We do not succeed fully, but to the extent that is possible, that is our objective.

House of Commons Debates, 21 June 1951

Words written on a page can do little to fully describe the place of indigenous peoples in Canada's state-run health care system. Any descriptions are mere sketches of aspects of Aboriginal peoples' roles in the hospitals, nursing stations, mission hospitals, and other care institutions Canada employed to deliver care to Native peoples at various times. Perhaps the most obvious way Aboriginal peoples were involved in Canada's formal health care system was as patients. Even before Canadian provinces created a nationwide medical services system after the Second World War, the Department of Indian Affairs, and later the Department of National Health and Welfare, ran an extensive Indian

Health Services (IHS) to ensure that Indians, Inuit, and even the Métis population was accessed by nurses and doctors. From its inception in 1945 until the 1970s, IHS was primarily concerned with public health issues. Many Aboriginal people in Canada were patients in this system. Sometimes they were sick and treated in their home communities; other times, they were removed and placed in Indian Health Service or public hospitals far from their home territories. This essay does not focus on the mostly untold story of those patients, despite the need for such accounts. Instead, it seeks to introduce and describe a more hidden aspect of Aboriginal involvement in Canada's Indian Health Services: the role of Aboriginal peoples as caregivers, especially as nurses and nursing aides.

Important research has already been completed on historical aspects of Aboriginal health, and even the Indian Health Services. Similarly, new research into the history of nursing in Canada is beginning to analyze relationships between specific ethnic groups, including Aboriginal peoples, and the nursing profession, as well as issues in remote-region nursing. For example, nursing historian Kathryn McPherson has emphasized the need to study the social history of nursing at the juncture of the concepts of race, class, and gender.[1] In keeping with this idea, other works exist pertaining to the colonial nature of publicly funded health care in Aboriginal communities. To date, much of the existing literature in this wide field focuses on describing the work of individual IHS nurses and doctors (either as memoirs or analyses of their careers) or the impact of public health services on Aboriginal communities, past and present. Older literature providing an excellent overview of Indian health in Canada includes that by C.R. Maundrell (1941) and G. Graham-Cumming (1967).[2] Noteworthy contemporary works focusing on the relationships between Aboriginal peoples and health care delivery include Sally Weaver's *Medicine and Politics Among the Grand River Iroquois* (1972); T. Kue Young's work on the impact of the IHS on the Central Subarctic (1988); Waldram, Herring, and Young's excellent overview, *Aboriginal Health in Canada* (1995); and Mary-Ellen Kelm's *Colonizing Bodies* (1998), to name the most prominent.[3]

Clearly, the literary field involving both subjects, 'Aboriginal health' and 'nursing' together, is very wide. However, a recent review of literature by Leipert and Reutter (1998) related to the field of nursing practice in northern and isolated settings, and by extension, Aboriginal peoples, suggests that much of the literature is fragmented and spread among various disciplines, making the summarizing of this body of information difficult.[4] As a result, the research presented here attempts to draw together ideas from a variety of sources to inform its approach.

What this study hopes to contribute is a preliminary description, rather than a theoretical analysis, of Aboriginal involvement in public health care delivery and the context of that work. Although existing histories of the IHS often interpret the system as an instrument of colonial thought and offer compelling evidence of its dominating and victimizing actions, this essay refocuses attention on documenting and describing the specific ranges and roles of Aboriginal peoples within the service to deepen understanding of indigenous histories. Aboriginal involvement in health care work increased during a period in Canadian history when Aboriginal people had little control over Indian health policy and procedure. It was also a time when Aboriginal people were primarily perceived by the outside world as recipients of, not active participants in, these services. Yet active they were.

Roles of Aboriginal Peoples in the Federal Indian Health Services System

Archival records are not rich sources of information in this field. Since most Aboriginal peoples did not occupy professional positions within the Indian Health Services, their names were rarely recorded, and they did not feature prominently in administrative correspondence. Similarly, historic public service employment data distinguish neither Native employees nor their exact jobs within the federal service. Yet, here and there, records do exist that show how they permeated the entire system – not only as patients but also as workers. Oral history, photographs, and biographies of Aboriginal people whose careers served the federal government are far richer sources of information on this topic. These sources corroborate what Ponting and Gibbins point out: "status Indians and other Natives have been virtually "ghettoized" within ... the federal Public Service, in general. That is, they have been concentrated in the lowest level of the bureaucracy in menial jobs where their knowledge of, and sensitivity to, their people had no bearing on the actions of decision-makers."[5]

That said, despite their lower-level employment status within the federal system, specifically what type of work did Aboriginal peoples do? How did they eventually come to be trained and serve as nursing assistants, practical nurses, or even registered nurses within the Indian Health Services system? This study seeks a preliminary answer to these questions, searching for evidence in events that took place in the north-western region of Canada, and primarily the western subarctic.[6] Once these roles have been identified, our ability to interpret, theorize, and analyze their function can be more meaningful. It is openly recognized here that much more work needs to be done on this subject.

The main sources available for this study include the annual reports of the Indian Health Service and material from the Record Group 29, representing the records of the Department of National Health and Welfare as held both at Library and Archives Canada and Yukon Archives in Whitehorse, Yukon Territory. In addition, papers from Record Group 85, Northern Affairs program (Ottawa), and the North-west Territories Council contain related material. The most valuable sources included publications of the Charles Camsell Indian Hospital, printed by the Department of Indian Affairs, and nurse biographies collected by the Indian and Inuit Nurses of Canada.[7] Last but certainly not least, oral history corroborates some of the information found in the photographic record from this time period. Far from representing the final answers to these questions, the stories and views noted here seek to open up this topic for discussion and to present a summary of information that in the past has existed in a fragmented form.

Overall, the piecemeal efforts of the Canadian state to involve Aboriginal peoples as health care workers, ranging from orderlies and practical nurses to registered nurses and community health aides, reveal its lack of commitment to devolving the responsibility for the actual formal practice of health care to Aboriginal communities in this time period. Such devolution did not occur until the 1980s, following pressure from the communities themselves. Just as health care is now recognized as deeply rooted in culture, it is also a highly political activity. For most of its initial years, Indian Health Services operated in a top-down manner: expertise was perceived to lie with the administrators and not with those directly affected by and involved in the treatment of the sick and their families. The attitudes that permeated the IHS reflected the general integrationist attitudes toward Aboriginal peoples that permeated Canadian government and society between 1945 and the 1970s. The creation of universal health care in Canada also worked against further federal commitment to involvement in Aboriginal health care. Despite that, Aboriginal peoples did play important roles in the IHS, as the examples presented here illustrate. Their work formed a nearly invisible backbone and significant interface with the Aboriginal patients in the system. For these reasons alone, highlighting their work in the IHS is significant.

Indian Health Services: Overview

The structure and function of Indian Health Services reveal the context in which many Aboriginal peoples were exposed to professions in formal health care – and in which some were educated and employed as caregivers. Up to 1945, the Indian Affairs Branch handled the delivery of medical care to Indian peoples, and sporadically Métis and Inuit, through federally operated Indian hospitals, mission hospitals, and a field complement of medical officers and field nurses. Until 1945, Aboriginal populations in the southern provinces were served primarily by the federal Indian hospitals. Northern locations, like the Northwest Territories, were served entirely by mission hospitals funded through Indian Affairs.

This began to change in 1945. As Waldram, Herring, and Young ably describe, the Indian Health Services was launched in 1945 under the auspices of the new federal Department of National Health and Welfare.[8] This new bureaucratic body, the IHS, represented a consolidation and reorganization of health services delivered to Canada's indigenous communities. The new Department of National Health and Welfare, and the IHS, represented attempts by the federal government to prioritize public health care services for all Canadians after the war, and remove direct responsibility for health care from Indian Affairs.[9] The director of the Indian Health Services throughout most of this period, from 1939 to 1965, was Dr Percy E. Moore.

The purpose and goals of Indian Health Services were publicly stated in its annual reports. First and foremost, the IHS sought "to provide a complete health service for these [Status Indian and Inuit] peoples," based on a moral, rather than legal, imperative. More directly, "Canada's

Indian Health Service ... has arisen, not from legislative obligation, but rather as a moral undertaking to succor the less fortunate and to raise the standard of health generally."[10] A second goal was to "improve assimilation" of Indian peoples by supporting provisions against ill health and thereby eventually encouraging their economic independence.[11] The lack of interest in traditional Aboriginal health practices lasted through the 1960s. Their aim was also to "correct" in indigenous communities the so-called incorrect health practices of the past: "It is not as if we were merely trying to replace ignorance with correct attitudes and knowledge. We are trying to introduce new attitudes and practices to people who already have strong feelings and traditions about sickness and its treatment, however erroneous these may be."[12]

Lastly, IHS made clear that its primary interest was in public health: "Public health education and practice has been the keynote of Indian Health Services, the avowed purpose being to forestall disease and detect it in the earliest stages."[13] This was not a surprising priority, given that tuberculosis among Aboriginal peoples at this time had an incidence rate more than ten times that of the non-Aboriginal Canadian population, and represented a significant public health threat in the southern regions of Canada.[14] In 1951–2, 75 per cent of IHS hospital beds were occupied by tuberculous patients.[15]

In keeping with these ideals, the IHS-operated hospitals, nursing stations, health centres, and clinics, and employed an army of medical officers and nurses to staff them. Commitment to the creation and expansion of the IHS increased rather dramatically in the post-war years, as evidenced by the relative growth in facilities and staff:

Table 7.1 Facility and staff growth

Year	IHS hospitals	Nursing stations (excluding health centres or clinics)	Nursing staff (field and hospital)
1946–47	18	22	119
1951–52	18	30	275
1961–62	19	43	696
1970	14	64	Not available

Source: Department of National Health and Welfare, Indian Health Services annual reports

Despite the growth in facilities such as nursing stations, clinics, and health centres during the post-war decades, the federal government was always interested in sharing its care of Aboriginal patients with already-existing provincial facilities. Its implied aim was to avoid the creation of a separate health care system for either registered Indian peoples or other Aboriginal groups. In its own words, "over and above the facilities operated by the Indian Health Services, arrangements are made for the treatment of persons of native status at several hundreds of general and special hospitals."[16] The hope was that eventually Indian and other Aboriginal communities would take over their own service delivery: "As groups become able to obtain these services through their own resources, they are encouraged to do so."[17]

Growth in facilities and staffing continued up until the 1970s. After this date, government restructuring, the establishment of universal health care, and the declining need for tuberculosis control saw the federal government retreat from its commitment to Indian Health Services. By the 1970s little interest remained within the federal government to pursue this service to any large extent since, as T. Kue Young notes, "With the removal of financial barriers to health care, the problem of Indian health services was deemed by many to be solved."[18] Nursing stations, however, were always viewed as the foundation of the system. These facilities, serving Aboriginal people directly, remained concentrated in more remote and northern areas.[19]

Administration of IHS was centred in Ottawa, and changed in structure a number of times between its inception in 1945 through the 1970s. In 1962, the IHS was reorganized and subsumed under the auspices of a new branch: Medical Services. Medical Services represented the amalgamation of several federal medical services arms, including IHS, servicing Canadians outside the domain of provincial programs. Almost from its beginning, however, Indian Health Services fell under the control of a director, who oversaw the branch's activities in the various regions and zones across Canada. For example, in 1960, Canada was subdivided into five regions or administrative units, at that time subdivided into twenty-two zones. Each region and zone featured its own administrative office. The purpose of this system appears to have been to facilitate the challenge of addressing the different health care needs of Aboriginal communities across Canada. At that time, north-

western Canada, including northern Manitoba, Saskatchewan, Alberta,
British Columbia, the Yukon Territory, and Northwest Territories were
represented by four of the five regions. Eastern Canada was subsumed
under a single region until 1966.[20]

Two aspects of this bureaucracy are significant to the training and
role of Aboriginal peoples as health care workers in the IHS. First,
hiring for positions within the IHS was vetted through this highly
centralized service. Decision-making followed hierarchical lines, and
Indian health policy was devised primarily in Ottawa, far from the
realities of bush life experienced by most of the recipients of Ottawa's
services. Decision- and policy-makers were urbanites and military men
and women. Between 1945 and at least the 1960s, many of the bureaucrats, administrators, physicians, and nurses working for the IHS had
a military background. Second, with its shaky commitment to Aboriginal health care provision from the start, and the further erosion of
that commitment into the 1970s, the IHS and its federal department
had little interest in launching ventures that would set unwanted
precedents in terms of their deeper involvement in Aboriginal-specific
health care services.

Training Aboriginal Nurses and Health Care Staff

Given that specially created Indian Health Services facilities existed
mostly in Canada's middle north or subarctic regions where provincial
and territorial services were either thinly spread or not available, the
question arises as to who staffed these facilities. Many of the hospitals
and nursing stations were in or near Aboriginal communities. Not surprisingly, the nursing and medical staff in these facilities were almost
exclusively non-Aboriginal. Support staff, on the other hand, appears
to have been local and mostly Aboriginal. This pattern of employment
continued throughout the 1950s and 1960s despite a recognized
shortage of nurses to work in IHS facilities. For example, in 1953–54,
Indian Health Services annual reports mention for the first time its
Aboriginal staff. That year, 167 "Indians and Eskimos" were employed, and up to 250 worked on an hourly basis. Earlier archival
records of Aboriginal workers in Indian Affairs hospital facilities suggest men and women worked as support staff, and some young women

were trained as "ward maids" and employed there in exchange for room, board, and fifteen dollars per month.[21]

Yet after the Second World War, the federal government launched a number of initiatives to train or encourage Aboriginal people to assume paraprofessional or professional positions within the IHS facilities. As early as 1939, small and inconsistent efforts were made to train Native peoples in nursing positions via federally supported hospitals, and later as nurse's aides and orderlies and in other technical positions. Mission hospitals supported by Indian Affairs seem to have initiated training efforts, while later IHS hospitals and provincial institutes offered additional opportunities. By the 1960s, the IHS involved local community members in its mission by training them as community health aides, sanitation aides, and Native health workers.

The IHS system was not the only system offering training in nursing to Aboriginal people. Before the First World War, enterprising Native women sought out professionally accredited nurse training in various public facilities, and graduated successfully. Although financing advanced education was a challenge for these women, some were able to achieve their registered nurse designation through their own efforts. For example, Charlotte Monture of the Six Nations reserve graduated with honours as a registered nurse in 1914. Mrs Monture financed her nurse training by taking on a variety of jobs following her graduation from secondary school, and took her training in the United States at the New Rochelle Hospital School of Nursing in New Rochelle, New York. Following graduation, she worked in New York state as a public health nurse, returning to her home reserve in 1921 to marry, raise a family, and continue nursing part-time at the Indian hospital there, Lady Willingdon Hospital.[22]

Attending nurse training programs in the United States was not an unusual strategy for Aboriginal women in this time period, since some programs in Canada refused to allow non-White individuals to enroll. In her discussion of nurse training in Canada between the 1940s and 1960s, historian Kathryn McPherson reveals how older patterns of nurse training and work kept it the domain of White women, despite the fact that the need for graduate nurses expanded dramatically during and after the war. Although racial and ethnic barriers facing non-White women attempting to enter the nursing profession began eroding gradually in this time period, and the Canadian Nurses Association in

1944 reaffirmed its commitment to "support the principle that there be no discrimination in the selection of students for enrolment into schools of nursing," the reality was that some nurse training programs and provincial associations were less than keen on accepting non-White members into their midst. According to McPherson, minority women who did enter Canadian nurse training programs found that their small numbers and the ongoing prejudice made their experience a painful one.[23] In contrast, programs in the United States were open to women of colour. As a result, some First Nations women left Canadian programs for those in the United States. For example, Wilma Major, of Ojibway-European descent, left hospital training in Ontario for a program in Chicago, where she "was just another minority."[24] As Jean Cuthand Goodwill, herself an Aboriginal nurse, noted in 1989: Aboriginal nurses "have faced discrimination and lack of support in the Canadian educational and health care system" and many lacked the financial ability to pursue higher education.[25]

Other First Nations women graduated from Canadian institutions, before the end of the Second World War. Elizabeth Hill graduated from the Ottawa Civic Hospital in 1933, and subsequently worked at both the Fort Qu'Appelle Indian Hospital (Saskatchewan), and the Lady Willingdon Hospital on the Six Nations reserve. Ruth Porter, in turn, graduated from Victoria Hospital in London, Ontario, in 1941 and after working for some time at that facility moved to the Lady Willingdon Hospital as well. Lastly, Irene Desjarlais of Saskatchewan travelled to Brandon, Manitoba, to receive her RN Diploma via the Brandon General Hospital in 1945. Mrs Desjarlais' career was long, and included working as head nurse at the Fort Qu'Appelle Indian Hospital starting in 1953, and eventually assuming the nurse-in-charge and then assistant zone nursing officer positions within the Medical Services Branch in the 1970s.[26] After the war, others followed in the footsteps of these women and entered nurse training at various provincial institutions.

One of Canada's most prominent First Nations nurses was Jean Cuthand Goodwill. Like the other women described above, she sought her accreditation through a public program: Holy Family Hospital in Prince Albert, Saskatchewan. Graduating in 1954, she became the first Aboriginal person to finish a nursing program in Saskatchewan. She, too, began her career at the Indian Hospital in Fort Qu'Appelle, and subsequently accepted the position of head nurse at the IHS La Ronge nursing station in northern Saskatchewan. Mrs Goodwill later served in many important leadership roles, including as a member of the board of directors of the Canadian Public Health Association, as nursing consultant for the Medical Services Division, and as special adviser to the minister of National Health and Welfare.[27]

A common thread in the experiences of these First Nations registered nurses is that many of them, although trained in public schools of nursing, eventually took up employment in Indian Health Services facilities, either in Indian hospitals or in field nursing work. Whether they were drawn to the IHS positions because of the connection to Aboriginal communities and patients, or whether this trend represents a vagary of their relative visibility in the IHS system is unclear. Perhaps many Aboriginal RNs took positions in provincial service, thereby becoming invisible to the federal archival record. Mrs Willy Hodgson from Sandy Lake reserve in Saskatchewan, for example, boarded a bus to Manitoba at age eighteen to study nursing. She graduated from the Manitoba School of Nursing in 1956 and married that same year. Marriage to a military man saw her life involve moving from military base to military base across Canada. During that time she often acted as a translator for English physicians working with Cree-speaking patients, a role she viewed as her way to serve the social good. Her life work was completed outside the realm of the IHS.[28]

Federally supported initiatives were also important in drawing Aboriginal peoples as labour into the formal health care system. For example, an early initiative emerged in the Northwest Territories in 1939, supported by the Northwest Territories Council; upper level federal government representatives, including the director of the Indian Affairs Branch, Dr H.W. McGill; Indian Affairs medical officers; and church leaders. In that year, the Council struck a committee composed of Dr Millar, Dr P.E. Moore, Dr W.L. Falconer, Mr P. Phelan, and Director McGill, in order to devise a program for training young Native girls as nursing aides in the various NWT mission hospitals. The course received official endorsement from the NWT Council in October 1941.

The idea to create a Native nurse training program was not revolutionary at this time. The Indian Affairs Branch had already established the practice of employing Native peoples in its hospitals in service positions in the laundry and kitchen, and even on hospital wards as "ward maids." Similarly, mission hospitals were training individuals under their care in various nursing techniques. In fact, the plan to formalize a Native nurse training program in the NWT derived from a practice already in place at the Aklavik "All Saints" Anglican hospital. The plan was thoroughly debated by the committee for over a year, but warmly received by all parties involved in the discussion as a way of encouraging employment for young Native women. It was also viewed as a way of improving community health, should the trainees return to their homes. In his endorsement of this plan, Dr Ross Millar, Director of Medical Services for the Indian Affairs Branch, stated in November 1939:

> Concerning the scheme of training certain of the native girls while they are in the hospital ... I think that this is a splendid scheme and the more such girls can be trained in the rudiments of nursing, the better the medical and health conditions should become in the districts to which they return after their training. These girls could be known as experienced nurses rather than graduate nurses, because that is the term that is in general use throughout the country where they are of great assistance both to the surrounding inhabitants and to the visiting doctor, if any ... Such girls, however, would be in a higher class than the home nursing group, because it would be advisable to train them more or less in operating room procedure and ... partially trained dispenser of medicine.[29]

The Roman Catholic Church endorsed the scheme as a way to improve the lives of the Native trainees, but underscored that endorsement with an assimilationist rationale. Bishop Turquetil, O.M.I., in Montreal viewed the program as an opportunity; in his words, "there can be no question of considering their [Native girls'] training at the hospital as a chance to get married to white men, and so to give a better chance to these girls."[30] This same attitude was reflected in the views of Dr Millar, who believed that such training would be especially beneficial to "half-breed" girls, who he believed were "more intellectual" and "would be infinitely better off as hospital ward maids than in returning to their native environment."[31]

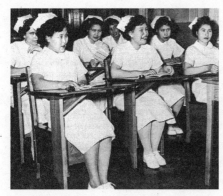

7.1 The original caption for the 1954 picture reads: "A group of girls taking training as ward aides at St Ann's Hospital, Fort Smith. In the front row are the first three Eskimo girls to take the course, and behind them are a German D.P. and three Indian girls. In addition to their practical work, they learn anatomy, physiology, ethics and hygiene." Photo taken from Charles Camsell Pictorial Review, Department of Indian Affairs, 1954.

Despite initial enthusiasm for the development of such a training program, Indian Affairs was cautious about providing any financial support. Indian Affairs was, at this time, responsible for the funding of mission hospitals in the Northwest Territories, and was anticipated to fund the training program. Dr H.W. McGill, director of the Indian Affairs Branch, was not in favour of paying tuition grants for the training of students, and the committee emphasized that "the scheme as outlined should not entail the expenditure of government funds."[32] This was later confirmed by the deputy superintendent of Indian Affairs, T.R.L. MacInnes, who feared that too much official recognition of the program might lead to Indian Affairs being called upon to bear the financial burden of such a venture, something it was not eager to do. In the end, Indian Affairs supported the program in principle, and agreed to supply any needed books and materials.[33] Significantly, the committee did endorse the expenditure of government funds for Aboriginal students displaying exceptional talent and potential to complete a course leading to a registered nursing diploma. Such students would be identified and moved to an institution where the higher education program was offered.[34]

The training program was officially launched in October 1941, and the mission hospitals in Aklavik, Fort Simpson, Fort Smith, and the Resolution Indian Residential School were enlisted to participate. The intention was to involve registered Indian, Inuit, as well as 'half-breed' girls in the training, and the participating missions would assume responsibility together with the attendant physicians for overseeing the program. The Indian residential schools in the district, as well as the hospitals themselves, would serve as the recruiting grounds for students.[35] In some respects, it is not surprising that the Northwest Territories was chosen as the location to launch such training. The region was relatively inaccessible; had an Aboriginal population suffering terribly from tuberculosis; and boasted one of the highest ratios of hospital beds per capita: four times that of British Columbia, which had the highest hospital bed complement of the provinces.[36]

The training, in this case, consisted of teaching students many of the skills taught to non-Aboriginal practical nurses, or nursing assistants. The idea was to teach: "elements of dietry [sic] and plain cooking, take temperatures, do simple dressings, make up dressings, give enemas, properly make beds and give sponge or bed baths. They should also understand the use of simple cathartics and have some knowledge of the proper use of simple remedies which are used in every home, such as the application of mustard, the use of pneumonia jackets and they should also be taught the elements of hygiene with particular regard to preventing the spread of tuberculosis in the home and out at camps."[37]

Dr H.W. McGill, himself a trained physician, added that students could be "taught to make beds, prepare hot-water bottles and assist in the preparation of meals for patients."[38] His vision for the role of Native nurse aides was minimalist. It is impossible to tell from the records used in this research what the exact program of instruction came to be, but it appears that since the program was controlled by the various mission hospitals and their attending medical officers, training varied locally. It is also clear that training did not involve the employment of any indigenous or local healing practices.

Upon completion of their training, which lasted between eighteen months and three years, students would receive an unofficial certificate, signed by the medical officer in charge of their program. It appears that girls as young as nine years of age were accepted into this training system, as were young adult women. In December 1941, the first graduates were awarded their certificates from the Fort Smith hospital. Dr J.A. Urquhart, physician attending this Roman Catholic mission hospital proclaimed, "with this group, the experiment can be considered an unqualified success."[39] The Fort Smith hospital was one of the larger facilities in the Northwest Territories, featuring a forty-three-bed capacity as well as laboratory facilities, second in size only to the Anglican hospital in Aklavik.[40]

This early program, characterized by lack of solid federal support, low expectations, and a piecemeal approach, could be viewed as the pattern for things to come in the field of Aboriginal nurse training until the 1970s. Programs that followed within the IHS were equally unsystematic, and focused primarily on training aides and helpers, rather than seeking to promote full certification of Native nurses, although some Native women were successful in achieving their registered nurse credential.

Just after the Second World War, the IHS also trained Native nursing aides informally. Mrs Muriel Innes, a young girl from Cowessess First Nation in Saskatchewan, gained her nurse's aide training informally at the IHS nursing station in Lac La Ronge in northern Saskatchewan. Following the death of her mother, her father took work at the Lac La Ronge fish processing plant, moving Innes to the nursing station so she could begin to work there. She remained at the nursing station for two years, receiving her aide's training from the IHS nurse stationed there. Her work ranged from preparing linens and bandages and sterilizing equipment to watching the outpost while the nurse was away. She recalled how the nurses at the La Ronge outpost had difficulty communicating with the Cree-speaking patients, and that the nursing station cook, a local woman, was used as a translator. Innes herself felt the nurses whom she worked with were very dedicated but noted these women never really integrated into the local community, as their workload was heavy and time-consuming. Following her work in La Ronge, Innes transferred to the federal Indian hospital at Prince Rupert to continue her nursing aide work.[41] The extent to which IHS trained and hired nurse's aides in this informal manner is unclear.

What is clear, however, is that more formal practical nurse and nurse's aide training programs were spearheaded in IHS hospitals in the 1950s. (Evidence for these initiatives is scanty; with additional research, perhaps more information will come to light.) In 1955, for example, the Coqualeetza Indian Hospital located in British Columbia began running a formal Practical Nurse Training Program in affiliation with the Vancouver Vocational Institute. Three trainees at a time were placed

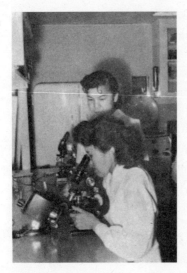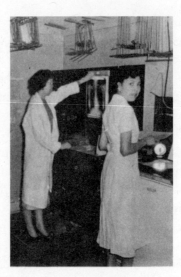

7.2 Aboriginal technical staff working in Charles Camsell Indian
Hospital in 1957. Photo taken from Charles Camsell Pictorial
Review, Department of Indian Affairs, 1957.

in the hospital for a two-month internship to gain experience in tuberculosis and pediatric nursing. Although non-Native women were involved in this training program, according to the Indian Health Services,
"The course is becoming increasingly popular with Indian girls." The
IHS assisted Aboriginal applicants with short-term jobs to "provide the
initial experience and helping to put the Indian on an equal starting
basis with the white girl."[42] A version of the practical nurse training
program spearheaded in the Northwest Territories continued into the
1950s as well. St Ann's Hospital in Fort Smith offered training to Inuit,
Indian, and non-Native 'outsiders' in 1954, as the photograph, published originally by Dr Percy E. Moore,[43] demonstrates.

   Similar ventures were initiated in other IHS hospitals. In general,
the idea seems to have been that non-Native women were the most desirable for hire in these hospitals, but that Native women could at least
be introduced to nursing careers. Between 1959 and 1961 IHS annual
reports make several mentions of the value of exposing Aboriginal
school students, recovering hospital patients, and others falling under
federal guidance to health care work. In 1959, the directorate was

pleased to report that it "continued to participate in programs where medical, nursing and physiotherapy students came for a period of experience and Indian girls were screened to assess their suitability as student practical nurses." That same year, eight "Indian girls" from the Qu'Appelle Diocesan School for Girls were entertained at a dinner and shown films while "opportunities in nursing and related fields were discussed."[44]

In the 1950s and 1960s, patients in IHS hospitals – often making long-term recoveries from tuberculosis – were also encouraged to take up employment in the hospital facilities. Although archival records documenting this trend are slim, the directorate of IHS did state openly that, "as soon as our patients are able, they engage in rehabilitation employment around the hospital. This is carried out on a selective basis."[45] Photographs from the Charles Camsell Indian Hospital during the mid-1950s reveal that its Aboriginal patients were actively being trained and employed as orderlies, attendants, X-ray and lab technicians, and nurse's aides. In-house training in the Charles Camsell Hospital allowed patients and other Aboriginal trainees to acquire their skills on-the-job and classes were held right in the hospital, as the following photo reveals.

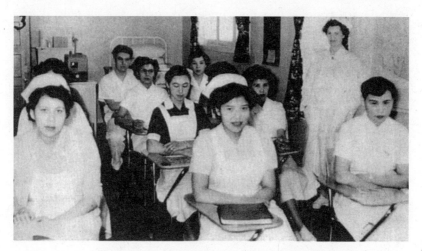

7.3 Young trainees in the class of Mrs Rapley at Charles Camsell Indian Hospital, 1956. Photo taken from Charles Camsell Pictorial Review, Department of Indian Affairs, 1956.

In 1961, from the IHS perspective, "Every effort is made to hire Indians and Eskimos. About 15% of the staff are from these ethnic groups. There are as yet no Indian or Eskimo physicians, but there are a few fully trained and registered public health nurses and many more native ward aides. The male native staff serves mainly as technicians, maintenance men, drivers, etc. although in 1961 the first Indian Sanitarian qualified."[46]

Training and recruiting Aboriginal workers through IHS facilities appears to have been the main tactic used by the Department of National Health and Welfare to create an Aboriginal workforce in health care fields. These efforts were sporadic and unsystematic, as illustrated by the foregoing examples. This lack of a cohesive approach might in part be attributed to the federal government's resistance to creating a separate or segregated Aboriginal health care system. The principle consistently expressed by the Department of National Health and Welfare through the IHS was that, "It is not desirable to maintain hospitals purely for Indians if this can be avoided as this tends to perpetuate ideas about Indians being a peculiar people distinct from other Canadians." This sentiment, coupled with a deeply rooted perception that Aboriginal peoples were somehow behind in their ability to acquire training and employment at higher levels, did much to undermine any formal nurse training programs under the auspices of the federal government. As expressed by the IHS directorate about northwestern Aboriginal communities: "The majority of the present adult Indian population is still employable only in the more humble occupations and consequently can only enjoy a low economic level of existence in our modern western society."[47] Nursing in Aboriginal communities and in IHS hospitals was viewed as difficult, demanding, and highly specialized work, something the Aboriginal population was perceived as not ready or able to take on in any professional capacity, with the exception of the occasional unusually talented individual. In fact, most training offered through the federal effort was training for what was perceived at the time to be general work. In federal health care facilities, tuberculosis was seen as a vehicle for training Aboriginal people. From the Saskatchewan region in the IHS system, the view was expressed that, "while one would hope that Tuberculosis will eventually be eradicated, nevertheless the disease has served as a medium for the academic training of a great many Indians."[48]

Beginning in the 1960s, the IHS began to focus more on community health in its training of Aboriginal health care workers and less on training individuals to take on nurses' duties. Indian policy in the 1960s emphasized "community development" and the Department of National Health and Welfare's IHS initiated programs that trained Aboriginal peoples to take on public health service responsibilities within their own communities rather than within IHS facilities. Such programs included the creation of health and welfare committees in Native communities, the training of Native health workers (1961) – individuals located in a community who could become assistants and helpers to IHS public health nurses as either sanitation aides or community health aides – and the later development of the Indian health liaison officer program (1969). For the IHS, "great stress is now being laid on involving the people themselves in discussing and planning solutions of their problems."[49]

The most prominent of the community-based health training initiative was the Native health worker program. A pilot of this program was run in 1960 under the guise of "sanitation aide" training. It involved training twenty-nine delegates, men and women from the Ohsweken reserve near Brantford in southern Ontario. Chosen by their individual band councils, these individuals received training at the Lady Willingdon IHS Hospital in issues related to sanitation. With assistance from a regional sanitarian and health educator, the workshop aimed to educate those attending in ways of improving sanitation on reserves. The workshop was well received by the participants, and the IHS concluded, "we have learned that the workshop technique, an unknown quantity in this particular setting, is a workable and effective method of stimulating interest in and action on local problems."[50]

The community health auxiliary (CHA) course, launched in 1961, became the more prominent of the two Native health worker programs. In that year, the first course for CHAS was held in Norway House, in northern Manitoba, co-sponsored by the Department of Indian Affairs and the Medical Services Branch. As with the sanitation aides, local band councils selected the individuals who attended. The first class consisted of four women and seven men. The program, which lasted several months, was held in the trainees' own communities as well as at the Indian hospital at Norway House. As a group, the students were introduced to basic health knowledge, germ theory, nutrition, and first aid. They were also sent into the field to observe conditions in Native communities and gain experience in the holding of public meetings. Following this general education, the men and women were split up: the women, to be trained in public health nursing techniques; and the men, in practical sanitation.[51] It seems that community health worker training programs continued to be held from that date forward.

The IHS records throughout this time period emphasize the difficult challenges facing those working in that system, and their heroic efforts to improve health care delivery to Aboriginal communities in Canada's northwest. The fact that the IHS system, with its imposition of an "outside" health care structure and staff on Aboriginal communities, was not working perfectly was not often articulated. But it was recognized that the creation of community health worker training programs could serve as the answer to the ills of the IHS system, since there was a growing realization that: "For years, doctors, nurses and others have been attempting to inculcate public health concepts into Indians and Eskimos with disappointingly meager results ... Telling has not worked."[52] Surprisingly, the IHS recognized that "planned change does not stem from a standard pattern [of health care] proposed at the national level ... people for whom the program is intended must be involved in the planning and implementation."[53] As a result of these realizations, community health worker training was launched with the aim of bridging the perceived culture gap between Medical Services' personnel and their Aboriginal clients.[54] Despite the efforts to include Aboriginal peoples in the IHS system at the community level, prejudice remained among IHS staff. Nursing staff continued to believe in their expertise in health-related matters, and some only grudgingly conceded Aboriginal community health trainees had expertise on matters pertaining to their own communities. As an IHS adviser reflected, after participating in community health worker training, "there seems to be a need for more understanding on the part of the nurses of the culture of the natives ... also they should be aware of their own set of beliefs and attitudes."[55] In contrast, Aboriginal peoples responded enthusiastically to their involvement in community health worker training, stating, "why weren't we told this long ago?"[56]

The community health auxiliary program ran until the early 1970s, when problems began to emerge at the local level. According to the

Community Health Auxiliary Task Force Study of 1972, the work of the CHA required reorganization and needed to allow, among other things, opportunities for continuing education. In the words of one analyst at that time, the difficulty CHAs experienced was the result of several factors: "it became difficult to provide sufficient encouragement and support for the large number of new graduates. Other problems included a high turnover of nursing staff in some outlying areas, and an awakening interest in self-determination among many Indian bands ... the role of the Community Health Worker became confused and frustrating."[57]

The 1970s marked a period of intense debate in Canada over the nature of federal commitment and involvement with registered Indian peoples, as well as all Aboriginal groups generally. The issue of health care, and its formal delivery to Aboriginal communities, was very much part of many of the conversations held by Aboriginal leaders and government representatives at this time. It was always clear, however, that the federal government would only directly encourage the involvement of Aboriginal peoples in its medical services at the community level. The philosophy continued to prevail in Ottawa that Indian, Métis, and Inuit peoples should receive formal health care in the same manner as other Canadians and, at most, would control the administration.

In a policy memo of 2 December 1969, the director of medical services forecast to IHS that federal policy was heading toward increasing IHS presence in the northern regions of the country while simultaneously decreasing the federal presence in the southern provinces. The memo emphasized that in the south, "ways and means should be investigated to close out these clinics [IHS clinics] and arrangements made so that Indians would have access to conventional resources." In other regions, liaison arrangements with Aboriginal political organizations and bands would lead to these groups "taking over some of the administration of health services in their own areas."[58] The goal of Medical Services was to reduce its direct involvement in Aboriginal health care delivery. In the area of training, Medical Services only directly supported training for Native workers, community health workers, and community aides in both the south and the north. The long-held vision of Indian Health Services – that it was a service *for* Aboriginal peoples rather than a service they formed *part of* as workers and professionals – lasted well into the 1970s: in 1974, Native employment in the service was noted to be at an all-time high of 18 per cent of all staff (including general labour).[59]

♦♦♦

Indian Health Services, in all it incarnations within Canada's federal bureaucracy, played a noteworthy role in the training and employment of Aboriginal peoples between 1939 and 1975. The IHS ran a variety of training initiatives in attempts to hire Aboriginal labour into its health care system, not so much in the hopes of creating a class of professional health care workers, but rather to inculcate in Aboriginal community members some of the so-called basics of public health in an era when tuberculosis and sanitation were of enormous public health concern. Its efforts to train Native workers in health care fields were unsystematic and sporadic at best. Ultimately, these efforts did little to encourage Indigenous peoples to become professionals in this system on any large scale. The IHS seemed to favour the hiring of foreign nationals and non-Aboriginal registered nurses rather than develop an indigenous professional nursing class. Furthermore, between 1939 and the 1970s, IHS actions in the field of Aboriginal nurse training changed from having a hospital-based focus to emphasizing the training of community health workers. This change was gradual, and took place in the 1960s.

Although it is difficult to generalize about the experience of Aboriginal people working within the IHS from so few examples, those presented here do provide a window into the role of Aboriginal workers. The emerging general pattern reveals indigenous labour as concentrated in the lower levels of the health care hierarchy. Those who did enter upper levels in the IHS did so by struggling for a higher education that enabled them to gain professional designations. Government records suggest that Aboriginal peoples came to work in the IHS through a variety of avenues, including as patients in the system who were subsequently trained to assume IHS technical positions, as young people selected through the residential school system, or simply as individuals hired on at various IHS facilities as their labour was required. Oral history reveals that their reasons for working in IHS were also varied: some chose health care careers for the stability of a government wage job; some joined out of personal interest; some hospital patients were inspired by health care workers they encountered; and still others assumed IHS posts to be closer to family members who were hospitalized. As IHS cooks, technicians, orderlies, sanitarians, nurse's aides, practical nurses, community health workers, and even registered nurses, Aboriginal peoples represented an important interface between the IHS and the communities targeted by that service. These workers were the translators, the caretakers, the comforters, and the helpers of Aboriginal patients in a system over which their own communities had little control. How this state of affairs represents further evidence of Canada's internal colonization of its Aboriginal populations should be the subject of future discussion and debate beyond the scope of this essay. In fact, rather than interpretation through the lens of Aboriginal colonization and domination by a bureaucratic apparatus, the varied roles of Aboriginal workers within Indian Health Services might as readily represent evidence of what Anishinaabe scholar Gerald Vizenor refers to as "native transmotion" – the movement of indigenous peoples through and between the power structures created by the state, and an example of their "absence" in history, as these same communities avoid detection within the state system as a whole.[60] The interpretive stance offered by scholars such as Vizenor extends analysis of these stories beyond debates between Native agency and the victimry inherently ascribed to the colonized in colonial theory. Such deconstruction of Aboriginal histories within the context of non-indigenous state systems is much needed.

Finally, the history of Aboriginal health care worker training, as illustrated through the IHS, gives insight into the attitudes of the federal service toward the training of Aboriginal people in health care fields. It also reveals aspects of the history behind contemporary devolution of health care responsibilities to Aboriginal communities. At a time when many studies have been directed toward understanding Indian residential schools and their impact as institutions on the social landscape of Aboriginal Canada, it seems that the social and political history of state-driven health care institutions in Indigenous communities deserves the same kind of attention. The history of Native nurse training by the federal government goes a long way to explain the inefficacy of that system, and provides a baseline for the evaluation and understanding of contemporary Aboriginal-controlled health services.

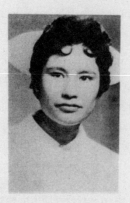

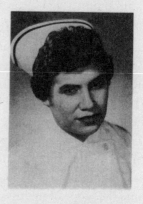

Miss Mariella Willier, R.N.,
a member of the Camsell
nursing staff, is a treaty Indian
of the Lesser Slave Agency,
Sucker Creek Band. She is seen
below at the General Hospital
graduation exercises.

Miss Isabel Crowchief, a member
of the Blackfoot Indian Band at
Gleichen, Alberta, graduated from
the Vegreville Hospital in 1959. She
joined the Camsell staff in September.

Scholarship for University Study

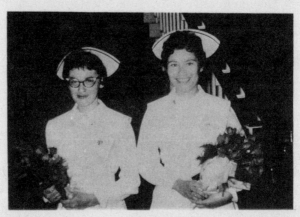

Miss Lillian George from the Yukon is pictured at the left with Miss
Mariella Willier at the General Hospital 1959 graduation exercises in
Edmonton. Lillian received a University Scholarship from the General
Hospital. She plans to attend University in the fall to study for her
Bachelor of Nursing degree.

7.4 Aboriginal girls graduate with distinction.

NOTES

1 Kathryn McPherson, *Bedside Matters: The Transformation of Canadian Nursing, 1900–1990* (Toronto: Oxford University Press, 1996), 12.

2 C. Richard Maundrell, "Indian Health, 1867–1940," unpublished MA thesis (Kingston: Queen's University, 1941). Maundrell's thesis is a descriptive work addressing the primary health issues facing Indian Affairs in its attempts to administer the health care of Indian reserve communities between 1867 and 1940. G. Graham-Cumming, "Health of the Original Canadians, 1867–1967," *Medical Services Journal of Canada* 23, 2 (1967): 115–166. Graham-Cumming reviews the health concerns in Aboriginal communities from a governmental perspective, and also provides an overview history of the administrative development of Indian Health Services. Both pieces provide important federal governmental points of view on primary issues in Aboriginal health at mid-century.

3 Sally M. Weaver, *Medicine and Politics Among the Grand River Iroquois* (Ottawa: National Museum of Man, 1972); T. Kue Young, *Health Care and Cultural Change: The Indian Experience in the Central Subarctic* (Toronto: University of Toronto Press, 1988); James B. Waldram, D. Ann Herring, and T. Kue Young, *Aboriginal Health in Canada: Historical, Cultural and Epidemiological Perspectives* (Toronto: University of Toronto Press, 1995); Mary-Ellen Kelm, *Colonizing Bodies* (Vancouver: UBC Press, 1998). Weaver's work represents a sociological analysis of medical acculturation on the Six Nations reserve. Her work contains a noteworthy description of the reserve's medical services. Young's piece describes the development of Indian Health Services in the western subarctic, while Waldram et al. provides an overarching history of Indian health and medical services provided to Aboriginal communities from contact through the late twentieth century. Finally, Kelm's work represents a case study of the work of Indian Affairs and Indian Health Services in British Columbia between 1900 and 1950. Kelm argues that the federally supported system aided and affirmed colonial relations between Aboriginal communities and the government, in addition to supporting the position of dominance the federal government has always maintained over Aboriginal peoples, ultimately illustrating how notions of Aboriginal "health" have been influenced by this process.

4 Beverly Leipert and Linda Reutter, "Women's Health and Community Health Nursing Practice in Geographically Isolated Settings: A Canadian Perspective," *Health Care for Women International* 19 (1998): 575–588.

5 J. Rick Ponting and Roger Gibbins, *Out of Irrelevance: A Socio-political Introduction to Indian Affairs in Canada* (Toronto: Butterworths, 1980), 140.

6 See T. Kue Young, *Health Care and Cultural Change: the Indian Experience in the Central Subarctic* (Toronto: University of Toronto Press, 1988), chap. 1 and 2. Northwestern Canada or 'western subarctic' here includes the region west of Hudson Bay, including the northern prairie provinces, the Northwest Territories, and the Yukon Territory. Young refers to the western subarctic as a region that has no precise boundaries, but includes lands south of the arctic tundra tree-line, and coinciding with the boreal forest and zone of discontinuous permafrost of the central and western provinces to the northern territories and Alaska (Young, 1988, 9). The Indian Health Services (IHS) was most active in this region since in southern areas provincial institutions took over the care of indigenous patients. The IHS focused its attention on serving indigenous populations in areas where no provincial services were available, generally the middle and far north.

7 The association is now known as the Aboriginal Nurses Association of Canada.

8 Waldram, Herring, and Young, *Aboriginal Health in Canada: Historical, Cultural and Epidemiological Perspectives* (Toronto: University of Toronto Press, 1995), 163.

9 Young, *Health Care and Cultural Change*, 90–91.

10 Dept. of National Health and Welfare, Annual Report, 1949–50, 80.

11 Dept. of National Health and Welfare, Annual Report, 1947–48, 41.

12 Canada's Health and Welfare, vol. 16, no. 2, 1961, "Indian and Northern Health Services," Supplement no. 38, n.p.

13 Dept. of National Health and Welfare, Annual Report, 1951–52, 49.

14 Dept. of National Health and Welfare, Annual Report, Indian Health Services, 1949–50, 82.

15 Ibid., 50.

16 Department of National Health and Welfare, Annual Report, Indian Health Services, 1948–49, 107. See also Canada's Health and Welfare, vol. 16, no. 2, 1961, "Indian and Northern Health Services," Supplement no. 38.

17 Dept. of National Health and Welfare, Annual Report, Indian Health Services, 1953–54, 42.

18 Young, *Health Care and Cultural Change*, 91.

19 Waldram, Herring, and Young, *Aboriginal Health in Canada*, 165.

20 See Dept. of National Health and Welfare, Indian Health Services and Medical Services Annual Reports, 1945, 1971.

21 Yukon Archives, Whitehorse, RG 85, C-1-a, vol. 791, file 6210. Extracts from the Minutes of the One Hundred and Thirty-Second Session of the Northwest Territories Council, 20 October 1941, Dr P.E. Moore on record.

22 Indian and Inuit Nurses of Canada, "Special Awards," in *Newsletter* 1, 1: 2–3.

23 Kathryn McPherson, *Bedside Matters*, 205, 209, 210–211.

24 Quoted in Ibid., 213.

25 Jean Cuthand Goodwill, "Indian and Inuit Nurses of Canada," in *Saskatchewan Indian*, March 1989, 14–18. Accessed at http://www.sicc.sk.ca/saskindian/a89 mar14.htm on 3 April 2004. Other First Nations women went even further abroad than the United States. Martha Soonias, originally of the Red Pheasant reserve, attended a "mothercraft" course in Toronto before leaving for New Zealand, where she qualified as a registered midwife. She returned to Canada to assume a nursing position at the new Battleford Indian Hospital in 1948. See Canada, House of Commons Debates, Fourth Session, Twenty-First Parliament, vol. V, 1951, (Ottawa: Queen's Printer, 1952), 4453, statement of MP Mr Bater, 12 June 1951.

26 Indian and Inuit Nurses of Canada, "Special Awards," in *Newsletter*, 1, 1: 3–4.

27 See Indian Women, *Saskatchewan Indian*, March 1989, 12. Also, "Jean Cuthand Goodwill, Nurse," in *Celebrating Women's Achievements, Canadian Women in Science*. Accessed at http://www.nlc-bnc.ca/2/12/h12-406-e.html on 26 May 2003.

28 Bruce Dyck, "Willy Hodgson, 1935–2003: The Nurse from Sandy Lake Reserve," *Globe and Mail*, 28 March 2003, R5.

29 Yukon Archives, Whitehorse, RG 85, C-1-a, vol. 791, file 6210, Dr Ross Millar, director of medical services, Department of Pensions and National Health, to R.A. Gibson, deputy commissioner, Northwest Territories Branch, Department of Mines and Resources, 28 November 1939.

30 Yukon Archives, Whitehorse, RG 85, C-1-a, vol. 791, file 6210, Extract from Bishop Turquetil's letter of 19 February 1940 to Mr R.A. Gibson, deputy commissioner, Northwest Territories Branch.

31 Yukon Archives, Whitehorse, RG 85, C-1-a, vol. 791, file 6210, Extract from the Minutes of the One Hundred and Thirty-Second Session of the Northwest Territories Council, 2 October 1941, 3.

32 Yukon Archives, Whitehorse, RG 85, C-1-a, vol. 791, file 6210, Proceedings of the Committee Authorized by Minute of the Northwest Territories Council Meeting of 9 October 1941 to Consider the Training of Indian Girls in the Hospitals of the Northwest Territories, 3.

33 Yukon Archives, Whitehorse, RG 85, C-1-a, vol. 791, file 6210, Extracts from the Minutes of the One Hundred and Thirty-Seventh Session of the Northwest Territories Council, 23 December 1941.

34 Yukon Archives, Whitehorse, RG 85, C-1-a, vol. 791, file 6210, Proceedings of

the Committee Authorized by Minute of the Northwest Territories Council Meeting of 9 October 1941 to Consider the Training of Indian Girls in the Hospitals of the Northwest Territories, 3.

35 A brief mention of the program and the need to co-operate with the schools is made by G.J. Wherrett, responsible for surveying health conditions in the arctic in 1945. See G.J. Wherrett, "Survey of Health Conditions and Medical and Hospital Services in the North West Territories (Part I, Arctic Survey)," in *The Canadian Journal of Economics and Political Science* 11 (1945), 49–60, 57.

36 Wherrett, "Survey of Health Conditions," 55.

37 Yukon Archives, Whitehorse, RG 85, C-1-a, vol. 791, file 6210, probably Dr J.A. Urquhart to R.A. Gibson, Director, Lands Parks and Forests Branch, Department of Mines and Resources, 19 February 1940.

38 Yukon Archives, Whitehorse, RG 85, C-1-a, vol. 791, file 6210, Proceedings of the Committee Authorized by Minute of the Northwest Territories Council Meeting of 9 October 1941 to Consider the Training of Indian Girls in the Hospitals of the Northwest Territories, 1.

39 Yukon Archives, Whitehorse, RG 85, C-1-a, vol. 791, file 6210, Dr J.A. Urquhart to R.A. Gibson, Director, Land and Parks and Forests Branch, Department of Mines and Resources, 8 December 1941. This group of 'graduates' had clearly already been in some sort of training program devised by the Fort Smith mission hospital, and were awarded their 'certificate' as soon as the document was given government endorsement. The example stands to reveal that Aboriginal "nurse" training occurred in an informal manner in remote locations before government-sponsored initiatives became prominent.

40 G.J. Wherrett, "Survey of Health Conditions," 49–60, 55.

41 Personal communication with Muriel Innes, 1 May 1999, Saskatoon, SK.

42 Ottawa, Indian and Northern Health Services, Directorate Report, 1960, 13.

43 Percy E. Moore, "Health for Indians and Eskimos," in *Canadian Geographical Journal* 48 (June 1954): 216–221. Photograph on 220.

44 Ottawa, Indian and Northern Health Services, Directorate Report, 1959, 2 and 13.

45 Ottawa, Indian and Northern Health Services, Directorate Report, 1960, 44.

46 Ottawa, Indian and Northern Health Services, Directorate Report, 1961, 9.

47 Ottawa, Indian and Northern Health Services, Directorate Report, 1960, 41.

48 Ibid., 44.

49 Ottawa, Indian and Northern Health Services, Directorate Report, 1961, 9.

50 Paul Roach, "Sanitation Workshop for Indians," in *Canada's Health and Welfare* (May 1960): 2–3, 3.

51 Alice K. Smith, "Indian and Eskimo Health Auxiliaries." In Roy J. Shephard and S. Itoh, eds., *Circumpolar Health, Proceedings of the 3rd International Symposium*, 591–5; 591–2 (Toronto: University of Toronto Press, 1974).

52 Ethel G. Martens, "Culture and Communications – Training Indians and Eskimos as Community Health Workers," in *Canadian Journal of Public Health* 57, 11 (November 1966): 495–503, 495.

53 Ibid., 497.

54 Ibid., 502.

55 Ibid.

56 Ibid.

57 Smith, "Indian and Eskimo Health Auxiliaries," 592.

58 Ottawa, National Archives of Canada, RG 29, vol. 3053, Interim Box 41, file 853-1-1, pt. 2, Memorandum, Director General, Medical Services, 2 December 1969.

59 Ottawa, Indian Claims and Historical Research Centre, Medical Services overview, February 1978, 23, table 13.

60 Gerald Vizenor, *Fugitive Poses: Native American Indian Scenes of Absence and Presence* (Lincoln: University of Nebraska Press, 1998), 15 and 181. In his conclusion, Vizenor emphatically announces, "we, as natives of this continent, are the presence, transmotion and stories of survivance." In his work he challenges the ability of narratives of dominance, such as those inspired by colonial theory, to reflect and interpret indigenous realities and epistemologies.

8

+++++

Conflict and Resistance to Paternalism: Nursing with the Grenfell Mission Stations in Newfoundland and Labrador, 1939–81

HEIDI COOMBS-THORNE

In October of 1959, W.A. Paddon, physician with the Grenfell Mission in North West River, wrote to his colleague in St Anthony disclosing his frustrations with the behaviour of one of the nurses. The nurse in question was Dorothy Jupp,[1] a senior Grenfell nurse who had been employed in district nursing in Labrador since 1938. Apparently, Jupp had neglected to report an outbreak of measles, mumps, and pneumonia in her community during which time two children died. Paddon argued that Jupp should have contacted him via radio; he could have advised her and evacuated her worse cases, which may have changed the tragic outcome. He proceeded to criticize Jupp's professionalism as a nurse and stated, "This is the sort of thing that has bothered me for some years with her. She is absolutely independent. She does not consider herself a part of the medical team and she does not seem to want any help or advice about cases. I am sure she thinks of herself as a Doctor rather than a Nurse."[2] Paddon wanted Jupp removed from his district of northern Labrador.

This episode was the culmination of several years of friction between Paddon and Jupp. Paddon was the physician at North West River and had medical jurisdiction over the northern section of the Labrador Coast. Jupp was a nurse in his district and therefore, according to the structure of the Grenfell Mission came under his authority. However, Paddon was only occasionally present in the communities where nurses practised; he was primarily based at the hospital at North West River and would travel throughout the district at certain intervals during the year. As a result, his medical authority in coastal communities was arbitrary and was really only a dominant factor when he himself was present. Under this form of health care provision, the nurse had a significant amount of responsibility and had to rely on her own judgment on a daily basis. With the lack of qualified physicians in remote areas of northern Newfoundland and Labrador, the Grenfell nurse was sometimes required to perform health-related duties for which she had not been formally trained.

The Jupp-Paddon conflict highlights several themes concerning the negotiation of professional boundaries within the Grenfell Mission. First, the Mission often attracted women with strong personalities to work in its Newfoundland and Labrador establishment. These women were usually thrilled with the level of responsibility that nursing with the Mission offered, especially on the nursing stations. However, the nurses' position in the Mission was of a contradictory nature: they practised with a significant amount of professional independence, but they were still situated within a paternalistic medical system. They were expected to use their own judgment to provide appropriate health care to local residents, but they were also expected to refer and defer to a physician whenever necessary. Second, although most nurses were apprehensive and nervous at the start of their Grenfell careers – especially with the prospect of so much responsibility on the stations – as they met the demands of nursing in the unforgiving coastal environment, they became increasingly confident in themselves and their abilities. Third, nurses on the stations sometimes came into conflict with physicians in the process of performing their duties, especially when the physician felt they had overstepped the boundaries of their profession. With their acquired confidence, some nurses became proactive in resisting and challenging the gender-based medical hierarchy of the Grenfell Mission. Taken together, this chapter argues that as nurses met the challenges they faced on the nursing stations and negotiated their professional boundaries, they came into conflict with male physicians and administrators and sometimes developed the confidence to resist the dominant paternalism of the Grenfell medical institution.

Background

The Grenfell Mission was established in 1893 as a paternalistic system of health care intended to reach people living in communities along hundreds of miles of rugged coastline in northern Newfoundland and Labrador. In 1892, Wilfred Thomason Grenfell travelled to the Coast with the British Mission to Deep Sea Fishermen to provide medical care to fishermen and their families. The conditions the young medical graduate witnessed in Labrador provided him with the opportunity to combine "the aspirations of a young medical man ... with ... a desire for adventure and definite Christian work."[3] The poverty and hardship that he observed among those families inspired him to return the following year and establish the first of many Mission buildings on the Coast – the hospital in Battle Harbour. From that moment on, Grenfell spent the rest of his life providing medical care to the people of the Coast, recruiting a range of volunteers and employees, and raising money through philanthropic channels to support the operation.

Although the Grenfell Mission unquestionably provided essential medical care to people in need, strong class-based assumptions of local inferiority underlay the institution and the services it provided. The people of northern Newfoundland and Labrador were considered to be economically and socially disadvantaged according to British middle-class standards. Known as 'livyers,' these people were working-class fishermen and labourers who were descended from generations of Newfoundland fishing families. Although there were resident Innu and Inuit living in the territory as well, until the mid-twentieth century the Mission focused most of its efforts on the white Anglo-Saxon population and only occasionally came into contact with Native peoples in certain parts of Labrador.[4] It is unique that the Mission focused so exclusively on the local white population and this is a theme that should be explored further in Grenfell historical research, which until recently has been primarily concerned with the history of Wilfred Grenfell himself.[5] The Mission did not necessarily overlook the Aboriginal population; indeed, Grenfell took many opportunities to pose with Native children for publicity purposes. And the Mission became more concerned with the health of Aboriginal peoples after Newfoundland became a Canadian province in 1949. But the focus of its attention between 1893 and 1949 was the white population. And despite the fact that these people were white Anglo-Saxon, the Mission viewed them as different, inferior, and requiring social and moral uplift.[6] It displayed colonial attitudes of English cultural superiority based on class distinctions and a desire to 'civilize' a 'backwards' corner of the British Empire. In her thesis, "Nursing for the Grenfell Mission: Maternalism and Moral Reform in Northern Newfoundland and Labrador, 1894–1938," Jill Perry argues that Grenfell nurses were central to this reform agenda because they represented the female embodiment of the 'superior' middle-class culture. Not only did they perform a myriad of essential health-related duties in isolated areas but they also performed a range of social reform duties in an attempt to 'civilize' local society. So, although nursing with the Grenfell Mission in Newfoundland and Labrador was "an exceptional female work experience,"[7] it was rationalized by the institution according to a conservative gender ideology that emphasized the maternalist qualities that trained nurses brought to the Coast.

The Grenfell Mission recognized the necessity of bringing medical care to the people of northern Newfoundland and Labrador, but Grenfell and his successors considered it "impossible and impractical to have trained surgeons available on [the] coast."[8] Therefore, they established nursing stations in the larger communities and hired nurses to provide health care services to those areas.[9] The Mission relied heavily on nurses and recognized that "the main care and diagnosis of serious illness [depended] ... on the nurse in the outlying district in a small nursing station who [was] intimately connected with the people and [saw] a case early."[10] This situation was not unique to the Grenfell Mission. Indeed, recent studies in Canadian nursing history have highlighted similar cases in other rural parts of the country where nurses performed medical duties due to the lack of a qualified physician.[11] In their article, "Medical Services to Settlers: The Gestation and Establishment of a Nursing Service in Quebec, 1932–1943," Nicole Rousseau and Johanne Daigle survey the establishment of nurses' dispensaries in remote areas of Quebec and argue that these nurses often performed non-nursing medical duties out of necessity.[12] Perry makes a similar argument in her thesis and points out that "a closer examination of the medical work undertaken by Grenfell nurses calls into question the usual professional divisions" between nurses and physicians.[13] Perry's analysis is more sophisticated than Rousseau and

Daigle's in that she tempers the opportunities for nurses to perform medical duties with the maternalist expectations of the Grenfell institution. Rousseau and Daigle's approach to outpost nursing tends to overemphasize the opportunities for nurses to fill the role of physician in such circumstances and threatens to skew the historical realities of nursing in an outpost. Most of the nurses' responsibilities with the Grenfell Mission consisted of established nursing duties (which were admittedly of an uncertain nature, being defined in direct relation to the shifting definitions of medical duties), child and maternal health, and public health nursing. The occasional emergency case required immediate attention, quick-thinking, and sometimes exceptional first-aid abilities, but would not usually constitute formal medicine. With the Grenfell Mission, if a nurse had a patient whose medical needs were beyond her training or skill, she was expected to contact the nearest physician via radio-telegraph for advice. If the patient required medical attention, arrangements were made for either the patient to be transported to the physician or the physician to visit the patient at the station. The real challenge that Grenfell nurses faced on the stations had less to do with the frequency or complexity of the medical duties that they performed and more to do with the level of responsibility they held as the only health professionals in their regions.

Nursing as a profession has suffered problems of identity and definition, exemplified by the nursing struggle to gain the respectable status of a 'profession.' Part of this problem stems from the difficulty for nursing to establish definite boundaries. Historically, nurses have often accepted the "discarded" responsibilities of physicians, and have passed their own nursing responsibilities on to nursing assistants.[14] The nursing profession shifts its boundaries according to those of the medical profession, so the boundaries that establish what nursing is are blurred.[15] Sarah Jane Growe also discusses nursing boundaries in her study, *Who Cares? The Crisis in Canadian Nursing*. She points out that developments in medicine changed (and continue to change) the duties of nurses as well as the relationship between physicians and nurses. As medicine became more complicated nurses inherited certain duties, such as taking blood pressure, previously performed by physicians only; consequently, nursing "derives its professional identity almost entirely from controlling medical acts."[16] In addition to shifting boundaries, health care in the twentieth century has also been char-

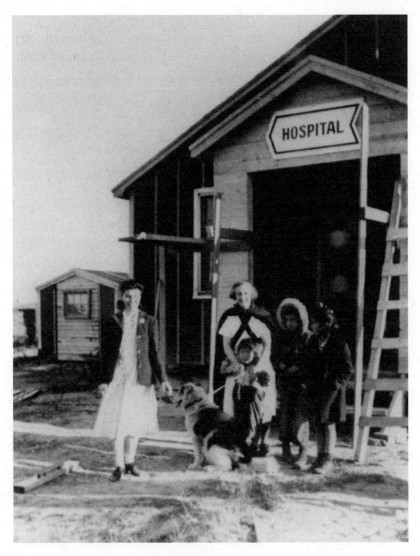

8.1 Annie Rhodes at Hamilton Village in the 1930s.

acterized by a gendered division of the professional responsibilities of
nurses and physicians. The role of the (female) nurse was strictly defined
according to the dictates of the (male) medical profession. And even in
the Grenfell Mission, which afforded nurses the opportunity to perform
duties that would not have been acceptable in a more formal hospital
environment, it was the medical profession that determined what

behaviour was appropriate for their nurses. However, the demands of nursing in isolated regions of Labrador challenged the conventional distinctions between nursing and practising medicine since the Grenfell nurse was sometimes called upon to perform duties traditionally reserved for the medical profession.

The nurses who served on these isolated stations were independent women who were eager to challenge themselves and to extend the boundaries of their strict hospital training. They worked in remote areas, independent from direct medical authority, and faced challenges on a daily basis. Nurses were attracted to the responsibility involved in district nursing and many candidates requested to be posted either on a station or in a small district. The secretaries of the Grenfell Association of Great Britain and Ireland (GAGBI), who were involved with recruiting and interviewing incoming staff, took note of a candidate's desire to work on a nursing station rather than a hospital.[17] The Mission also evaluated applicants according to their perceived suitability for station nursing versus hospital nursing. When Lesley Diack[18] applied to the Mission in 1949, the secretary for the GAGBI reported, "I would recommend her for a nursing station rather than a hospital as I think her common sense, age and experience are best suited for the former."[19] Diack certainly had extensive nursing experience in the field and was a prime candidate for a nursing station.[20] The nurse on a station was usually the only health professional in the area; the nearest doctor was sometimes hundreds of miles away,[21] and the nurse was sometimes required to perform duties for which she had not been formally trained. However, as they met with success on the stations, they became increasingly confident Grenfell staff members, most notably as a result of the responsibility they held rather than the frequency or complexity of 'medical' duties they performed, and became proactive in challenging the paternalist establishment.

Duties on a Nursing Station

En route to Newfoundland to begin her contract with the Grenfell Mission, Genevieve Brown met a Newfoundland Outport Nursing and Industrial Association (NONIA) nurse who was assigned to an adjoining district on the island.[22] The nurse informed Brown that in outport

Newfoundland, nurses were expected to perform a variety of duties, including "midwifery, dental extraction, suturing wounds, diagnosing cases, prescribing medication, nursing the sick, and acting as social workers in addition to a few other things."[23] Brown began to wonder if she had read the contract properly before she signed it. However, the reality was that Grenfell nurses provided a range of services in northern Newfoundland and Labrador, especially if they were posted to a station rather than a hospital – although it must be reiterated that most of the duties on the station could be defined as nursing rather than practicing medicine. And even when a nurse approached the dominion of the physician, she was still under the surveillance of the medical hierarchy. In some cases, average nursing skills were not sufficient to meet local health care needs, and previous historians have focused on such situations in interpreting rural nursing history. However, the true challenge of nursing with the Grenfell Mission lay not with the nurses' performance of medical duties, but with the unpredictable nature of the work and the level of responsibility with which the nurses carried out their work. For example, at the prospect of treating an influx of patients – "a sea of aches and pains, cuts and infections and people calling me from every doorway" – Alice Phillips "began to get uneasy. Most of the wounds were old, infected and neglected, and never before had [she] to make so many decisions by [herself] so hastily."[24] In terms of direct health care, the station nurse's responsibilities involved: (1) standard nursing duties, (2) operating the dispensary, (3) midwifery, (4) public health, and (5) first aid and dentistry.[25] In the context of these responsibilities, nurses developed the confidence and the desire to challenge the paternalistic authority of the Grenfell Mission.

Standard nursing duties involved those activities concerned with the patient's physical and emotional comfort and health, especially organizing, regulating and cleaning the patient's immediate environment; maintaining a sterile environment and controlling the spread of communicable disease; selecting and preparing sterile instruments and supplies; observing the patient, and reporting and recording observations; maintaining patient records; checking the patient's temperature, pulse, blood pressure, and respiration; assisting the patient with his or her dietary needs, personal hygiene, and elimination; assisting the patient with his or her posture, exercise, rest, and sleep; providing diversion, occupation, and recreation for the patient; and admitting and discharging the patient.[26] Regardless of the level of professional independence experienced by Grenfell nurses on the stations, performance of these standard nursing duties accounted for most of the nurses' daily work schedules. At any given moment, each hospital and station housed a number of in-patients – children and adults at various stages of illness and convalescence – for which the nurse was responsible in terms of these standard nursing duties. Mabel Hainsworth described the demands of administering antibiotics to a patient at Harrington Harbour Hospital where there was no night staff: "There is a patient on ... Penicillin, and evidently it is the rule here, to have no night staff, but one of the day staff to stay up to give the 11 pm dose and then get up & come down in your dressing gown to give the 3 am dose & then be on duty at 7 am in time for the 7 am dose, but I told Miss Hewitt that I could not do that, she said she had always done it, so I said, I would not do it, so I went on nights, & that does not suit her ... I came on duty at 8 pm and remain on until 10 am to help make all the beds, so I do not see why Miss Hewitt should be run off her feet."[27]

Operating the dispensary and treating outpatients, sometimes referred to as holding clinics, at the nursing stations and answering sick calls in the community also demanded much of the nurses' professional time. Occasionally the demands of treating outpatients were so overwhelming that some nurses would close the clinic on a Sunday and refuse to answer the door, except for emergencies. And in situations where a nurse was hired specifically for public health, she would sometimes restrict the clinic to three days a week in order to focus on health visiting for the remainder of the week.[28] Operating the dispensary, holding clinics, and treating patients in their homes[29] involved listening to the patients describe their symptoms, deciding on the best method of treatment, and taking the necessary steps toward that treatment. The three options available to the nurse were: (1) prescribing the necessary medication, such as aspirins, cascaras, and soda-bicarbonate,[30] and sending the patient home; (2) admitting the patient into the station for short- or long-term care and observation; and (3) providing first aid if necessary and sending emergency cases that were beyond her abilities to the nearest physician. It was while treating outpatients that the Grenfell nurses experienced the most professional autonomy. With no physician present on the station, it was the nurse's responsibility to see every case that came in the door, determine each patient's needs, and take the necessary steps. Even in the smaller hospitals (Harrington Harbour, Cartwright, and North West River), if the staff physician was away on a medical trip, which could last for several weeks at a time, it became the nurse's responsibility to see everyone who came to the hospital for care. As a result, nurses on the stations and in smaller hospitals took part in the diagnosis of patients to a greater degree than nurses in larger, more conventional western hospitals. Furthermore, the nurses often performed emergency first aid at various levels of difficulty, especially cleaning and suturing lacerations of arms or legs and treating septic fingers and abscesses. These types of accidents – whether associated with the fishery, the lumber industry, hunting and trapping, or the everyday business of life in rural areas – occurred to varying degrees in all communities in northern Newfoundland and Labrador.[31] Regarding emergency first aid, Nurse Ivy Durley commented that "sewing up axe wounds, opening abscesses comes fairly easily, in fact when you find yourself the one to do it, it almost seems as if you have been doing it always before. I suppose it is because we have watched it done so often."[32] Durley enjoyed the work but also felt "there [was] a good deal of anxiety in having the full responsibility."[33]

Nurses from Britain were especially useful on the isolated nursing stations of the Grenfell Mission due to the great need for midwives to assist local women in childbirth: according to one British nurse who worked with the Mission, "a lot of the work was midwifery."[34] The GAGBI recruited nurses who had full midwifery training (in the form of certification through the Central Midwives Board (CMB) in Britain) to fill the nursing station posts.[35] Midwives certified under the CMB provided prenatal care, abdominal examinations, and guidance and assistance during labour and delivery; they also often held antenatal and postnatal clinics for mothers.[36] Obstetrical work (prenatal and postnatal care, and deliveries) was routine for Grenfell nurses who were posted to the stations. During the year June 1946 – May 1947, Iris Mitchener had eighteen obstetrical admissions to the station (including twelve deliveries – nine were normal deliveries, two were forceps deliveries, and one was a stillbirth), which accounted for 24 per cent of in-patient admissions. She also attended five deliveries in the mothers' homes, and conducted ninety-six prenatal and twenty-three postnatal visits in the Forteau area.[37] The reports from other nursing

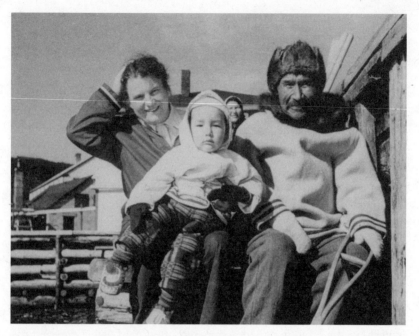

8.2 Ivy Durley with Aboriginal man and child.

stations also underline the prevalence of obstetrical work: for example, in 1950–51, obstetrical cases accounted for 79 per cent of the patients admitted to the nursing station at Mutton Bay, 64 per cent at Forteau, and 51 per cent at Mary's Harbour (which was also a centre for convalescent tuberculosis patients at that time).[38] Patricia Cowley had so many maternity cases at the beginning of one month at Port Saunders that "it was like the caplin coming in."[39] Obstetrical work was also unpredictable, since the start of a woman's labour could only be approximated and the length of time for the delivery was always unknown. Dorothy Jupp testified to an autumn rush of deliveries in her *Among the Deep Sea Fishers* article, "Five Babies in Six Days." By the time she got to the last delivery, "[their] supply of sterile goods had been used up, but the kitchen oven was pressed into emergency service and [they] soon had enough to use."[40] They also ran out of room for the babies and had to put two in a cot, one at each end.

The Grenfell nurses had extensive public health duties in northern Newfoundland and Labrador. The Mission did not hire any nurses under contract as 'public health nurses' until 1958; before that time it relied on nurses posted at the stations to conduct this work. The nurses would take lengthy immunizing trips around the communities in the region to administer large-scale vaccinations, especially for infectious and childhood diseases – diphtheria, pertussis (whooping cough), and tetanus (DPT). In the 1950s, with the prominence of consumption as a leading cause of death on the Coast and the vaccine Bacillus Calmette-Guérin (BCG) newly available, concern shifted to addressing tuberculosis. In 1953, Sheila Rawlings travelled with the Newfoundland Tuberculosis Association on an immunizing trip around White Bay, with plans to make similar rounds of the Flowers Cove area during the winter.[41] The Mission also administered BCG to local children via the hospital ship *Gould*, which visited fifty settlements in 1956 and administered 1500 doses of the vaccine.[42] The 1950s also witnessed epidemic polio in Newfoundland and Labrador, and a resultant widespread immunization campaign. Public health became "a very important part of [the] work on the Coast. It [meant] spending some time on the district, travelling by dog team and plane, giving injections, visiting the sick, seeing to anti-natal [*sic*] and pre-natal [*sic*] mothers, etc. etc."[43] Nurses held child welfare clinics, promoted public health among the residents, and performed follow-up checks on tuberculosis patients. During the early-1960s, the Mission became interested in organized health education and hired Caitlin Williams to deliver a series of six lectures on hygiene and health principles at Spotted Islands. However, her duties were not limited to these lectures. Being the only trained nurse in the area, Williams had to divide her time between "supplying medical care, preparing the lectures, visits to neighbouring settlements for clinics and public health rounds, answering emergency calls and tending to the major and minor ills of the crews of visiting schooners."[44]

Dental hygiene was a widespread problem in northern Newfoundland and Labrador during the mid–twentieth century, largely due to the paucity of professional dental services and the local diet of "potatoes, white bread, milkless tea with molasses, not to mention the numerous candies."[45] As a result, nurses on the stations frequently performed dental extractions, even though they had not received formal training in this area and most nurses approached their first extractions with apprehension.[46] However, despite their lack of preparation and early trepidation regarding dentistry, nurses on the stations performed many extractions over the course of their contracts. Within months of arriving at Flowers Cove, Durley had already pulled "dozens of teeth" and felt quite used to it. She facetiously told the secretary of the GAGBI: "My good strong arms have served me well on the men's back molars."[47] Diack became so adept at "hauling teeth" that she extracted one of her own, and was "agreeably surprised to find how painlessly [she] extracted teeth."[48] In terms of comparable statistics, during the year 1950–51, dental extractions on the nursing stations totaled 612 at Flowers Cove, 566 at Roddickton, 419 at Forteau, 129 at Mutton Bay, and 103 at Mary's Harbour.[49] These figures do not represent extractions performed exclusively by the nurses since the Grenfell Mission also hired dentists who were based out of the hospitals and visited the nursing stations on a yearly basis.[50] However, the availability of dentists was not consistent and although the hospitals at St Anthony and Harrington Harbour usually had resident dentists, North West River and Cartwright and their outlying settlements were not always so fortunate.[51] In 1948, E. Terry Hunt was hired as the dentist at St Anthony, but he had to divide his time between that hospital and North West River and Cartwright.[52] At each of these hospitals, Hunt was also required to travel to the smaller communities in outlying areas. Considering the infrequency and short duration of the dentists' visits and the poor condition of local teeth, it is safe to assume that the station nurses performed many dental extractions.

When trained nurses arrived at a Grenfell station, most of them had little idea of the responsibility and health-related demands they would face. In a 2004 interview, retired Grenfell nurse Margaret Campbell[53] recalled that she had entered the Mission as a respectful junior member of staff, but "by the time you're running a nursing station you've got the whole town on your doorstep and you either sink or swim."[54] Campbell was initially nervous about her posting to a station rather than a hospital: "I was almost quaking in my shoes."[55] On the station, Campbell became responsible for mixing poultices, which she had never done before and which caused her much worry. She also took over the housekeeping duties at North West River, which she did not expect. However, years of nursing on a station helped her develop confidence in her abilities and in her ability to cope with the unexpected. In a similar fashion, the feisty Diack was astonished by the necessity of her performing certain duties and, early in her tenure she even ques-

tioned the wisdom of giving nurses so much physician-related responsibility early in her tenure with the Grenfell Mission.[56] However, once
she adjusted to the extra-professional demands associated with Grenfell
nursing she became confident in her role and proactive in her position.
By the end of her career, Diack had become one of the most outspo-
ken nurses with regard to the subordinate position of nurses within the
Grenfell Mission.

Providing health care to isolated regions of coastal Labrador was
a physically demanding experience for the Grenfell nurse. Even with
the four hospitals and five nursing stations that were operating by
1949, the Grenfell Mission still faced innumerable challenges in bringing health care to people in the outlying areas that were many miles
from a health care centre. All nurses and physicians on the Coast were
required to travel long distances by foot, boat, dogsled, or snowmo-
bile, often in hazardous conditions. Such geographical and elemental
conditions had a direct impact on the experience of working with the
Grenfell Mission. Their unique and adventurous travel experiences in-
cited much attention in the nurses' writings and Perry points out that
many Grenfell nurses were thrilled with the prospect of "pushing the
boundaries of what was considered suitable behaviour for women"
and were proud to confront weather that was "'not fit for a woman.'"[57]
Personal memoirs and magazine articles abound with stories of thrilling
trips on swinging komatiks in blinding snowstorms. In some instances
the nurse would transport a patient to the nearest hospital for the doctor's
attention, often facing complications under poor weather conditions.
Bessie Banfill, a Canadian nurse stationed at Mutton Bay in 1942–43,
described one such trip: "At four-thirty, like a thunderbolt from the
blue, a blizzard came swooping down on us … Here we were and here
we stayed until two o'clock the next afternoon. An emergency patient
being rushed to a doctor, death facing him … no means of communication with land, and frequent treatments requiring a sterile needle and
syringe! A swaying wood stove and a sliding basin in which to boil my
sterile equipment did not help matters."[58]

In the unforgiving terrain of northern Newfoundland and Labrador,
the Grenfell nurse was not only personally challenged by the hazards
of travel but also professionally challenged by having to perform emergency medical duties under extreme circumstances.

Conflict with Paternalism

As demonstrated by the Jupp-Paddon controversy described at the beginning of this chapter, the Grenfell nurse sometimes came into conflict with the physicians as she met the demands of a nursing station. However, Grenfell nurses did not often realize their own strength and abilities until they had some experience on the Coast. Campbell admitted that during her first two years with the Grenfell Mission she did not realize how valuable she was, but after a year on leave she returned to Labrador with a new attitude, stating, "I knew I could come back on my own terms."[59] Her early years nursing with the Mission taught her that the organization needed her, needed her abilities, and needed her services. This helped her become more self-confident and more assertive in negotiating her position with the Grenfell Mission. Jupp's independence developed over years of living and nursing is extremely isolated circumstances; she was stationed in some of the most northern communities in Labrador. As a result, Jupp learned self-reliance. On the stations, Grenfell nurses did not know what kinds of cases were going to come through the door, but they knew they had to deal with whatever came their way. Furthermore, although most stations, by the middle of the twentieth century, were equipped with radio-telegraphs to assist with communications, the nurses sometimes could not reach a physician for advice if he was away on a medical trip. The pressures on a lone nurse in the often snowbound communities of northern Labrador can only be imagined. Years of dealing with unexpected medical situations helped to develop Jupp's confidence in her own abilities and this, in turn, encouraged her independent nature that so offended Paddon. One of Paddon's main criticisms of Jupp was that, in his estimation, she was "absolutely independent" and she did not want interference or assistance from other medical personnel.[60] This section discusses the circumstances in which nurses came into conflict with physicians, especially in terms of the negotiation of professional boundaries, the perception of physicians' disregard of the nurses' abilities, and the perception of physicians' lack of respect for the nurses and their abilities.

Grenfell nurses occasionally became unhappy in the Mission hospitals, where they took direct orders from the physician in charge and where they were required to follow formal medical procedure.

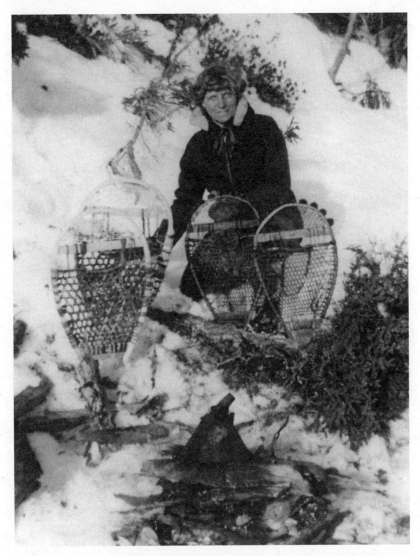

8.3 Jo Lutley in the woods with snowshoes.

Hospital nursing was perceived as the primary cause of friction between Jupp and Paddon. From 1951–59, Jupp nursed in Nain, a larger health care centre in northern Labrador. She had a tremendous amount of independence from medical authority and after years of nursing by herself on isolated stations she also had a great deal of confidence in her abilities. Although she was under the supervision of

Paddon, he was stationed at North West River and so did not work
with Jupp on a daily basis in a strict hospital setting. He disagreed with
many of her methods in running the station but found it difficult to
supervise her under the circumstances. The situation peaked in June
1959 when Paddon sent his concerns to Gordon Thomas, medical
superintendent of the Grenfell Mission. Paddon insisted upon the
removal of Jupp from the hospital and he recommended that:

(a) [she] take a refresher course in Hospital procedure in Great
    Britain, or Canada, preparatory to returning to Nain, or,
(b) [t]hat [she] put in 6 months around St Anthony Hospital
    for refresher work in Hospital procedure, or,
(c) [she] be transferred to a smaller station.[61]

Paddon's criticisms at this point were composed, at least on the sur-
face. He informed Jupp that he felt that the problem stemmed from
her unhappiness with hospital work and in-patient care. He intimated
to her that she would be all right in a small station, on her own,
and/or in district work. Jupp perceived "the hospital" as the only
source of disagreement between herself and Paddon and she was certain their professional relationship would improve if she were transferred to a station in his district. However, Paddon's criticisms of
Jupp ran much deeper. In October 1959 he informed his colleagues in
the Grenfell Mission, "I do not think she can be depended on to take
any responsibility, without the very closest supervision. I doubt that
she is well enough informed medically – even if she were willing to be
co-operative."[62]

At this point in her career, Jupp had been nursing in remote
communities of Newfoundland and Labrador for twenty-three years
and had been in Nain since 1951. She was an eminently qualified
nurse, she knew the people of northern Labrador, and she had even
learned to speak their language. Charles Curtis, who was then medical
superintendent of the Grenfell Mission, appreciated her value to the
organization; he disagreed with Paddon's assessment, and defended her
to Paddon in the fall of 1958:

I saw Dr Paddon in New York in November and he told me
frankly that he didn't wish you back at Nain. Most of his

reasons I thought were not justified, and I told him that as long
as he was in charge of Nain station he and the nurse must get
along well together ... that when you were at St Mary's River
you did excellent service and that you were a pioneer nurse under
the most extraordinarily difficult conditions in the early days at
Hope Simpson. I told Dr Paddon frankly my opinion of you and
told him that I would do everything possible to see that you had
a station on this Mission but ... it would be unwise for you to
go to Nain.[63]

Thomas was also in favour of keeping Jupp on staff in northern
Labrador and he even recommended her transfer to Hebron, knowing
that Paddon would disagree.[64] The crux of the conflict between Jupp
and Paddon revolved around her independence from his direct
authority and became manifested in the nature of "station" versus
"hospital" work. Jupp disliked hospital work and in June 1959 she
threatened to resign rather than transfer to a hospital: "I have decided
to return to England as soon as I can, unless I can get a post on the
Labrador only ... I do not feel inclined to go into a Hospital, and as
you intimated in your letter, you felt I would be happier in a District
Nursing place."[65] It is difficult to determine the degree to which hospital structure or routine was the root of the problem between Jupp
and Paddon. What is significant is that both of them perceived their
disagreement as stemming from hospital work – Paddon emphasized
that Jupp did not sufficiently understand hospital procedure and Jupp
stated that she was happier working alone on the stations. However,
although she preferred station work, Jupp had trained as a hospital
nurse and would have been familiar with its respective protocol. Why
did such a disagreement erupt between the nurse and physician? Is it
possible that Jupp had become so accustomed to the independent
nature of nursing on the stations that she genuinely lost the ability to
meld into the hospital structure? Did Jupp purposely cause problems
for Paddon because she was unhappy with her duties there and wished
for even more professional independence? Or was Paddon the source
of the conflict? Did he resent the independence that the woman exerted
and her lack of regard for male authority? In any instance, it is clear
that Jupp had become highly qualified for station work and was uncomfortable nursing within the formal medical hierarchy that defined

the hospital experience. Furthermore, from the perspective of the physicians, it was only Paddon who experienced outright conflict with Jupp; both Curtis and Thomas appreciated her contribution to the medical services of northern Labrador and, because of this support, Jupp won the battle against Paddon..

Several nurses voiced complaints regarding Paddon's disregard for their abilities and their authority, a disregard that was even obvious in the presence of patients. However, most of the complaints regarding physician conduct of nurses did not reach official channels. It is oral histories that provide a window into the nurse-physician relationship not evidenced in official documents. In an August 2004 interview, Campbell commented on "a considerable element of staff abuse" toward the nurses.[66] The expectation level placed on nurses was enormous, especially on the stations; but the Mission did not acknowledge that level of expectation. In remembering her days nursing at Happy Valley, Campbell recalled, "we were totally reliable and ... managed extremely well ... but the minute something went wrong ..."[67] She also remembered "being let down more than once in front of patients" by Paddon.[68] According to Campbell, many of the nurses felt overworked and underappreciated by the authoritarian attitude of the Grenfell Mission. The boundaries between traditional nursing and medical work – in other words, the boundaries of Grenfell nursing – were so blurred that Campbell doubted if the Mission authorities actually realized what they expected of their nurses and what their nurses did in providing essential health services to the people of Newfoundland and Labrador.

It was not only with Paddon that the Grenfell nurses came into conflict; another clash occurred between Diack and Thomas. Diack was stationed at Forteau for two years. She began her tenure there in optimistic spirits and felt that she was fulfilling her destiny. Many of her patients through the winter were emergency deliveries and in one case, Diack had to manually remove the placenta of a woman who had just given birth, a procedure that required her first attempt at giving an anaesthetic. The life of the mother was clearly in her hands and the ordeal caused Diack a great deal of stress. However, her second winter in Forteau brought her "the greatest trial of all, that of dealing with a paranoid personality in isolated circumstances."[69] Very little is known about this situation except what Diack describes in her memoirs: "the paranoid stirred up more and more trouble, it was like having a poison pen maniac in our midst. I was so alone with it all, and it was so intangible, that at times it was difficult even to be sure of my own judgment. That others doubted it was made plain on one of the doctor's rare visits, and the more I tried to convince him of the horror of the situation, the more powerless I felt to convey one half of it."[70] The doctor did not entirely trust the judgment of Diack in this situation. He remained wary of her diagnosis and his lack of support contributed significantly to her problems and unhappiness in the community. However, the situation was resolved when "finally no-one could doubt the diagnosis or fail to certify."[71] The doctor himself gave the final diagnosis and, tired from the strain of her ordeal, Diack requested a six-month leave.[72]

Jupp, Campbell, and Diack also expressed frustrations over the physicians' lack of respect for their health care abilities. However, sometimes (especially in the hospitals rather than the stations) the physician's lack of respect concerned a nurse's professional evaluation of other staff members. Unlike the Jupp-Paddon conflict, which concerned the nurse's approach to her health care duties, the disagreement between Paddon and Jayne Allen[73] centred on the physician's respect – or, more accurately, lack of respect – for Allen's evaluation of another Grenfell nurse. In 1973, Allen confided to the GAGBI that "Dr Paddon kicked below the belt again."[74] The matter surrounded the appointment of a nurse at North West River of whom Allen did not approve. Allen was head nurse there and did not want to work with that nurse in a health care environment. However, Paddon did not ask for Allen's opinion on this matter, an appointment that would fundamentally affect her position as head nurse of the hospital; he was insistent on the appointment. Allen sent several letters to the secretary of the GAGBI, pouring out her frustrations with the situation and her opposition to the appointment. According to Allen, the nurse in question had suffered from previous mental health problems; she approached Paddon about her concerns and related to the secretary that "he was not very helpful, he said he felt humiliated and that he knew nothing about all her previous problems."[75] Allen stated that she would resign from the Mission if this appointment went through.

Resistance to Paternalism

Threatening resignation was one method that Grenfell nurses employed in their attempts to influence their professional circumstances and to resist the paternalistic authority of male physicians and the Grenfell institution itself. They also questioned their subordinate positions within the Mission and petitioned the Grenfell administration to intervene on their behalf. Many of the nurses had joined the Mission specifically to have charge of a health care facility and one nurse resigned her post at Harrington Harbour when the Mission could not secure for her a nursing station.[76] By nursing for years in such remote regions, meeting extraordinary demands, and performing tasks they had never imagined, many Grenfell nurses developed confidence in their abilities to deliver health care and to cope with unexpected circumstances. They also gained an appreciation for their own individual value to the Grenfell Mission and as they realized their value, some tried to use this awareness to their advantage. As the Allen example demonstrated, if a Grenfell nurse was unhappy with her working environment, she would threaten resignation – and usually, in such cases, the Mission negotiated with the nurse to reach a viable solution.

Jupp asserted herself with the Grenfell Mission by threatening resignation if she was not posted to a Labrador station. With experience nursing in both Newfoundland and Labrador, she grew to prefer the lifestyle north of North West River and northern Labrador. She spent several years among the Innu and Inuit and even learned their language in order to communicate with them. When Paddon attempted to send her to Englee, she was incredibly persistent in her refusal to transfer. While he was determined to keep Jupp out of northern Labrador, she was just as determined to remain. And she succeeded. Although Paddon demanded her removal from Nain and wanted her transferred to another district completely, the other Grenfell physicians appreciated her importance to the region and supported her wish to stay. Because Jupp had been so determined to remain in northern Labrador and threatened resignation if she was transferred, the Mission found a compromise. Jupp was sent to Hebron and then Makkovik for a short tenure and was transferred back to Nain in 1965, where she remained until her retirement in 1974.[77]

Diack also threatened resignation from the Mission when she felt that she was being taken advantage of by the authorities. Diack's assertion usually took the form of letters and more letters to anyone who would listen. A main complaint was the terse manner in which the Mission transferred nurses on a moment's notice, along with the fact that nurses never knew they would be stationed on the Coast. Diack was introduced to the Mission's sudden transfers during her first summer, when she was stationed at Spotted Islands:

> Then, all unexpectedly, one midnight, a familiar siren blew. It was the *Maraval*. I got a boat and went on board. 'Are you packed ready?' asked Dr Paddon. I said 'No! What for?' Apparently I was to proceed to St Mary's River on the *Maraval*, to relieve Miss Jupp while she went over to St Anthony for a holiday. Dr Paddon said all the Mission radio-telephones had been buzzing with instructions for several days, he couldn't think why I hadn't heard. I murmured that, not having an R.T., I was a little out of ear-shot. 'Anyway,' said Dr Paddon, 'when can you be ready? The *Maraval*'s in a hurry, she's wanted back.'[78]

This narrative highlights Diack's interpretation of the somewhat inconsiderate nature of staff transfers on the Coast. Not only did Paddon expect her to have heard the instructions over a radio-telephone, which the Spotted Islands station did not possess, but he also expected "several days" to be enough time for her to close up the station and leave a community that had been her home through the summer. Although Diack found this first experience with staff shuffling upsetting, she was still new to the Coast and had not yet developed her confidence and assertiveness in negotiating with the Mission, and therefore did not protest to the Grenfell administration. However, five years later, she contacted Thomas to complain about the Association's tendency to transfer nurses to different communities with very little notice or consideration.[79] In 1954, before she signed a new contract with the Mission, Diack told Seabrook that she would only serve under a two-year contract for Forteau and demanded the clause in writing. When the Mission ignored her demand, she returned her contract unsigned and stated that she was not prepared to return to the

Coast with a contract that could send her "just anywhere."[80] Compared to her first summer on the Coast, Diack had become much more assertive in negotiating with the Mission, especially in terms of the unpredictable nature of staff shuffling.

Despite her pleas for Forteau, Diack was sent to Flowers Cove, the busiest nursing station on the Coast. Her term at Flowers Cove was characterized by tremendous overwork and frustration with the lack of nursing staff – her co-worker was often 'borrowed' by St Anthony to substitute for nurses on holiday. Diack's frustration peaked in July 1955 when the Canadian nurse at Forteau took her second holiday in less than two years and Diack was asked to take on her maternity cases. The Canadian nurses were hired through Canada's Grenfell Labrador Medical Mission (GLMM) under one-year contracts and could negotiate an annual holiday. But British nurses were hired under two- and three-year contracts, making holidays much more difficult to attain. The situation prompted Diack to compose a list of recommendations for the Grenfell Mission concerning the shortage of nurses. She argued for higher salaries, holidays, and equality of contracts for nurses, regardless of nationality. She also pointed out the constant strain of nursing in a station:

> There is never a single day in the year when we can relax and know that we wont [sic] be disturbed, never a single night when we can go to bed and shut the door and <u>know</u> that we can stay there till the morning ...
>
> Neither Dr Curtis nor Dr Thomas have ever spent even one winter alone on the Coast and I dont [sic] think either of them have the slightest idea as to what that really means. I dont [sic] mean the isolation only, but the fact that there is no-one to turn to for help, that whatever comes, however tired or short of sleep one may be, one must still go on. Dr Thomas always laughs and says the nursing stn nurses always spend all their time sleeping when they get to St Anthony, but it doesn't seem to have occurred to anyone that that could be a sign of being over-done![81]

Diack recognized an imbalance between the physicians and nurses with regard to coastal work. The hospital physicians did not experience the same feelings of isolation and the gravity of responsibility that the station nurses felt because they were not alone on the stations for any length of time. Furthermore, in the hospitals, the physicians had a large support staff. Diack's arguments regarding the shortage of nurses, their low salaries, and their lack of holidays reflected an acute awareness of nurses' professional, economic, and social demands that the Grenfell Mission, clinging to its missionary agenda (at least where the nurses were concerned), was failing to acknowledge.

Regardless of her two-year contract for Flowers Cove and her protests at being transferred yet again, Diack was sent to Mary's Harbour. She viewed this transfer as a demotion, since Mary's Harbour was less busy than Flowers Cove and provided less opportunity for medical work. She wrote a letter of protest to Thomas concerning the breach of her contract, addressing him in the familiar as "Gordie," rather than the formal "Dr Thomas," but she found no friends within the Mission hierarchy. Diack was clearly discontent at Mary's Harbour and pleaded to Thomas, "I do not like it here, in fact I dislike it intensely."[82] She became increasingly frustrated at her treatment and at her lack of power within the organization, and she vocalized these frustrations in letters to Seabrook and Thomas and to the Grenfell Mission board of governors. After several sudden station transfers and years of dealing with nursing shortages and unpredictable orders from the Grenfell Mission, Diack became disillusioned and acutely aware of her authoritative limitations as a woman within a paternalistic organization. The realities of nursing on the Labrador Coast, the nursing shortages, and the inequality of contracts and holidays for Grenfell nurses encouraged her to campaign for better labour rights and equality for northern Newfoundland and Labrador's nurses. Diack composed "Recommendations for Consideration by the Directors of the International Grenfell Association" – which included holidays for nurses, equality of contracts, and an improvement in nurses' salaries – and took her professional complaints to the highest level of the Grenfell Mission.[83] Through such action, Diack became one of the most professionally assertive nurses with the Grenfell Mission.

+++

The position of 'nurse' with the Grenfell Mission in northern Newfoundland and Labrador was of a contradictory nature. On the nursing station, where she was removed from direct medical supervision, the nurse held a position of authority. But that authority was tempered by her subordinate position within the medical hierarchy of the Grenfell Mission and by the expectation that she would contact the nearest physician in circumstances that were, according to the medical profession, beyond her expertise. As a result, conflict sometimes erupted between a nurse and a physician through the negotiation of ambiguously defined professional boundaries, especially if the physician felt the nurse was not consulting him or deferring to him in an appropriate manner. In the meantime, many of the women who nursed on the stations of the Grenfell Mission, like Dorothy Jupp, Lesley Diack, and Margaret Campbell, learned to trust their own abilities, embraced the challenges they faced, and developed a strong sense of professional self-confidence. The Jupp-Paddon conflict of 1959 demonstrated how tense relations between the physicians and nurses could become when the nurses exerted too much independence. After years of nursing by themselves on isolated stations, the nurses gained an appreciation for their professional abilities and also for their ability to cope with unexpected medical situations. They developed a great deal of confidence in themselves and became more inclined to disagree with Grenfell authority and stand up for themselves in conflicts with physicians. Diack took this a step further and became a vocal advocate for nurses' rights and benefits in the Grenfell Mission. As these nurses met the challenges of nursing in northern Newfoundland and Labrador and developed confidence in their own abilities, they expanded their practice into the medical realm, came into conflict with physicians, and resisted the male authority of the Grenfell institution.

NOTES

The author would like to thank Linda Kealey, Myra Rutherdale, and the anonymous reviewers for their helpful suggestions. This research has been funded by the Hannah Institute for the History of Medicine (Associated Medical Services), the Hugh John Flemming Fellowship at the University of New Brunswick, and the SSHRC/NSERC-funded interdisciplinary research project "Coasts Under Stress: The Impact of Social and Environmental Restructuring on Environmental and Human Health, 2000–2005."

1 Dorothy Jupp was a British nurse born in London. She attended Mayday Hospital in London for her nurse and midwifery training. She left England in 1938

and became a district nurse for the Labrador Development Company in Port Hope Simpson, Labrador. When the Second World War started, Jupp's work with the lumber company came to an end and she was offered a job with the Grenfell Mission at their station at Mary's Harbour. See International Grenfell Association (IGA) Archives, Box "Dorothy Jupp," File "Dorothy Maud Jupp," Document: "Dorothy Jupp, 1909–1986."

2 Provincial Archives of Newfoundland and Labrador (PANL), MG 372 Gordon Thomas Collection, Box 32, File "Dorothy Jupp, 1959–1961," letter from W.A. Paddon to Gordon Thomas, 31 October 1959.

3 Grenfell, *The Grenfell Association for Aiding Philanthropic Work*, ([Ottawa: Grenfell Association of Ottawa], 1908), 3.

4 This is in contrast with many Canadian examples of outpost nursing in which health care establishments focused on white women nursing in Aboriginal communities. For example, in "Nursing and Native Peoples in Northern Saskatchewan: 1930s–1950s," Laurie Meijer Drees and Lesley McBain argue that federal support for Status Indian health care was not clearly defined and that a policy of health care "sharing" between the federal and provincial governments often created problems for the nurse, who was unsure where treatment responsibilities lay and who was reimbursing the station for drugs and treatments. In addition to standard health care provision, the outpost nurse in northern Saskatchewan engaged in public health education and nutrition counselling and attempted to instil conformity and discipline in patients. The outpost nurses in Saskatchewan were part of a colonialist imposition of white, middle-class values on Aboriginal populations in the forms of structured Western medicine. See Laurie Meijer Drees and Lesley McBain, "Nursing and Native Peoples in Northern Saskatchewan: 1930s–1950s," in *Canadian Bulletin of Medical History* (*CBMH*) 18, no.1 (2001). Kathryn McPherson also explores the theme of colonizing functions in the provision of health care to Aboriginal communities in her article, "Nursing and Colonization: The Work of Indian Health Service Nurses in Manitoba, 1945–1970." McPherson found that the restructuring of the Indian Health Services (IHS) in 1945 brought increased resources for meeting the health needs of Aboriginal peoples but did not separate IHS from its earlier colonizing functions. Nurses in rural areas of Manitoba sometimes found their professional obligations compromised by colonialist government policies. Kathryn McPherson, "Nursing and Colonization: The Work of Indian Health Service Nurses in Manitoba, 1945–1970." In Georgina Feldberg, Molly Ladd-Taylor, Alison Li, and Kathryn McPherson, eds., *Women Health and Nation: Canada and the United States Since 1945* (Montreal & Kingston: McGill-Queen's University Press, 2003).

5 See, for example, Iona Bulgin, "Mapping the Self in the 'Utmost Purple Rim': Published Labrador Memoirs of Four Grenfell Nurses," PhD dissertation (St John's: Memorial University of Newfoundland, 2001), and Jill Samfya Perry, "Nursing for the Grenfell Mission: Maternalism and Moral Reform in Northern Newfoundland and Labrador, 1894–1938," MA thesis (St John's: Memorial University of Newfoundland, 1997).

6 Quoted in Perry, "Nursing for the Grenfell Mission," 18.

7 Perry, "Nursing for the Grenfell Mission," 61.

8 Charles S. Curtis, "Medical Work," in *Among the Deep Sea Fishers* 44, no. 3 (October 1946): 81.

9 Similar circumstances inspired the creation of nursing stations throughout the Prairies and the Red Cross outposts throughout rural Ontario. See Jayne Elliott, "Blurring the Boundaries of Space: Shaping Nursing Lives at the Red Cross Outposts in Ontario, 1922–1945," in *CBMH* 21, no. 2 (2004): 303–325.

10 Curtis, "Medical Work," 81.

11 For example, Jayne Elliott discovered that nurses performed many nursing, medical and non-medical duties in her study of Red Cross outpost nurses in rural Ontario. See Elliott, "Blurring the Boundaries of Space."

12 Nicole Rousseau and Johanne Daigle, "Medical Service to Settlers: The Gestation and Establishment of a Nursing Service in Quebec, 1932–1943," in *Nursing History Review* 8 (2000): 96–116. See also Victoria Page Sparkes Belbin, "Midwifery and Rural Newfoundland Health Care 1920–1950: A Case Study of Myra Bennett, Nurse Midwife." Honours essay (Memorial University of Newfoundland, 1996). In both studies, the system of nursing-based health care was created by the government because physicians refused to practice (or were not enlisted to practice for financial reasons) in rural areas. The reasons for the lack of physicians in areas of Newfoundland and Labrador were twofold: doctors did not want to practice in such remote areas, and the Mission could not justify increasing their expenses by stationing physicians in these regions, especially when there were so many trained nurses available. This is a common theme in the historiography of rural medicine, especially in terms of the challenge that rural nursing presented to the traditional gendered division of health care provision. Within the context of the Grenfell Mission, class and gender intersected to create a situation in which nurses viewed themselves as socially superior to local working-class culture (their patients) but simultaneously professionally secondary to male authority and the paternalistic institution.

13 Perry, "Nursing for the Grenfell Mission," 74.

14 Janet Muff, "Of Images and Ideals: A Look at Socialization and Sexism in Nurs-

NURSING WITH THE GRENFELL MISSION STATIONS   237

ing." In Anne Hudson Jones, ed., *Images of Nurses: Perspectives from History, Art, and Literature*, 202 (Philadelphia: University of Pennsylvania Press, 1988).

15 In *Bedside Matters: The Transformation of Canadian Nursing, 1900–1990*, Kathryn McPherson examines five generations of nurses in Canada, beginning with the pioneer nurses of the late nineteenth century and concluding with the emergence of the politically aware nurse – the militant unionist. She explores how each generation faced challenges associated with a gendered-construction of nursing unique to their period. McPherson also emphasizes the difficulties these generations of Canadian nurses have had in establishing the boundaries of their profession. See McPherson, *Bedside Matters*.

16 Sarah Jane Growe, *Who Cares? The Crisis in Canadian Nursing* (Toronto: McClelland & Stewart, 1991), 103.

17 For example, see PANL, MG 63, Box 53, File 1235 "Maureen McQuade, Nurse: 1971," note by Shirley Yates, 1 April 1971; and Box 65, File 1562 "Christine Short, Nurse: 1974–1975," note by Shirley Yates, 30 September 1974.

18 Lesley Molloy Diack was born in 1910 in Simla, India, of British nationality. She attended nursing school at East Suffolk and Ipswich Hospital and practised nursing from the time of her graduation in 1932 to the outbreak of the Second World War. Diack served as Sister and assistant matron with the Territorial Army Nursing Service for the duration of the war and was mostly stationed overseas in France, Iceland, North Africa, and India. After the war she returned to nursing in Britain. But during her war experience Diack had discovered "what it meant to feel really fulfilled: to be part of something that demanded all that one had to give." She also learned that she "enjoyed the roving life" and after a couple of years back in Britain she began inquiring into positions for overseas nursing service. See Lesley Diack, *Labrador Nurse* (London: Victor Gollancz, 1962), 9.

19 PANL, MG 63 International Grenfell Association (IGA) Collection, Box 34, File 710 "Lesley Molloy Diack, Nurse: 1946–1970," note by Betty Seabrook, 5 April 1949.

20 Diack served as Sister and assistant matron with the Territorial Army Nursing Service during the Second World War and was stationed overseas in France, Iceland, North Africa, and India.

21 There were three physicians who had authority over the station nurses who were spread throughout the isolated communities of Newfoundland and Labrador – the medical superintendent of the Grenfell Mission was at the St Anthony hospital with a physician at the North West River hospital (with authority over Labrador north of Cartwright) and a physician at the Harrington Harbour hospital, located in Quebec (the "Canadian Labrador").

22 The Newfoundland Outport Nursing and Industrial Association was created in
   1919 (originally as the Outport Nursing Scheme) as a means to provide health
   care services to people in rural areas by posting trained midwives in the outport
   communities. See Joyce Nevitt, *White Caps and Black Bands: Nursing in Newfoundland to 1934*, (St John's: Jesperson Press, 1978), 127–45.

23 International Grenfell Association (IGA) Archives, Genevieve Fink Brown Collection, MG 93.4, Box "Diaries and Letters," Unpublished essay "The Labrador
   Lure," n.d., 2.

24 IGA Archives, Box 97, File 151 "Diaries and Letters," transcript of letter from
   Alice Phillips to Jean [Phillips], [1943?].

25 Some of the non-health-related duties that nurses performed on the stations included domestic chores, administration, animal care, gardening, and bottling
   preserves.

26 See Bertha Harmer and Virginia Henderson, *Textbook of the Principles and
   Practice of Nursing*, 4th ed., (New York: The Macmillan Company, 1939).

27 PANL, MG 63, Box 41, File 913 "Mabel Lilian Hainsworth, Nurse: 1949–1977,"
   letter from Hainsworth to Seabrook, 9 January 1949.

28 PANL, MG 63, Box 51, File 1174 "MacQuiens (Rawlings) Sheila, Nurse: 1953–
   1975," letter from Seabrook to Rawlings, 14 September 1967.

29 Nurses usually visited patients in their homes in cases of influenza or pneumonia. See PANL, MG 63, Box 27, File 520 "Bridge (Currant) Ethel, Nurse: 1935–
   1974," letter from Currant to Spalding, 26 February 1939.

30 PANL, MG 63, Box 23, File 428 "Barnard, Mary Penelope, Nurse: 1934–1978,"
   "LABRADOR: An Account of a Summer Spent at a Grenfell Mission Station,"
   n.d.

31 In her reference letter for a Grenfell nurse, Betty Seabrook commented that the
   nurse had been stationed in a lumber community, and therefore had experience
   treating "many serious accidents there with the electric saw-cutters and other
   equipment." See PANL, MG 63, Box 32, File 656 "Cowley, Patricia," letter from
   Seabrook to Miss Peebles (matron, Brook Hospital London), 2 December 1968.

32 PANL, MG 63, Box 35, File 738 "Durley, Ivy Constance, Nurse: 1947–1981,"
   letter from Durley to Seabrook, 16 November 1947.

33 PANL, MG 63, Box 35, File 738 "Durley," letter from Durley to Seabrook, 4 April
   1948.

34 Margaret Campbell, Telephone interview, August 2004.

35 Between 1902 and 1926, education for midwifery was three months and focused
   exclusively on labour. In 1926, the program was expanded to twelve months and
   included training in antenatal and postnatal care. In 1936, the program was in-

creased to two years (with one year remission for trained nurses) and in 1938 it was divided into two parts: Part I consisted of theoretical training and focused on abnormal deliveries while Part II was six months in length and included three months of practical experience on the district. Since 1968, training has been in single format across Britain. See E.A. Bent, "The Growth and Development of Midwifery," in Peta Allan and Moya Jolly, eds., *Nursing, Midwifery and Health Visiting since 1900* (London: Faber and Faber, 1982), 191–2. The CMB was a product of the Midwives Act of 1902, which was created "to secure better training of midwives and to regulate their practice." The Act prohibited anyone to use the title *midwife* if she was not certified, and in 1910 it prohibited anyone from practising who did not have a certificate from the CMB. The board approved the courses of training, established examinations and regulations for practice, and maintained a register of practising midwives in Britain. See Robert Stevens, "The Midwives Act 1902: An Historical Landmark," in *Midwives* 5, no. 11 (2002): 370. See also, Jean Towler and Joan Bramall, *Midwives in History and Society* (London: Croom Helm, 1986).

36 By requiring that British nurses could only work on nursing stations if they were certified by the CMB, the GAGBI ensured a strong supply of such midwifery services, which were severely lacking in northern Newfoundland and Labrador. British nurses without midwifery training could also work with the Mission, but were posted to hospitals rather than nursing stations. See PANL, MG 63, Box 56, File 1313 "Newton (Ormerod), Margaret, Nurse: 1944–1975," letter from Ormerod to Spalding, 24 May 1944. See also Mary Laetitia Flieger, "Midwifery in Great Britain," in *The American Journal of Nursing* 28, no. 12 (1928): 1195–8.

37 Iris F. Mitchener, "Forteau Facts," in *Among the Deep Sea Fishers* 45, no. 3 (October 1947): 68–71.

38 [Charles S. Curtis], "The Superintendent Reports," in *Among the Deep Sea Fishers* 49, no. 3 (October 1951): 69–71.

39 PANL, MG 63, Box 32, File 656 "Cowley, Patricia, Nurse: 1963–1980," letter from Cowley to Seabrook, 14 March 1966.

40 Dorothy M. Jupp, "Five Babies in Six Days," in *Among the Deep Sea Fishers* 47, no. 4 (January 1950): 116.

41 PANL, MG 63, Box 45, File 1008 "Hughes, Winifred Helena Rose, née Burgess, Nurse: 1945–1975," letter from Burgess to Seabrook, 22 August 1953.

42 Charles S. Curtis, "Air Era: Report of the Superintendent for 1956," in *Among the Deep Sea Fishers* 54, no. 4 (January 1957): 105. Tuberculosis was especially problematic among Native communities in Labrador, and the public health

nurses frequently conducted follow-up tuberculosis checks along the coast. See
PANL, MG 63, Box 68, File 1616 "Stephens, Mary Kiese Jean, Nurse: 1958–
1977," "Public Health Nursing in Northern Labrador, Past, Present and Future,"
November 1961.

43 PANL, MG 63, Box 30, File 619 "Clark, Jean May Deller, Nurse: 1958–1978,"
letter from Seabrook to Clark, 5 May 1961.

44 PANL, MG 63, Box 75, File 1798 "Williams, Kathleen, Nurse: 1962–1977,"
"Spotted Islands, Summer 1963."

45 PANL, MG 63, Box 66, File 1585, Folder 3 "Smith, Jean Battinson, Nurse: 1943–
80," letter from Smith to Spalding, 12 June 1945.

46 Some nurses, such as Lydia Veitch and Sheila Fortescue, who trained and/or
worked in England during the Second World War did acquire experience ex-
tracting teeth during their employment. Veitch was stationed at Harrington Harbour during the war, while the hospital was without a resident physician. She
noted how valuable her previous dental experience was while she was extract-
ing teeth there in 1944–45. See PANL, MG 63, Box 72, File 1710 "Lydia Veitch,
Nurse: 1944," letter from Veitch to Spalding, 8 February 1945. Fortescue trained
at the Prince of Wales General Hospital and was employed there during the war,
where she acquired dental experience as a junior casualty Sister. See PANL, MG
63, Box 37, File 805 "Sheila Mary Fortescue, Nurse: 1951–56," note by
Seabrook, 11 October 1948.

47 PANL, MG 63, Box 35, File 738 "Durley, Ivy Constance, Nurse: 1947–81," letter from Durley to Seabrook, 16 November 1947.

48 Diack, *Labrador Nurse*, 95.

49 Charles S. Curtis, "The Superintendent Reports," in *Among the Deep Sea Fishers* 49, 3 (October 1951): 70–1.

50 During the year 1950–51, the Mission had an American dentist on staff at
St Anthony, Dr Alexander T. Andrews. See Eleanor J. Cushman, "Our Staff,"
in *Among the Deep Sea Fishers* 48, 2 (July 1950): 43.

51 In 1955, Betty Seabrook noted that North West River and Cartwright has been
without a dentist for six years. See Betty Seabrook, "A Return Visit to the Coast
(concluded)," in *Among the Deep Sea Fishers* 53, 4 (January 1955): 113.

52 Eleanor J. Cushman, "Our Staff," in *Among the Deep Sea Fishers* 46, 3 (October 1948): 80.

53 This is a pseudonym to protect the identity of the nurse who agreed to an interview in August 2004. Campbell was a British nurse, born in Manchester. She
studied nursing at St Bartholomew's Hospital, London, became state registered

in 1958, and earned her certificate from the Midwifery Board in 1959. Campbell joined the Grenfell Mission in 1960. See Margaret Campbell, Telephone interview, August 2004.

54 Campbell, Telephone interview, August 2004.

55 Campbell, Telephone interview, August 2004.

56 PANL, MG 63, Box 34, File 710 "Lesley Molloy Diack, Nurse: 1946–1970," letter from Lesley Diack to Betty Seabrook, 14 August 1950.

57 Perry, "Nursing for the Grenfell Mission," 91.

58 Bessie Banfill, "Night Watch," in *Among the Deep Sea Fishers* 47, no. 2 (July 1949): 44.

59 Campbell, Telephone interview, August 2004.

60 PANL, MG 372, Box 32, File "Dorothy Jupp 1959–1961," letter from W.A. Paddon to Gordon Thomas, 31 October 1959.

61 PANL, MG 372, Box 32, File "Dorothy Jupp 1959–1961," letter from W.A. Paddon to Dorothy Jupp, 2 June 1959.

62 PANL, MG 372, Box 32, File "Dorothy Jupp 1959–1961," letter from W.A. Paddon to Gordon Thomas, 31 October 1959.

63 PANL, MG 372, Box 32, File "Dorothy Jupp 1959–1961," letter from Charles S. Curtis to Dorothy Jupp, 19 March 1959.

64 PANL, MG 372, Box 32, File "Dorothy Jupp 1959–1961," letter from Gordon W. Thomas to Charles S. Curtis, 6 July 1959.

65 IGA Archives, File "Makkovik, Miss Jupp," letter from Dorothy Jupp to Tony Paddon, 28 June 1959.

66 Campbell, Telephone interview, August 2004.

67 Campbell, Telephone interview, August 2004.

68 Campbell, Telephone interview, August 2004.

69 Diack, *Labrador Nurse*, 44.

70 Ibid., 144–145.

71 Ibid., 145.

72 Bulgin, "Mapping the Self," 257.

73 Pseudonym.

74 PANL, MG 63, Box 66, File 1595 "[Jayne Allen], Nurse: 1965 1980," letter from Jayne Allen to Shirley Yates, 13 May 1973.

75 PANL, MG 63, Box 66, File 1595 "[Jaybe Allen], Nurse: 1965–1980," letter from Jayne Allen to Shirley Yates, 2 August 1973.

76 See PANL, MG 372, Box 35, File "Harrington: 1958–1962," letter from D.G. Hodd to Jean DuMont, 1 July 1960.

77 IGA Archives, Box: Dorothy Jupp, "Dorothy Jupp 1909–1986."

78 Diack, *Labrador Nurse*, 8.

79 Her letter aptly describes the emotional attachment a nurse could develop with the people of the community in which she practised: "out on the Nursing Stations we get our roots down deep among a particular group of people and their needs and their problems and it is very hard indeed to have to leave and start all over again, particularly out here where, on the N. Stns anyway, our only recreation is in the work, and where it takes most of a year: 1 To get to know the people, and 2 For them to know and have confidence in a new nurse." This letter also testified to the community-based challenge the Grenfell nurse faced in Labrador. In order to provide the people with quality health care she had to earn their trust and confidence. See PANL, MG 372, Box 35, File "Mary's Harbour 1955–62," letter from Lesley Diack to Gordon Thomas, 20 October 1955.

80 PANL, MG 63, File 710 "Lesley Molloy Diack, Nurse: 1946–1970," letter from Lesley Diack to Betty Seabrook, 12 January 1954.

81 PANL, MG 63, File 710 "Lesley Molloy Diack, Nurse: 1946–1970," letter from Lesley Diack to Betty Seabrook, 26 April 1956.

82 PANL, MG 63, File 710 "Lesley Molloy Diack, Nurse: 1946–1970," letter from Lesley Diack to Gordon Thomas, 20 October 1955.

83 PANL, MG 63, File 710 "Lesley Molloy Diack, Nurse: 1946–1970," Document: "Recommendations for Consideration by the Directors of the International Grenfell Association."

Part Four

Northern Nursing, Natives, and Newcomers

9

+ + + + +

A Negotiated Process: Outpost Nursing Under
the Red Cross in Ontario, 1922–84

JAYNE ELLIOTT

Nurse Audrey Woodget believed that her work in the North during the 1960s provided "Seldom a Dull Moment."[1] Most stories of nursing in outlying regions of Canada contain examples of the high drama and unusual events that nurses experienced, typically as young women, attending to the health and medical needs of people who called on their services.[2] Hailed as "pioneers in every sense of the word," outpost, outport, and district nurses have been acclaimed for their success in caring for patients under difficult circumstances, for pushing the boundaries of "appropriate" feminine behaviour, and for helping to lay the foundation of government involvement in Canadian health care.[3]

Many of the adventures they had and the challenges that they faced resulted from the degree of independence demanded of them as medical and health care practitioners. Nurses in general obtained marketable skills from their education, but those choosing employment in isolated areas added the potential for travel and adventure as well as the ability to support themselves. As both practitioners and historians of outpost nursing attest, nurses were forced to rely on their own knowledge and expertise without close supervision from physicians. Particularly in the early to mid-twentieth century, living at an outpost provided nurses with a more independent lifestyle than young, single women on their own could often realize in urban centres, and one which was surely better than that experienced by many rural women teachers.[4] As the prime resource for skilled aid in areas where easy access to medical treatment was limited, outpost nurses gained some prestige – a status that they often maintained when they married and remained in their outpost communities.[5] Both in imagery and in practice then, the idea of autonomy has underlined the identity both claimed by and granted to outpost nurses everywhere.

Implicitly or otherwise, this independence is contrasted to the nature of nursing work in hospitals where, until recently, the vast majority of nurses were educated and where most nursing graduates could be found after the Second World War. As many historians and other scholars have pointed out, hospital nursing required nurses to conform within a highly regulated and hierarchically structured environment. Both students and graduates fell under the regular oversight of physicians, hospital administrators, and their own nursing supervisors.[6] Even social lives came under close scrutiny in times when graduate nurses as well as students lived in residences attached to hospitals. Nurses found independent decision-making much more difficult in a hospital setting, and their superiors did not consider it a desirable characteristic. As outpost nurses were warned, "When you return home, you will find it almost impossible to cope within the limited range of duties allowed in southern hospitals."[7]

The strong focus on independence that is found in accounts of nursing 'on the margins' also relates to ongoing efforts to define the status of nursing as a profession. Autonomous practice within a field of specialized, exclusive knowledge and within moral and self-regulating guidelines has been viewed as a hallmark of traditional professions, such as law and medicine.[8] Autonomy for nurses in this sense refers to the freedom to construct a practice, both individually and as a group, that is grounded in the knowledge and values of contemporary nursing education and that is recognized and valued as nursing work. Nursing leaders aspired to this kind of professional prestige in attempts to establish the uniqueness of nurses and their work in the health care field. But as British sociologist Celia Davies observed, "The question of whether nursing is or is not a profession appears with great regularity."[9] From the beginnings of organized nursing, struggles from registration to educational reform have been considered part of the quest to establish professional legitimacy, authority, and value.[10] Although many would argue that these debates have often been based to a large degree on a problematic (and perhaps out-dated) model of a profession, the sustained attempt to argue for a distinct body of expert knowledge and to control workplace practice in nursing has nevertheless engaged much effort.[11] Implicit within narratives of outpost nursing, therefore, is the understanding that the autonomous practice for which outpost nurses have often been celebrated reflects their closer proximity to this desired professional ideal than their colleagues in other branches of nursing could possibly obtain.

In this discussion, however, I want to pay closer attention to this concept of autonomy and to explore its dimensions with respect to the practice and the social lives of nurses in 'frontier' situations. This investigation is centred on one group of nurses who were employed by the Ontario Division of the Canadian Red Cross Society for its outpost program. Between 1922 and 1984, the Division hired nurses and nursing assistants to staff a total of forty-four medical outposts in remote settlements, primarily across the northern sections of the province. Despite their geographical isolation, these nurses were embedded within a matrix of relationships with supervisors, community residents, and local physicians. I am not denying that they attained some level of independence or that they often overcame severe challenges to care for their patients. I am arguing, however, that both their workplace and social autonomy were complicated by these social connections. Through an examination of Red Cross annual reports and nursing records, and government documents, and through oral interviews with former Ontario Red Cross outpost nurses, issues of gender, class, professionalism, and authority emerge. These factors had the potential to expand, sustain, or constrain both nurses' work and personal activities, helping to illustrate that outpost nursing with the Red Cross was, indeed, often a negotiated process.

This analysis builds on insights derived from recent writing in nursing history. Kathryn McPherson has demonstrated through her research on primarily institutional Canadian nursing how variables of gender, class, and ethnicity interacted to define the relational position of nurses within the health care system. Nurses were simultaneously subordinate to the male-dominated professions of medicine and hospital administration, superior to less-skilled working women, and in an ambiguous position in regard to their patients.[12] For nurses working in outlying areas, Meryn Stuart had earlier illustrated the gendered and class dimensions of the labour of a group of early public health nurses in Ontario.[13] In their attempts to carry out health demonstration projects in rural areas of the province, they could not directly challenge local doctors threatened by the autonomous nature of nursing work in the field. Instead, they were often compelled to enlist the help of their medical superiors from the public health department, subvert their ambitions, or find ways of quietly circumventing local medical authority. Jill Samfya Perry documented the extreme isolation and hard work that the nurses working with the International Grenfell Association faced, but she also pointed out that they were ultimately subject to the norms of contemporary feminine respectability as perceived by the Mission's male physician administrators. Too aggressive an independence could result in condemnation or dismissal.[14]

Nursing practice in outpost communities was also circumscribed by nurses' relations with patients and other community members. Perry demonstrated that Grenfell nurses often brought their own feelings of cultural superiority to their interactions with local residents, and that these attitudes sometimes caused patients to bypass the nurses and seek medical aid from traditional community healers.[15] Studies of the work of federal nurses located in Aboriginal communities in the rural and northern areas of Saskatchewan, Manitoba, and present-day Northwest Territories and Nunavut, have also deepened our understanding of how nurses participated as agents of 'civilization' at the same time as they were constrained within a specific societal context. Both McPherson and Judith Bender Zelmanovits suggested that professional nursing services were accepted more readily in indigenous communities where nurses were sensitive to cultural differences and were able to forge respectful alliances with local women.[16]

Red Cross Nurses in Ontario

Following the First World War, the Canadian Red Cross Society shifted its energy from wartime to peacetime activities. Several Divisions of the Red Cross in Canada developed a medical outpost program to aid settlers in remote sections of the country, but the one in Ontario evolved into the most complex of all. The Ontario Division's outpost program consisted of a chain of small hospitals and nursing stations administered from a central office in Toronto. The hospitals were located in towns with at least one resident physician and typically ranged in size from seven to twenty-five beds. They contained delivery and operating rooms, sometimes within the same space. The nursing stations, situated in districts without permanent doctors, were usually staffed by one nurse and a housekeeper, but also incorporated from one to five hospital beds, supposedly reserved for emergency use.

The outposts were one of several projects undertaken by the Red Cross that emerged out of a focus on the new public health, which now included an emphasis on individual behaviour and responsibilities.[17] Matters of health and disease became increasingly important to and vested in notions of civilization. Efforts at health reform, produced through gendered, raced, and classed processes, thus played into historical transformations of what it meant to be 'civilized.'[18] From its inception, Red Cross officers had viewed the program as a nation-building exercise, as the Society's contribution to the construction of "a strong, healthy, vigorous, virile nation" in which bringing up "a race of sound, healthy children ... would raise the whole status of our citizenship and our nationhood."[19]

The outpost nurses served as vital links in this program that connected ideals of good health with ideas of good citizenship. From 1922 to 1969, the Ontario Division hired 1,168 registered nurses and (after 1947) certified or registered nursing assistants to staff its outposts, of which 422 were listed as beginning work before 1945, and 746 after that date.[20] These nurses appeared to fit within the parameters of the third and fourth generation of nurses described by McPherson.[21] All were female, and most were likely white, native-born Canadians. The majority were employed as general duty nurses for the outpost hospitals, while the remainder staffed the nursing stations. The Red Cross medical directors preferred to send accredited public health nurses to the one-nurse outposts, but not enough could be found before the Second World War. Although approximately 85 per cent of the nurses hired between 1922 and 1945 were single, reliance on married nurses grew steadily following the war. When employment of married female nurses in Canada jumped from 5 per cent in 1941, to 25 per cent in 1951, and to 47 per cent a decade later, the Division's nursing workforce mirrored these trends.[22] At the end of the 1960s, married nurses outnumbered single, although no breakdown is possible between part-timers and those working full-time.

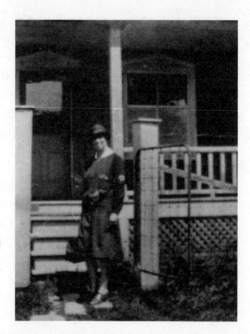

9.1 Red Cross Nurse Louise de
Kiriline in front of her outpost
hospital at Bonfield, Ontario.

Many Red Cross nurses expressed satisfaction with their outpost
experiences and the opportunities for independence that living and
working in remote environments presented. The Ontario Division furnished those posted to the nursing stations with a stable wage as well
as a 'home of their own,' offering a place to live that would likely have
been beyond the financial reach of most other single nurses, particularly before the Second World War. Part of nurse Louise de Kiriline's
pleasure in acquiring her position at the Bonfield outpost in 1927
stemmed from her delight "in having my own little house which I can
style as I please."[23]

All of the Red Cross nurses acquired diverse skills considered more
the province of physicians.[24] Without doctors always nearby, suturing wounds, administering anaesthesia, taking X-rays, and diagnosing
illnesses were tasks usually learned by doing – and hoping for the best.
Professional independence was, of course, a double-edged sword. For
example, attending women in childbirth formed a significant portion
of outpost nurses' work, but except for Newfoundland and parts of
Alberta, Canadian nurses had no distinct legal authority to deliver
babies.[25] Lack of official support for nurse-midwifery therefore prohibited advanced obstetrical nursing education in the country, and con-

sequently, confinements conducted on their own caused anxious moments for many nurses. Over time, however, most of the Red Cross nurses gained confidence and competence in their obstetrical skills. Maude Weaver's description of her actions at one childbirth revealed that she felt confident enough to pursue a course of treatment rivalling a physician's care. "[The woman] came in Sunday night having rather feeble 15 minute pains. That went on till 7 a.m. with no sign of increasing, so I gave her some quinine – and the pains speeded right up and she was all through by 8:20. Miss Sanderson [the previous nurse] had told me that last time she bled "like the devil" so I shot .5 cc pituitrin in her as soon as the baby was born and gave her a dram of Ergot. She bled quite a bit before the placenta was delivered, but her uterus contracted down right away and her pulse never went over 98 – then slowed down to 80 within an hour."[26]

Many nurses welcomed the variety of medical problems with which they were presented and their role in caring for patients. Constrained only by the guidelines of the Red Cross and local co-operation, those posted to the one-nurse stations made plans to formulate and administer the community health program in their districts. Nurse Gertrude LeRoy Miller recalled her enthusiasm as she settled into her outpost at Wilberforce: "I had been told that none of my predecessors had any training in Public Health Nursing, so it was up to me to set up a Public Health Program. What a challenge! Where should I begin? ... I could hardly wait to get started."[27]

C.S.A. had tried private duty nursing, but had not cared for it. For her, the attractions of outpost nursing included the variety, the responsibility, and the comradeship. "I enjoyed the outpost hospitals because at that time [in the 1950s] there was everything – emergency, operations, delivery of babies – you know, you had a lot of responsibilities."[28] "It was very simple the type of care we gave in some respects," C.S. stated, "yet it was complex because you had to do all kinds of things."[29]

In the following section, however, I will argue that independence for nurses under the Red Cross in Ontario, no matter how much it was desired or lauded, was not a straightforward matter. Instead, it was often determined through interactions with the differing groups of people with whom the nurses came in contact. Nursing supervisors from head office in Toronto may have visited nurses infrequently in the field, but they retained ultimate authority over employment and their postings. They also evaluated the impact of nursing behaviour and activities in the outpost communities on the reputation of the Red Cross. The nurses discovered that community members did not always accept the program of health education and advice that they offered, and as young, single women often working on their own, they found themselves under close moral surveillance and regulation. Finally, professional autonomy was bounded by the traditional hierarchical relationship between medicine and nursing to which they were expected to adhere, whether or not they worked directly under physicians' supervision.

Red Cross Nursing Supervisors

The Red Cross nursing supervisors provided the vital links that connected the Toronto office with the outposts and local hospital boards, and their first-hand assessments of the staff, buildings, and general conditions under which the outposts functioned guided the administration of the program. One of their primary roles was to advise and direct their staff in the field. They visited each outpost at least once a year, for two to three days at each destination, to assess their professional and personal capabilities as well as relationships between nurses and domestic personnel. Most of the time they appeared satisfied. Supervisor Ida Brand arrived at the Apsley outpost in 1945 at the precise moment that the nurse delivered a baby on her own, and "since the birth was a breech delivery and the nurse was successful in getting a living child, she was to be congratulated."[30] They especially prized any innovation that furthered the mission of health care in the community. Supervisor Isabel McEwen praised the "excellent" public health work that nurse Finnemore had undertaken in 1935 in Atikokan. Over and above all the immunization work accomplished, she had also arranged to dole out the daily dose of cod liver oil to passing schoolchildren whose mothers tended to be a bit "forgetful" on that account.[31] Reports of outright professional incompetence were rare. Only once did a supervisor reprimand the entire staff in one small hospital; poor account keeping and "carelessness" in burning a child's leg with a hot

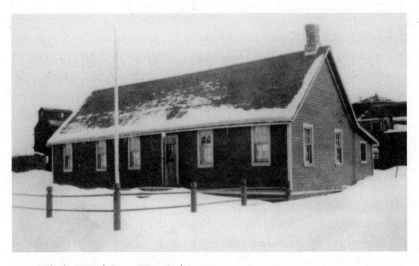

9.2 Atikokan Red Cross Hospital.

water bottle later became grounds for transferring the staff members to a larger outpost where they had less responsibility.[32]

Supervisors' recommendations and counsel appeared to be welcomed by the rank-and-file nurses.[33] Many isolated nurses at the nursing stations likely enjoyed the visits from their superiors, who, by virtue of gender and education, offered both some female company and intellectual stimulation on their rounds together. On a snowy night in 1935, supervisor McEwen accompanied nurse Dorothy Adams at Kakabeka Falls to the home of a baby with a high fever, helping her bathe the infant and apply a mustard poultice before leaving the reassured parents.[34] Many nurses asserted that "you always had support from them if you phoned with a problem."[35] J.F. always looked forward to Helen Singer's visits to the Matachewan nursing station in the 1950s. "I wasn't afraid of her coming up. I know some people would have been worried about it, but she was a wonderful person, very down to earth, [a] practical soul, and had good experience herself. She wasn't one of these theoretical types. She was good."[36]

Nonetheless, since the outposts were a visible marker of the Red Cross in the small towns and villages, the supervisors believed that the professional and personal behaviour of the nurses reflected on the organization. The rapport that the nurses developed with local residents was just as important to them as professional competence. Nurses who were well liked helped to encourage local use of outpost services. In a 1931 visit to Hornepayne, supervisor Maude Wilkinson found that nurse Gladys Taylor was a "great favourite in the community and doing excellent work."[37] Brand discovered in 1944 that, despite nurse Norma Tonkin's "youth and inexperience," she was "very friendly with the people" in Apsley; "the mothers chatted easily with her when they brought their babies in for weighing."[38] Harmonious relations among the nurses were also essential if the local population was to continue utilizing the outposts.[39] Problems of personal incompatibility, magnified by living and working in close quarters, prompted the movement of offending nurses. In 1942, supervisor Brand found the two in Jellicoe "most uncongenial," advising that a move for one was wise. The nurse's work was "above reproach, but her manner and attitude to [the] general public [was] most unfortunate."[40] The supervisors had the authority not only to hire the nurses but also to remove them. Wilkinson dismissed the new charge nurse in Thessalon in 1933 after confirming the suspicions of the local ladies' auxiliary regarding accounting irregularities in the fees collected from patients.[41] Despite the rumours and innuendo that brought the Thessalon hospital committee some bad publicity, supervisor Wilkinson was concerned to keep the whole issue quiet because of possible harm to the reputation of the Red Cross.[42]

Demonstrated efficient management of the outposts was another factor that the supervisors considered essential to the image of the organization. From their perspective, efficient operations included the degree to which the nurses managed the business affairs of the outposts. The most onerous duties fell on the charge nurses, who maintained the hospital's financial accounts, collected patients' bills, and sent a continuous stream of reports, patient statistics, and fee payments back to headquarters. Nurse Phillips may have been "kindness itself to the patients," but supervisor Brand could see that "one of her drawbacks ... [was] her [poor] aptitude for figures."[53] The ability to guide the work of the domestic staff was also important. Brand reported in 1944 that the nurse and the housekeeper in Apsley "appear to be quite congenial, but it remains to be seen as to [the nurse's] ability to direct the housekeeper to do efficiently the domestic work."[44] She later criticized the charge nurse at the Englehart hospital for the lack of direction given to both the nursing and domestic staff. "In fact, every department and every person appeared to be doing exactly as they chose," she regretted, and "the condition of the building certainly bore this out."[45]

Personal preferences of the nurses were rarely allowed to stand in the way of the supervisors' drive for efficient administration. Single nurses, for example, were expected to change posts willingly on demand, and these demands often came suddenly. B.T. declared that "[We] went where someone was needed and they phoned you the night before and boom, we went."[46] Possibly reflecting a lack of reliable communication, Dorothy Rowat Baxter recalled that in 1952, she found out about her moves when train or bus tickets arrived in the mail.[47] Most of the nurses appeared to comply but evidence exists of occasional resistance. Nurse Taylor's "[hinting] in a kindly way that a move from Hornepayne might precipitate her resigning from the staff" did not prevent the supervisor recommending a transfer should her services be needed elsewhere.[48] Undoubtedly, some of the single nurses were annoyed with the attitudes of the supervisors to the development of personal relationships. As several related, supervisors Brand and Singer transferred young nurses if they became interested in a local man. When one nurse became involved with the male secretary of the local Red Cross branch in Haliburton, supervisor Brand "promptly moved [her] up north," telling her that she "didn't want to marry an old fogey like that."[49] Miss Brand had not realized that the previous eighty-six-year-old man had recently been replaced by a much younger twenty-four-year-old. The nurse soon gave her notice and returned to Haliburton to marry the younger man. Although she and the young man, now her husband, can see the humour in the situation, the episode suggests a degree of control over the nurses that they may not have universally appreciated. According to nurse Marion Sedgwick, agreeing to a move was "the proper thing to do," but she also believed that the supervisors may have been trying to protect young women since some nurses did not always make good matches. "There's so little social life that [the nurses] often did find somebody [who] was totally inappropriate. You know, he looks fine up here, but in mother's living room in Toronto [he] might not," she stated. She thought, however, that "[their] aim was maybe too maternal."[50]

The supervisors may indeed have had their nurses' best interests at heart, but they were also undoubtedly aware that there was at least some ambivalence about these young, mostly single women serving on their own in areas populated by high numbers of men working in resource industries. Community surveillance and moral regulation served to constrict the personal lives of the nurses. Too much freedom and autonomy had the potential to make local residents uneasy. In February 1934, for example, nurse Maude Weaver endured a humiliating meeting with the local Atikokan hospital committee, which questioned both her time off and the suitability of entertaining friends in the outpost. In her support, the supervisor asserted that "the nurse should have the same privilege as any other homemaker in the district and in her time off duty when there were no patients [she] should not be criticized for having her friends in."[51] But nurse Weaver could not consider the outpost her home in the same manner as other homemakers saw their domestic environment. The principal role of the outposts and of the nurses themselves was to provide medical services to those in need. Both the community and the outpost directors insisted that institutional functions had to take primacy over household use. In the early 1930s, supervisor McEwen reprimanded a young Brand after she had transferred her living room in the Coe Hill outpost downstairs and placed the patients' rooms upstairs. The nurse argued that this "added to her convenience and comfort," but the supervisor agreed with the complaints from the townspeople that the outpost "was looking more like a nurse's home than a hospital proper."[52]

Moreover, the nurses themselves often realized that they were visible targets in their small communities and that their personal reputations were at stake. In 1948, supervisor Edith Chapman found that the entire staff at the Thessalon hospital was requesting a change. The nurses enjoyed the work within the hospital, but as she reported, "This town has become vicious; gossip runs rampant about everyone until the girls feel it is impossible for them to leave the building without starting further gossip. With the influx of men working in the construction camps, the town has become wide open and it has become unsafe for the girls to go out even in groups. On occasion when police protection has been needed at the hospital, it has been discovered on their arrival that the police themselves were in no condition to be of any help."[53]

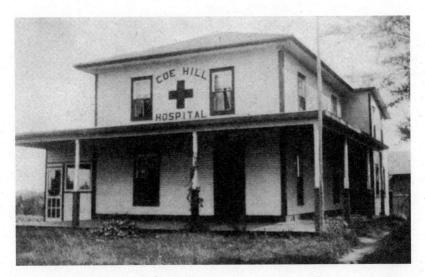

9.3 Coe Hill Red Cross Hospital.

Historians have suggested that the nursing uniform supplied a kind of personal security for young women who ventured into areas they would never have gone unaccompanied and in civilian dress. Red Cross supervisor Singer, too, asserted that over her many years of working in isolated districts, she never felt threatened by any men because she "always felt completely safe with [her] uniform on."[54] Even if this form of protection did not always hold up in practice, it was theoretically a means to present a "traditional asexual occupational image," helping to legitimate the entry of young women into the expanding field of nursing work, especially during the interwar period.[55]

Nonetheless, a close relationship between the public and private areas within the outpost could generate some discomfort around the sexuality and sexual safety of the nurses. As paid staff, housekeepers not only provided company for the nurses, but they also served as chaperones. Most lived in, but the supervisors were occasionally forced to hire married women who returned to their own families at the end of the day. Nurse Margaret Maclachlan recalled her first evening alone in the Armstrong outpost after her housekeeper had left. One of the two male in-patients assured her that no harm would come to her. "They were both ambulatory patients, they could have slaughtered me ... I thought it was darn decent of him," she related.[56] The comments made by the male patients indicate that they were aware of the specific personal concern Maclachlan might experience about being alone in the building. On her own in the nursing station, she would literally be sleeping in the next bedroom, possibly glimpsed going about her daily private routine, 'out of uniform' so to speak, thus perhaps destabilizing the implied professional "asexual" imagery of a nurse.

As long-term employees of the Red Cross in Ontario, and in concurrence with its goals, the nursing supervisors remained vigilant to issues and perceptions that threatened to undermine the reputation of the voluntary organization. They cared about the well-being of their nurses and were prepared to offer them substantial support for problems that they encountered in their outpost communities. Nonetheless, issues of professionalism and authority pervaded these relationships. The supervisors expected the nurses not only to maintain acceptable standards of nursing service but also to uphold the reputation of the Red Cross and to act as agents and promoters of its programs. Thus they evaluated the nurses' labour as well as their social activities within these parameters. Ultimately, for the nurses, continued employment with the Division depended upon acquiescing to the demands of those who employed them.

Outpost Nurses and the Community

The professional and personal independence of the Red Cross nurses was also shaped through relations with patients and other members of the communities in which the outposts were located. The ability to carry out their work was determined by the extent to which local residents sought out and accepted the premises of public health advice and education upon which the outpost project had been built. People did not always readily respond to the messages of health and hygiene in the manner anticipated by urban advocates of public health programs.[57] Scholars exploring the gendered, raced, and classed relationships between outpost nurses and aboriginal societies have provided some of the most insightful analyses in this area. American historian Emily K. Abel illuminated the restricted ability of the nurses working with the Bureau of Indian Affairs during the 1930s to provide medical

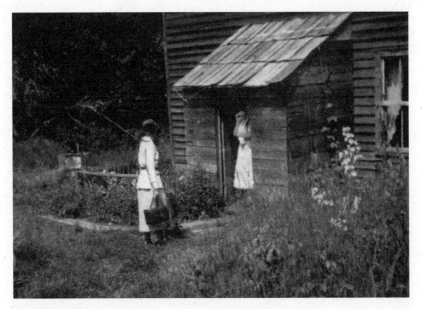

9.4 Red Cross nurse on a home visit in northern Ontario.

assistance on reservations. They were often confronted by the 'obstacles' of relatives, friends, and traditional healers of Native patients who comprehended medicine and healing from differing perspectives.[58] Zelmanovits has also paid particular attention to relationships between white, southern nurses and aboriginal midwives over childbirth in her study of the government outpost nursing stations in the Arctic and Subarctic regions of Canada.[59] At times the federal nurses were sidelined in local birthing rituals but on other occasions, both midwives and their clients eagerly sought their services.

The program of health and medical treatment, education, and advice brought by the Red Cross nurses represented the ideals of white, middle-class, and especially urban-based, North American medicine, which residents of small northern towns and villages often did not accept as relevant to their own lives. The capacity of the nurses to promote concepts of health and hygiene rested not only on the relationships that they developed within their districts, but also on both the ability and desire of community members to implement the health services offered. Just as teachers had to "be at [their] diplomatic best" within the community so, too, were nurses told to use tact to convince sometimes skeptical residents of the value of 'city' suggestions around health and hygiene.[60] Recognizing that urban-trained nurses planning on working in a rural community needed special preparation, nursing leaders advised them to make friends with farmers, become knowledgeable about their interests, and "be able to call a field of grain by its proper name."[61] Nurses felt they had to break through barriers of reserve in people who were sometimes wary of outsiders and who found health visitors a "somewhat dangerous innovation."[62] Differences of class and ethnicity could hinder effective communication. By 1926, the second nurse at the Lion's Head station happily reported that no longer did the "general public" feel that "the nurse was so remote from themselves that they could have nothing in common."[63]

Individual nurses sometimes recognized the disjunction between the conditions that confronted them and the sources of their own education. Prompted to wonder if textbook writers had gained their knowledge only through "hearsay," nurse Miller quickly dropped the health rule "sleeping with the windows open." Even in winter, many residents had only "quilts or cardboard in place of glass to keep out the cold."[64] Nevertheless, she began to question her capacity to handle her job when so many Wilberforce citizens rejected her efforts at health teaching, a fact made especially galling after a short course in New York exposed her to "how much more should and could be done." She was frustrated with the beliefs of the locals that "what was good enough for their parents was good enough for them."[65] Similarly, nurse M.R.M. was rebuffed by a father who told her that he did not see why his children had to use a toothbrush, since he had never used one. She contended that she intensely disliked going into people's homes. "I had no business going there ... I don't think they thought that just because I was young, in uniform and driving a car that I was any better than anyone else."[66] Along with other public health workers, both she and Jean Birch Williamson recognized that poverty had much to do with why they both believed home visits were intrusive. Williamson acknowledged that inviting herself into homes was "not something that I did too freely, especially if you knew the people were poor and you couldn't tell anyone to go and get their children's teeth fixed."[67] Other Red Cross nurses also realized that "it [was] impossible to get corrections unless ways and means are provided, so after one visit has been made, unless the nurse is arranging to have the work done, they can't see much use in going back."[68]

Expectations of a gendered solidarity between nurses and female community members made women and their families the prime targets of public health nursing programs. As McPherson argued about the work of the Indian Health Services nurses in northern Manitoba prior to 1970, "nurses stood as front-line service providers who boasted specific professional skills [but] to make that system work ... [they] were obliged to address local health needs ... often by forging gender-based bonds with local women."[69] Many of the Red Cross nurses testified to the willingness of community women to invite them into their homes for dinners and parties. To the chagrin of some men on local hospital committees, women residents preferred to put their fundraising toward comforts for the nurses, rather than toward such needs as a new roof for the outpost.[70] Evidence suggests, however, that most close friendships appear to have been made with the educated and middle-class women attached to families of teachers, industrial managers, and the ministry. At least one nurse confessed that she had little in common with the local and more-permanent residents.[71]

In matters of maternity care, local women continued to make choices that did not always meet the nurses' expectations and were often related to poverty.[72] Since women knew that the nurses could and would not refuse to help, 'emergency' births may have been a strategy used by some to obtain professional aid in the births of their children when they were unable or unwilling to pay a doctor. Nurse Miller was a bit dismayed as she hurried through a cold winter's night to the bedside of a labouring woman. She was told that "no doctor would be needed when they were able to get me!"[73] For many women, choosing to have their children at home better enabled them to look after older children. For others, financial considerations likely played a larger role in this decision. For example, the Division charged thirty dollars for the basic ward rate for a ten-day maternity package of delivery and postpartum care in 1927.[74] Physicians' fees would have added twenty-five dollars to the bill. In contrast, the Division charged five dollars for home confinements with the outpost nurse alone. Even then, many people could not see the need for medical intervention; if husbands could attend to birthing farm animals, one nurse complained, they believed they were "just as capable of attending their wives at such a time, for, after all, wasn't it just a natural process?"[75]

Nurses' attempts to deliver the mandated programs of public health placed them in an ambiguous position. On the one hand, as both Zelmanovits and Lesley McBain note in this book, outpost nurses can be viewed as agents of state colonization efforts that were, at best, insensitive to cultures constructed as different and, at worst, a means of assimilation.[76] On the other hand, some public health measures provided real benefits in the amelioration of certain diseases, and at an individual level, many nurses demonstrated a willingness to accommodate and work with notions of health and disease held by people in their communities. By virtue of their gender, class, ethnicity, and training, however, Red Cross nurses embodied the ideals of Western scientific medicine for the dissemination of public health measures. As employees of an organization that had found legitimacy for its peacetime activities through alignment with state-sanctioned ideas on health, the Red Cross nurses stood at the centre of that transition throughout remote districts of the province, whether or not they were fully convinced of its benefits in all situations. Nonetheless, the amount and kind of nursing work around education, advice, and treatment for health-related matters that the nurses were able to carry out depended on the willingness of local people to accept both the nurse herself and her role as health educator. Not all did, and the choices residents continued to make highlight the significant role of communities in shaping delivery of the nurses' mandated programs.

Physicians and Outpost Nurses

The isolated circumstances in which the Red Cross outpost nurses often worked contributed to the sense that they enjoyed a greater professional independence than their fellows in urban institutions. Whether or not a doctor was actually present in their communities, those employed with the Ontario Division nevertheless practised under the general authority of the nearest physician or medical officer of health. The nurses' professional activities were thus bounded by the relationships that they developed with these medical colleagues. Nurses and doctors had both been schooled in the culture of the hospital workplace whose structure replicated dominant societal relationships of power. Studies in nursing history have well demonstrated that successful nursing students quickly learned the discipline of loyalty and deference demanded by their superiors in the medical 'family,' and that physicians continued to shape the labour of graduates as their bedside assistants.[77]

The Division anticipated that its outpost nurses would adhere to the familiar gendered pattern of relations with any doctors with whom they came in contact and that they would "[honour] the formal line between nursing and medical prerogatives."[78] Indeed, the success of the outpost program depended on it. The outpost directors tried to reassure rural physicians that their nurses remained under constant medical oversight, insisting that "the service we are giving ... is incomplete without a doctor's supervision."[79] The nurse's first duty on taking up her position was to meet with the nearest physician and seek standing orders for patient treatment for the times when he was unavailable. Within a day of her arrival at Wilberforce, nurse Miller made an arduous two-hour drive to the village of Haliburton to introduce herself to the two doctors there.[80]

Many of the Division's nurses developed satisfactory relationships with their local physicians, and those who enjoyed co-operation and support from them were fortunate. Supervisor McEwen, for example, was pleased with the "excellent teamwork" between the physician and the Red Cross nurse in Hornepayne in the 1930s.[81] Miller was genuinely saddened to hear of the early and unexpected death of the physician with whom she had worked for four years: "I had lost such a wonderful friend on whom I had learned to depend so much," she wrote.[82] Donna Burnside's "adrenaline flipped up a little bit" when accident victims were brought into the Mindemoya hospital in the early 1950s, but her confidence in the availability and the capabilities of the local doctor helped quell her anxieties.[83] Collegial partnerships that encompassed feelings of mutual respect and trust helped to ease the potential professional isolation experienced by both the outpost nurses and their medical associates. Despite Miller's protestations that nurses did not diagnose, Dr Frain sought her opinion as to the cause of the condition in one of his patients.[84] Romance occasionally blossomed through these friendships. Nurse Eudora Watson spent five years in close collaboration with Dr Donald Dingwall during her post-ing in the 1930s as charge nurse of the Dryden hospital. She left the Division to marry the widowed physician.[85]

Deference to medical authority, however, was often complicated by the conditions of rural practice. Stuart illustrated in her research on a group of early rural public health nurses in Ontario that professional boundaries differentiating the work of nurses and physicians often "blurred and shifted" in remote areas. Nursing labour was made more difficult when physicians were "hostile and uncooperative, or simply indifferent."[86] Nurses with the Ontario Division also experienced the frustrations of working with medical men who had not kept pace with new knowledge, who feared competition to their own hard-won liveli-hood, or who, it was intimated, had problems with alcohol or mental illness. Physicians retained authority over the direction of patient care, and nurses concerned about its quality could do little about it. One charge nurse lost weight worrying over her neglected patients "with-out the power to suggest that they go out and get outside treatment and advice when needed."[87] Whether or not a nurse agreed with a physician's actions or medical expertise, professional etiquette de-manded that she keep a discreet silence, even if she believed that she was better informed about the necessary treatment. A nurse quietly complained to one supervisor over the physician's diagnosis in the death of a child; the doctor had prescribed for asthma, but the nurse was positive that the illness was diphtheria.[88] Another physician ap-peared to be popular in his community, but the staff saw him as "quite temperamental and with only fair technique in the operating room."[89] In some instances, nurses believed that they had to protect their patients from physicians whose medical expertise they considered questionable. In one outpost, a former Toronto Western Hospital stu-dent testified that nurses would wait until the last minute to call the physician for a delivery, hoping that it was too late and they could look after the women themselves.[90] Two other nurses whom I interviewed related 'off the record' that their surgeon attempted procedures in the 1960s and 70s that were far too complicated for their small hospital.

Some physicians were overtly uncongenial, fearing that nurses' community work encroached on their authority, their influence, and their income. Reinforcing the subordinate position that gender and occupation imposed on nurses, one urban medical man believed that public health nurses would be "happier if they had some actual nursing to do," and contended that they threatened to undermine the association between physicians and families on which he believed doctors' survival depended.[91] Immunizations appeared to be one of the more problematic issues. For example, the attempt by the provincial government to provide free toxoid for the mass immunization of schoolchildren against diphtheria represented, for many physicians, state interference in medical practice.[92] Doctors in rural areas perceived it as a threat to their economic well-being, in part because the procedure necessitated three separate trips to schoolchildren who were found only in small, widely scattered schools. Nurse Georgina Gladbach reported in frustration that she "gets less cooperation from [the doctor in Callander] than from any other physician"; she had not been able to persuade [him] to give toxoid in his municipalities "unless he is paid for it."[93] Other physicians appeared to resist the concept of public health nursing entirely. The nurses in Lion's Head, believing that the local physician resented the Red Cross moving into his area, complained that he "flies into rages with the nurse for no apparent reason [and] is not interested in public health." According to their reports throughout the 1930s, he immunized only those children whose parents could afford to pay, allowed children with infectious diseases to return to school without waiting for the quarantine period to expire, refused to co-operate with other physicians who offered free remedial operations, and did not think that it was the nurses' place to know about patients with tuberculosis, syphilis, or gonorrhea. Blaming the failed relationship on their own personalities and "much discouraged about the public health work," nurse after nurse requested a transfer, hoping that her successor would be able to break the impasse in the district.[94]

Personal problems of physicians also required tactful handling. Reading between the lines of the supervisors' reports, it appears that doctors struggled with alcoholism, mental illness, and possibly drug abuse. "The medical man is good when on the job but has regular bouts when he is not on duty," wrote McEwen on a visit to Beardmore.[95] She also regretted that in Hornepayne, "the medical situation is similar to that in so many other small centres [where] the one medical man has one bad fault, which means that he does not go near the hospital for days at a time." The extra demands on the nurse occurred

not just because of her added responsibilities in patient care, McEwencontinued, but attempting to quell the "great feeling of unrest" had
to be accomplished without irritating or antagonizing the doctor
"who is apt to think she is interfering with his practice."[96] In these
cases, nurses had to carry on as best as they could, diplomatically
buffering the discontent arising from disgruntled patients whose appointments were not kept or treatments begun. They were compelled
to use tact, engage in a great deal of diplomatic manoeuvring, and find
ways to "make [nursing] recommendations sound like nonrecom-
mendations." In what has been dubbed the 'doctor-nurse game,'
nurses needed to offer information in such a manner that appeared
not to threaten physician authority.[97] For example, when confronted
with patients she considered too sick for the outpost to handle, Marion
Sedgwick could "usually *cajole* [the doctors] into getting the patient
out to a larger centre." Despite her intimate knowledge of the condition of the patient and the depth of her experience, the necessary
coaxing of physicians suggests that direct communication from the
nurses would not have been welcomed. At the same time, Sedgwick
recognized that the success of these strategies rested ultimately on
physicians accepting the information that nurses had to offer. "It was
fine if you could boss the doctor," she continued, "but if you could-
n't boss him, you could be in deep trouble."[98] Nicely illuminating the
gendered power dynamics in play, her words also reveal that she understood the limits of the relationship.

Despite recognizing the need for circumspection in relations between doctors and patients, the Red Cross supervisors expected the
field nurses to monitor the use of the outpost hospitals. They admonished nursing staff to prevent physicians from admitting long-term or
non-emergency patients, from performing elective surgery beyond the
support capabilities of the outpost facilities, or from treating the outposts in any other way as their private hospitals. The nurses were thus
forced to negotiate the political minefield of gender and authority,
striking a delicate balance between acquiescing to the demands of local
doctors, with whom they often had to work closely, and acknowledging the wishes of their supervisors from head office, who employed
them. The nursing supervisors were aware of and sometimes sympathetic to the situation in which this placed the nurses. Brand reprimanded nurse Phillips at Hawk Junction for allowing the doctor to

conduct a post-mortem examination in the bathroom of the small hospital. She commented that "[the doctor] is very fond of the present staff – mainly because he has his way in everything. In Mrs Phillips' desire to keep things going smoothly, she has not disagreed with him in any particular."[99] Even though the status of the supervisors as nurse-managers provided them with substantial authority within the Division, both their gender and the fact that they were also nurses mitigated against their power to influence the behaviour of physicians in the community. Supervisor Brand was incensed at the chaos she found at the Atikokan outpost in 1944. The outpost was overfilled with workers with minor injuries, some of whom had outside privileges, and the physician could see nothing wrong with the staff nurse preparing to give up her own bed for a maternity case. Brand reported that the doctor had taken advantage of the nurses for too long, but confronting him produced only personal recriminations and threats to quit admitting any patients at all.

The interaction of gender and the power of physicians provided nurses with only a limited number of options to resolve these types of conflicts. Calling the facility a "blot on the reputation of Red Cross outpost hospitals," Brand's angry account revealed not only her frustration, but also her comprehension of the boundaries of her authority. "As long as we operate this outpost, and [the doctor] is still here, we shall have to choose between staffing the place with an efficient nurse who insists on operating the place properly – thereby incurring [the doctor's] displeasure – or staffing it with a nurse who likes [him] and takes all orders from him and who practically turns it into a home away from home for him."[100]

Implying in this exchange that the behaviour of the nurse was also at fault, Brand nevertheless realized the impossible situation in which the doctor's conduct placed her. Supervisors could only transfer nurses in the hope that a new staff member with a different combination of maturity and experience would resolve the situation. In extreme situations, where it appeared that both patient and staff safety were compromised, the only recourse was to close the outpost. In the late 1950s, the charge nurse of the Hornepayne hospital was frightened by the alleged neglect of several patients, which resulted in the death of one and only "luck" in the survival of another. She complained to Singer of what she believed was the physician's incompetence and what she saw as his total inconsideration of her staff as he pushed to build up a surgical practice for "mercenary" gain. Despite Singer's repeated attempts to reason with the doctor over the inadequacies of the facility for planned surgery, he refused to comply. Powerless to remove him, the supervisors had no choice but to shut the hospital when the nurses eventually resigned, leaving the citizens of Hornepayne temporarily without emergency medical facilities. A "discreet inquiry" of this doctor was planned, but physicians in administrative positions with the health department, the Ontario Hospital Services Commission, and the College of Physicians and Surgeons of Ontario who were aware of the case agreed with the Division's decision to publicize a "nursing shortage" as the official reason for closure.[101]

+++

With fewer resources at their disposal, Red Cross outpost nurses undertook a wider variety of duties and responsibilities than did their urban colleagues, and they both lived and worked without the close supervision encountered in institutional settings. They thus seemingly enjoyed an enhanced professional autonomy around which they could organize their work. However, as this essay has demonstrated, outpost nursing was complex – created and produced through a web of intricate social relationships of gender, race, class, and power. As fellow female colleagues, supervisors offered welcome support to workers in the field, but at the same time, were ever mindful that all nursing activities reflected well on the Red Cross in its search to become a legitimate peacetime organization involved in health care. Many patients sought out the medical acute-care services that the nurses provided, but were often unwilling or unable to meet the white, urban, middle-class standards of public health that the nurses promoted. Still politically subordinate to medical authority, the scope and character of the work that the nurses were able to carry out often depended on the co-operation and assistance that they received from local physicians. To meet the demands of these inter-professional relationships without alienating their superiors, the physicians, or the patients upon whom the outpost services depended brought nurses up against the limits of workplace autonomy and authority.

Nursing administrators and policy-makers today are still occupied with fixing professional status, and continue to formulate strategies to help identify and articulate the unique characteristics of nursing work within the health care system. A recent major Canadian study examined the nature of nurses practising in remote districts of the country. Outlining an interdisciplinary gulf between historical research and current social policy analysis and development, none of the references upon which the authors based their investigation acknowledged the growing body of literature on the history of rural nursing in Canada or elsewhere.[102] Their research identified problems around increased nursing responsibilities, the lack of adequate resources and infrastructure, the difficulties in maintaining standards of nursing practice, and the disparity between urban-based theory and rural realities – all factors that historians of outpost nursing have well outlined in their investigations of outpost nursing in the past. Although the final report noted that the "interconnections between rural nurses and their context was most apparent" and highlighted "the importance of community in shaping the nurses' work lives and everyday practices,"[103] the components of that context were not made clear. As this study has recognized in the case of the Red Cross outpost nurses, nursing work had to be continually negotiated and renegotiated within parameters determined by contexts of gender, race, and class, which shaped both ideologies and material practices of employers, community members, and physician colleagues, as well as those of the nurses themselves.

NOTES

I am grateful to the Social Sciences and Humanities Research Council of Canada for financial support of the research and writing of this article.

1 Audrey Woodget, "Seldom a Dull Moment." In J. Karen Scott with Joan E. Kieser, eds., *Northern Nurses: True Nursing Adventures from Canada's North*, 43–44 (Oakville, ON: Kokum Publications, 2002).

2 For autobiographical and biographical narratives, see Elliott Merrick, *Northern Nurse* (Halifax: Nimbus Publishing, 1942, reprinted 1994); B.J. Banfill, *Labrador Nurse* (Toronto: Ryerson Press, 1952); Irene Stewart, *These Were Our Yesterdays: A History of District Nursing in Alberta* (Altona, MB: D.W. Friesen and Sons, 1979); J. Karen Scott, *Northern Nurses II: More Nursing Adventures from Canada's North* (Oakville, ON: Kokum Publications, 2005). For accounts of outpost nursing services, see Sharon Richardson, "Frontier Health Care: Alberta's

District and Municipal Nursing Services, 1919 to 1976," in *Alberta History* (Winter 1998): 2–9; Laurie Meijer Drees and Lesley McBain, "Nursing and Native Peoples in Northern Saskatchewan: 1930s–1950s," in *Canadian Bulletin of Medical History/Bulletin canadien d'histoire de la médecine (CBMH/BCHM)* 18 (2001): 43–65; Nicole Rousseau and Johanne Daigle, "Medical Service to Settlers: The Gestation and Establishment of a Nursing Service in Quebec, 1932–1943," in *Nursing History Review* 8 (2000): 95–116.

3 For an overview of the field in Canada, see Dianne Dodd, Jayne Elliott, and Nicole Rousseau, "Outpost Nursing in Canada." In Christina Bates, Dianne Dodd, and Nicole Rousseau, eds., *On All Frontiers: Four Centuries of Canadian Nursing*, 139–52 (Ottawa: CMC and University of Ottawa Press, 2005).

4 Mary Anne Poutanen, "'Unless she gives better satisfaction': Teachers, Protestant Education, and Community in Rural Quebec, Lochaber and Gore District, 1863–1945," in *Historical Studies in Education* 15 (2003): 261–7; Paul J. Stortz and J. Donald Wilson, "Education on the Frontier: Schools, Teachers and Community Influence in North-Central British Columbia," in *Histoire Sociale/Social History* 26 (1993): 265–90; J. Donald Wilson, "'I Am Here to Help If You Need Me': British Columbia's Rural Teachers' Welfare Officer, 1928–1934," in *Journal of Canadian Studies* 25 (1990): 94–118.

5 Gertrude LeRoy Miller, *Mustard Plasters and Handcars: Through the Eyes of a Red Cross Outpost Nurse* (Toronto: Natural Heritage Books, 2000).

6 Kathryn McPherson, *Bedside Matters: The Transformation of Canadian Nursing, 1900–1990* (Oxford and New York: Oxford University Press, 1996); Susan M. Reverby, *Ordered to Care: The Dilemma of American Nursing, 1850–1945* (New York: Cambridge University Press, 1987); Barbara Melosh, *"The Physician's Hand": Work Culture and Conflict in American Nursing* (Philadelphia: Temple University Press, 1982).

7 J. Karen Scott, "Foreword," *Northern Nurses*, n.p.

8 Eliot Freidson, *Profession of Medicine: A Study of the Sociology of Applied Knowledge* (New York: Dodd, Mead and Co., 1970).

9 Celia Davies, *Gender and the Professional Predicament in Nursing* (Buckingham and Philadelphia: Open University Press, 1995), 133. For a brief outline of the complex nature of professional autonomy for nurses in Canada, see Bernard Blishen, *Doctors in Canada: The Changing World of Medical Practice* (Toronto: University of Toronto Press, 1991), 107–10. For other perspectives on nursing as a profession, see Fred E. Katz, "Nurses." In Amitai Etzioni, ed., *The Semi-Professions and Their Organization*, 54–81 (London: Collier-MacMillan, 1969);

Mary Kinnear, *In Subordination: Professional Women 1870–1970* (Montreal & Kingston: McGill-Queen's University Press, 1995).

10 For example, see Celia Davies, "Professionalizing Strategies as Time- and Culture-Bound: American and British Nursing, Circa 1893." In Ellen Condliffe Lagemann, ed., *Nursing History: New Perspectives, New Possibilities*, 47–63 (New York and London: Teachers College Press, 1983); Kate Gerrish, Mike McManus, and Peter Ashworth, "Creating What Sort of Professional? Master's Level Nurse Education as a Professionalizing Strategy," in *Nursing Inquiry* 10 (2003): 103–12.

11 These debates are far from over. For one example, see Sioban Nelson and Suzanne Gordon, eds., *The Complexities of Care: Nursing Reconsidered* (Ithica and London: Cornell University Press, 2006)

12 McPherson, *Bedside Matters*, 9–10.

13 Meryn Stuart, "Shifting Professional Boundaries: Gender Conflict in Public Health 1920–1925." In Dianne Dodd and Deborah Gorham, eds., *Caring and Curing: Historical Perspectives on Women and Healing in Canada*, 49–70 (Ottawa: University of Ottawa, 1994). See also her "'Half a Loaf is Better than No Bread': Public Health Nurses and Physicians in Ontario, 1920–1925," in *Nursing Research* 41 (January–February 1992): 21–7, as well as "Ideology and Experience: Public Health Nursing and the Ontario Rural Child Welfare Project, 1920–25," in *CBMH/BCHM* 6 (1989): 111–31.

14 Jill Samfya Perry, "Nursing for the Grenfell Mission: Maternal and Moral Reform in Northern Newfoundland and Labrador, 1894–1938," MA thesis (St John's: Memorial University, 1997).

15 Perry, "Nursing for the Grenfell Mission," 127, 138–9.

16 Judith Zelmanovits, "'Midwife Preferred': Maternity Care in Outpost Nursing Stations in Northern Canada, 1945–1988." In Georgina Feldberg, Molly Ladd-Taylor, Alison Li, and Kathryn McPherson, eds., *Women, Health and Nation: Canada and the United States since 1945*, 161–88 (Montreal & Kingston: McGill-Queen's University Press, 2003); Kathryn McPherson, "Nursing and Colonization: The Work of Indian Health Services Nurses in Manitoba, 1945–1970." In *Women, Health and Nation*, 223–46. For an American example, see Emily K. Abel, "'We Are Left So Much Alone to Work Out Our Own Problems': Nurses on American Indian Reservations during the 1930s," in *Nursing History Review* 4 (1996): 43–64.

17 Helen E. Harrison, "'In the Picture of Health': Portraits of Health, Disease and Citizenship in Canada's Public Health Advice Literature, 1920–1960," PhD dis-

sertation (Kingston: Queen's University, 2001); Judith Walzer Leavitt, *Typhoid Mary: Captive of the Public's Health* (Boston: Beacon, 1996). See also Elizabeth Toon, "Selling the Public on Public Health: The Commonwealth and Milbank Health Demonstrations and the Meaning of Community Health Education." In Ellen Condliffe Lagemann, ed., *Philanthropic Foundations: New Scholarship, New Possibilities*, 119–30 (Bloomington and Indianapolis: Indiana University Press, 1999).

18 Dorothy Porter, *Health, Civilization and the State* (London and New York: Routledge, 1999), 7.

19 *Canadian Red Cross Annual Report*, 1920, 31.

20 The figures quoted in the following section were based on staffing lists published in the Ontario Division's annual reports, but calculations from them can only be considered approximate. The outpost program continued until 1984, but since the reports stopped listing the names in 1969, I have obviously missed some nurses. For names that do not appear consecutively, I also have no way of knowing whether the nurse took a break from employment with the Division during the time that her name does not appear, or whether she was relieving somewhere else and missed being counted. Some married nurses may also have been counted twice because I was not able to correlate unmarried and married nurses.

21 McPherson, *Bedside Matters*, 115–29 and 205–19.

22 McPherson, *Bedside Matters*, 116, n.2 and 214. One source estimated that about 70 per cent of the almost 237,000 nurses employed in Canada by 1986 were married. Pat Armstrong, Jacqueline Choiniere, and Elaine Day, *Vital Signs: Nursing in Transition* (Toronto: Garamond Press, 1993), 10. The entry of married women into nursing was a North-American-wide phenomenon. For American rates, see Susan Rimby Leighow, "An 'Obligation to Participate': Married Nurses' Labor Force Participation in the 1950s." In Joanne Meyerowitz, ed., *Not June Cleaver: Women and Gender in Postwar America 1945–1960*, 38 (Philadelphia: Temple University Press, 1994).

23 Library and Archives Canada (LAC), Louise de Kiriline Lawrence papers, MG31, J18, Vol. 11, File 11-19, Letter to her mother, 19 November 1927. My translation from the original Swedish.

24 See Miller, *Mustard Plasters and Handcars*.

25 On nurse-midwifery's "'alegal'" status in Canada, see Zelmanovits, "'Midwife Preferred,'" 165 and 183, n. 22. For an examination of the laws pertaining to midwifery in Ontario, see Jutta Mason, "A History of Midwifery in Canada," in *Report of the Task Force on the Implementation of Midwifery in Ontario*, 1987, 206–9. Newfoundland followed the British system and chose to regulate

nurse-midwifery through courses of varying lengths. See Joyce Nevitt, *White Caps and Black Bands: Nursing in Newfoundland to 1934* (St. John's, NF: Jesperson Press, 1978); Edgar House, *The Way Out: The Story of NONIA, 1920–1990* (St. John's, NF: Creative Publishers, 1990). After 1919, nurses in Alberta were allowed to practise midwifery only in remote areas without physicians. See Sharon Richardson, "Political Women, Professional Nurses, and the Creation of Alberta's District Nursing Service, 1919–1925," in *Nursing History Review* 6 (1998): 25–50.

26 Letter from Maude Weaver to her sister, Gwennie, 1 November, likely 1933. Photocopy in possession of author. Her care of this patient was remarkably similar to that of Dr Harold Geggie, a rural physician who practised from 1911 to 1965. See Jayne Elliott, "'Endormez Moi!' An Early Twentieth-Century Obstetrical Practice in the Gatineau Valley, Quebec," MA thesis (Ottawa: Carleton University, 1997).

27 Miller, *Mustard Plasters and Handcars*, 25.

28 Telephone interview, C.S.A., 2 May 2000.

29 Telephone interview, C.S., 9 April 2000.

30 Ontario Zone, Canadian Red Cross Society, Mississauga (OZM), Hospitals Department Files, Apsley, 2–4 October 1945.

31 OZM, Hospitals Department Files, Atikokan, 8–9 January 1935.

32 OZM, Hospitals Department Files, Thessalon, 23 February 1932.

33 Letter from Barbara Jones to author, 11 May 2000.

34 OZM, Hospitals Department Files, Kakabeka Falls, 5–7 January 1935.

35 Telephone interview, Dorothy Bauer, 12 April 2000.

36 Interview, J.F., Ottawa, 15 February 2000.

37 OZM, Hospitals Department Files, Hornepayne, 14–15 March 1931.

38 OZM, Hospitals Department Files, Apsley, 21–23 October 1944.

39 For a similar attitude to nurses at the Grenfell Mission, see Perry, "Nursing for the Grenfell Mission," 104–6.

40 OZM, Hospitals Department Files, Jellicoe, 2–4 May 1942.

41 OZM, Hospitals Department Files, Thessalon, 19 July 1933.

42 OZM, Hospitals Department Files, Thessalon, 15 March 1934.

43 OZM, Hospitals Department Files, Hawk Junction, 15–17 June 1943.

44 OZM, Hospitals Department Files, Apsley, 21–23 October 1944.

45 OZM, Hospitals Department Files, Englehart, 21–24 January 1950.

46 Telephone interview, B.T., 6 June 2000.

47 Interview, Dorothy Baxter Rowat, Ottawa, 20 November 2003.

48 OZM, Hospitals Department Files, Hornepayne, 26 October 1936.

49 Telephone interview, Be.T., 5 March 2000.

50 Telephone interview, Marion Sedgwick, 28 March 2000.

51 OZM, Hospitals Department Files, Atikokan, 23–24 February 1934.

52 OZM, Hospitals Department Files, Coe Hill, likely 1932.

53 OZM, Hospitals and Department Files, Thessalon, 5–9 December 1948.

54 OZM, Fergus Cronin, "History of Red Cross Hospitals in Ontario," unpublished manuscript held at the Canadian Red Cross Society, Ontario Zone, Mississauga, 1981, 3:10.

55 For instance, see Kathryn McPherson, "'The Case of the Kissing Nurse': Femininity, Sexuality, and Canadian Nursing, 1900–1970." In Kathryn McPherson, Cecilia Morgan, and Nancy M. Forestell, eds., *Gendered Pasts: Historical Essays in Femininity and Masculinity in Canada*, 189–90 (Toronto: Oxford University Press, 1999). For a brief discussion of this same phenomenon outside North America, see Sheryl Nestel, "(Administering Angels: Colonial Nursing and the Extension of Empire," in *Journal of Medical Humanities* 19 (1998): 265. Not all nurses found the uniform to be protective. A New Brunswick Red Cross nurse wrote to her supervisor about a terrifying taxi ride she had experienced. The driver refused to take her where she wanted to go and instead headed out of town on a dark and lonely road. She managed to escape from the moving car, but when the driver pursued her, she kicked off her shoes and ran along the railway tracks until she reached the first house she saw. See Bronwyn McIntyre, *A History of Red Cross Outposts in New Brunswick, 1922–1975* (New Brunswick Division of the Canadian Red Cross Society, n.d.), 36–7.

56 Interview, Margaret Maclachlan, Cornwall, 10 February 2000.

57 Stuart, "Ideology and Experience," 118.

58 Abel, "'We Are Left So Much Alone to Work Out Our Own Problems," 46–9.

59 Zelmanovits, "'Midwife Preferred,'" 161–88.

60 Stortz and Wilson, "Education on the Frontier," 285.

61 N. Edna Howey, "The Rural Relationships of the Public Health Nurse," in *Canadian Public Health Journal* 26, 2 (1935): 94.

62 Adelaide Plumptre, "The Effect of a Red Cross Nursing Outpost on a Community," in *Canadian Red Cross Bulletin* (December 1926): 9.

63 Myrtle Scott, "The Changes in Attitude in the Community of Lion's Head Towards the Outpost from September 1925 to September 1926." In *Fifty Years of Service: A Profile of a Small Red Cross Branch in Ontario*, compiled by Maitland Warder, 17 (Lion's Head Red Cross Branch: Lion's Head, 1981).

64 Miller, *Mustard Plasters and Handcars*, 58–9.

65 Miller, *Mustard Plasters and Handcars*, 94.

66 Telephone interview, M.R.M., 30 March 2000.

67 Interview, Jean Birch Williamson, Mindemoya, 9 May 2000. Rural nurses in general were confronted with the realization that the effects of poverty thwarted their best efforts in health reform. See *Public Board of Health of Ontario Annual Reports*, 1927, 64; also Cynthia Comacchio Abeele, "'The Mothers of the Land Must Suffer': Child and Maternal Welfare in Rural and Outpost Ontario, 1918–1940," in *Ontario History* 80 (1988): 191.

68 Archives of Ontario (AO), RG 10, 30-A-3, Box 16, File 16.5, Public Health Nursing Field Reports, public health supervisor N.E. Howey's report on visit to Apsley, Wilberforce, Bancroft, Coe Hill, and Whitney, June 1935.

69 McPherson, "Nursing and Colonization," 240.

70 OZM, Hospital Department Files, Thessalon, 30 October 1924.

71 Interview, Margaret Maclachlan, 10 February 2000.

72 For other examples of women's choices in matters of health and medical care, see Denyse Baillargeon, "Care of Mothers and Infants in Montreal Between the Wars: The Visiting Nurses of Metropolitan Life, Les Gouttes de lait, and Assistance maternelle." In Dianne Dodd and Deborah Gorham, eds., *Caring and Curing: Historical Perspectives on Women and Healing in Canada*, 163–81 (Ottawa: University of Ottawa, 1994); Ellen Ross, *Love and Toil: Motherhood in Outcast London, 1870–1918* (New York & Oxford: Oxford University Press, 1993), 195–221.

73 Miller, *Mustard Plasters and Handcars*, 66.

74 OZM, Hospitals Department Files, Kirkland Lake, "Schedule of Rates for Red Cross Hospitals for 1927." For patients who did not qualify as indigent but who would have been hard pressed to pay even the basic rate, the fee could be reduced to fifteen dollars. It is not clear if these rates would have been the same for the smaller nursing outposts, but Gertrude LeRoy Miller noted the five-dollar rate for a home confinement with the nurse at Wilberforce in the early 1930s.

75 Miller, *Mustard Plasters and Handcars*, 160.

76 See also Mary-Ellen Kelm, *Colonizing Bodies: Aboriginal Health and Healing in British Columbia, 1900–50* (Vancouver: UBC Press, 1998), and many of the articles in Katie Pickles and Myra Rutherdale, eds. *Contact Zones: Aboriginal and Settler Women in Canada's Colonial Past* (Vancouver: UBC Press, 2005).

77 For examples, see McPherson, *Bedside Matters*; 15–16; Reverby, *Ordered to Care*, 30–76.

78 Melosh, *"The Physician's Hand,"* 114.

79 Maude Wilkinson, "The Rural Community and the Nursing Outpost," in *Public Health Journal* 17 (1926): 580.

80 It is unknown how many other nurses followed this procedure or, indeed, how possible it was for them to do so, especially in areas like Atikokan with no roads and only the railway telegraph line available for outside communication.

81 OZM, Hospitals Department Files, Hornepayne, McEwen, 15 June 1935.

82 Miller, *Mustard Plasters and Handcars*, 174.

83 Telephone interview, Donna Burnside, 20 July 2000.

84 Miller, *Mustard Plasters and Handcars*, 156.

85 "Dr Donald G. Dingwall's Career at Dryden," *The Glengarry News*, 6 June 1957, 6, col. 4 & 5.

86 Stuart, "Shifting Professional Boundaries," 58. My research on this section closely parallels Stuart's discussion on relations between rural physicians and the early public health nurses she studied.

87 OZM, Hospitals Department Files, 14–15 June 1935.

88 AO, RG10, 30-A-3, Box 16, File 16.10, Public Health Field Reports, Lion's Head, 3–5 June 1936.

89 OZM, Hospitals Department Files, Hawk Junction, McEwen, 18–19 May 1942.

90 Personal communication from J.S., Toronto Western Hospital (TWH) graduate of 1958, 24 March 2000. From 1952 until the hospital school of nursing closed in the early 1970s, nursing students from TWH were sent to the Red Cross outposts in Ontario for one month of outpost experience.

91 A.M. Jeffrey, "How the Private Physician Looks at Public Health Nursing," in *The Canadian Nurse* 29 (1933): 33–4.

92 Jay Cassel, "Public Health in Canada." In Dorothy Porter, ed., *The History of Public Health and the Modern State*, 294 (London: Wellcome Institute Series in the History of Medicine, 1994). The Ontario government supplied physicians with diphtheria antitoxin from the late 1890s on, and the toxoid following 1910.

93 AO, RG 10, 30-A-3, Box 16, File 16.7, Public Health Nursing Field Reports, Callander, 27 November 1935.

94 AO, RG 10, 30-A-3, Box 16, File 16.10, Public Health Field Reports, Lion's Head, 21–22 May 1934; 3–5 June 1936; 4–6 April 1939.

95 OZM, Hospitals Department Files, Beardmore, 13 November 1945.

96 OZM, Hospitals Department Files, Hornepayne, McEwen, 14–16 November 1945.

97 See Thetis M. Group and Joan I. Roberts, *Nursing, Physician Control and the Medical Monopoly* (Bloomington and Indianapolis: Indiana University Press, 2001), 165–8 and 195; McPherson, *Bedside Matters*, 240. The primary source upon which their discussions are based is a classic article by Leonard Stein, "The

Doctor-Nurse Game," in *Archives of General Psychiatry* 16 (1967): 699–703. For another example of the "game," see Stuart, "Shifting Professional Boundaries," 63–4.

98 Telephone interview, Marion Sedgwick, 28 March 2000. Emphasis mine.

99 OZM, Hospitals Department Files, Hawk Junction, 15–17 June 1953.

100 OZM, Hospitals Department Files, Atikokan, 15–17 June 1944.

101 AO, RG 10-154, MS6041, Hospitals and Institutions Central Files, Letter to Helen Singer from charge nurse, 10 October 1959; Report on Hornepayne from Singer, 4–6 November 1959; Report on Hornepayne from Irma McCallum, 14–17 November 1959; Memo from Dr J.B. Neilson, commissioner of the OHSC, 21 November 1959.

102 Martha L.P. MacLeod, J. Roger Pitblado, Judith C. Kulig, Marian Knock, and Norma J. Stewart, "The Nature of Nursing Practice in Rural and Remote Canada," in *Canadian Nurse* 100 (June 2004): 27–31.

103 Martha L.P. MacLeod et al, "The Nature of Nursing Practice in Rural and Remote Canada," Final Report to Canadian Health Services Research Foundation (14 September 2004), 13. Accessed at www.chsrf.ca/final_research/ogc/pdf/macleod_final.pdf on 11 December 2008.

10

+++++

Caring, Curing, and Socialization: The Ambiguities of
Nursing in Northern Saskatchewan, 1944–57

LESLEY McBAIN

That day at Norma Redbird's was the first time I really began
wondering about a lot of things. Someone was lying and I wasn't
sure who. Miss Jackson (nursing instructor) told us that part of
Indian culture was close family ties, and that was why they lived
in such cramped quarters ... Bullshit! They were poor. They had
no jobs. And nothing to do all day but watch reruns. And nothing
to do tomorrow either. No prospects. I had never seen or tasted
poverty before and it scared me ... what did she know about
Indians or family ties, or poverty or culture? All that garbage
about rumpus rooms and fruit cellars ... me standing there with
my Canada Food Guide and sunburned nose, telling them their
house was dirty or their food disgusting. Who the hell did I
think I was?[1]

The excerpt from *The Occupation of Heather Rose* draws on the personal observations of playwright Wendy Lill. The play illustrates the
poverty and despair of the native population and the demoralization
of the non-Aboriginal individual as seen through the eyes of an ide-
alistic, although reflective, southern nurse.[2] When asked how successful she had been in bringing change to the northern community
where she worked, another nurse expressed similar feelings: "I don't
think you should try and change it [Indian lifestyle], I think you
should try and help them and I don't think the Indian people want

white people's houses. I think they think we're crazy, scrubbing and working all the time when you can sweep the dirt down between the boards and in the summer you just move your tent around. I think a lot of them resent it because then they feel they have to work and do things and it's not their way. They want to sit around and visit and do whatever they please."[3]

Although the above quotes are from two very different sources, they both speak to the fact that introducing health care to northern, predominantly Aboriginal communities involved more than providing care. Health care services were based on humanitarian need and a genuine concern for people's welfare in remote northern areas of Canada,[4] but they also served the needs of the state[5] by drawing the primarily Aboriginal population into mainstream Canada, a complex process for both patients and nurses.

There is little argument that the goal of the Canadian state following the Second World War was to dismantle and refashion Aboriginal people's societies, with the expectation that they would be assimilated into Canadian society.[6] In Northern Saskatchewan, nursing was one of many institutions introduced into the region to modernize and improve people's lives. But inappropriate programs and inadequate support from the south hindered the process of modernization in the north, and resulted in a colonial relationship between the two regions. Nurses played an ambiguous role: they cared and cured, but they also contributed to changing the way people lived in order to improve their health. The question is: what was involved in the socialization process and what role did the nurses play in shaping the region? In particular, did their socialization activities reinforce the colonial-like relations that had emerged? Based on these questions, the purpose of this essay is to examine the role of nurses as harbingers of social change in Northern Saskatchewan between 1944 and 1957.

I begin with a brief historical overview of the study area, and the sources of data used in the research. Second, I situate the essay within the theoretical frameworks pertaining to various dimensions of colonialism.[7] Third, I present empirical evidence to highlight the contradictory nature of nursing practices and illustrate the dual role that nurses played as agents of change and also as recipients of the same colonial attitudes exhibited by government administrators toward the region in general.

Prior to the onset of large-scale resource development following the Second World War, residents of Northern Saskatchewan experienced little exposure to modern industrial development. Early excursions into the area associated with the fur trade brought about few changes as the activity was integrated into existing ways of life. However, trading did influence where and how people lived, and included economic domination by the Hudson's Bay Company (HBC) and psychological domination by the churches. By the early 1900s, interest and government involvement in the region included yearly visits by a single RCMP officer and an Indian agent. Even the period between the two world wars saw only a handful of provincial and federal civil employees become permanent residents in the area.[8] Following the Second World War, the region's relative isolation changed dramatically when growing energy demands, the "roads to resources" program, and government economic and social programs were introduced to northern residents. The proliferation and scale at which post-war institutions and programs were implemented was vastly different from what had taken place previously, and affected almost every aspect of life in the north.[9]

When Northern Saskatchewan became formalized as a region in 1944, living conditions for the population – primarily of Aboriginal descent – were appalling. Educational and medical facilities were lacking. There was little decent housing, communication and transportation systems were inadequate, and there was an almost complete absence of government-run social services. It is into this landscape of hardship that public health nurses were introduced.

Data Sources and Interpretation

This research is based on two archival collections that document the experiences of nurses working at nursing stations located in Northern Saskatchewan. The first collection consists of letters written between nurses working at outpost hospitals in Northern Saskatchewan and their supervisors in Regina from 1944 to the mid-1950s. These documents are housed in the Saskatchewan Archives at the University of Saskatchewan in Saskatoon. The records show that twenty public health nurses worked at the nursing posts between 1944 and 1957, with only eight in the north at any given time.

The second source of information is thirty-four taped interviews conducted by Joy Duncan in the mid-1970s. Ms Duncan secured a Canada Council grant, travelled across the country, and recorded the experiences of nurses who worked in the outpost hospital system. Ms Duncan donated all of the materials to the Glenbow Museum in Calgary.

Theoretical Framework: Colonialism in Canada

Finding an appropriate framework that guides inquiry into northern Canada has plagued the research process, leaving researchers to use conventional theories and make adjustments along the way.[10] The continuing absence of a model, however, is not necessarily detrimental because no single framework can adequately explain the complex situation for individual communities.[11] In Northern Saskatchewan, attempts to modernize the region involved the introduction of a number of under-resourced institutions and programs that left the territory and its people in a subordinate position to those in the south. Therefore, I combine aspects of two 'made-in-Canada' variations of colonialism – internal and bureaucratic – to examine the outcome of modernization more closely.

There are numerous definitions of colonialism. According to Johnston, colonialism is "the establishment and maintenance of rule, for an extended period of time, by a sovereign power over a subordinate and alien people."[12] Laliberte et al. define colonialism as "the various economic, political, and social policies by which an imperial power maintains or extends its control over other areas or peoples."[13] A similar definition is provided by geographers Knox and Marston, who define the process as "the establishment and maintenance of political and legal domination by a state over a separate and alien society."[14] Wilkins describes colonialism as "the establishment of domination over a geographically external political unit most often inhabited by people of a different race or culture."[15] These definitions provide a helpful framework for exploring colonial relations, particularly at the international level. Yet, they do not begin to reflect the multiple forms of colonialism. Willems-Braun argues that there really is "no global theory of colonial culture, only localized theories and historically specific accounts that provide insights into colonial practices."[16] Furthermore, colonization takes place on a number of levels with many dimensions of oppression involved in the subjugation of people.[17]

These models of colonialism are used most often to explain the economic and social-welfare disparities between developed and less-developed countries. Application of such frameworks to the relationship that evolved between the Canadian state and Aboriginal peoples and their communities can be problematic, because the social and political patterns in Canada differ from those of Third World countries. Furthermore, some Aboriginal individuals take exception to being thought of as 'colonized' because it portrays them as victims, and does not account for differences between various 'colonial' voices (e.g., Slezkine).[18] Conversely, there are those who believe that Aboriginal peoples in Canada were "unquestioningly colonized," resulting in their marginalization within Canadian society.[19]

The majority of the population in Northern Saskatchewan is of Aboriginal descent, which, as Wilkins points out, raises different questions with respect to colonialism.[20] Therefore, the Aboriginal peoples who are a majority in the region are critical to any discussion of colonialism. However, I extend the discussion to show how internal colonial processes also affected non-Aboriginal peoples (i.e., the nurses). By doing so, I join the increasing number of scholars who are examining the notion of internal colonialism in Canada in an effort to find an appropriate theoretical model that fits the history and circumstances of northern regions.[21] To explore dimensions of colonialism within the northern Canadian milieu, I draw from the work of David Quiring and Toby Morantz, who speak to different dimensions of colonialism.[22]

Quiring's research pertains directly to Northern Saskatchewan. His comprehensive study examines the various agencies such as the churches, fur traders, and governments that, over time, tried to control Northern Saskatchewan. The Co-operative Commonwealth Federation (CCF) government was elected to power in 1944 with the expectation that social programs would be extended to the north and conditions for the area's residents would improve. Consequently, a considerable effort was put into modernizing the region, which included replacing the traditional Aboriginal way of life with new and different ways of living. Change did take place in the region, but the government failed to address the overall needs of the people, leaving them vulnerable and with little power to compete with a foreign infrastructure. As a result, a colonial relationship between Northern and Southern Saskatchewan emerged that continues to the present.[23] Quiring's claim that government support and/or inappropriate programs resulted in the subordination of the north is also supported by Morantz's model of internal colonialism.[24]

In her research focused on the James Bay Cree of northern Quebec, Morantz distinguishes three models of colonialism: settler, civilizing (i.e., missionary), and state. Settler colonialism was most applicable to events in southern Canada where domination took place by force resulting in gradual appropriation of tribal lands, and emasculation of leaders.[25] According to Morantz, civilizing or missionary colonialism involved the (impossible) objective of total destruction and reconstruction of societies and cultures. State colonialism occurred when colonial governments administered territory through indirect rule. There are no sharp divisions among the three categories but various combinations of the historical models are found across Canada.

The concept of bureaucratic colonialism is based on the governance structures of state colonialism, *minus* the settlers. It was neither settlers nor capitalism that lead to subordination of (in Morantz's case) the Cree people, but rather the combination of low-quality versions of southern-style Canadian services such as education, health and welfare, and government management that were introduced into Aboriginal communities in the 1950s. Morantz argues that the contradictions of colonialism were exacerbated by various government agencies responsible for social engineering, and cites the worst example of bureaucratic colonialism as the government's ineffectiveness and frugality in providing the resources for Indian people to live as they saw fit. In the end, bureaucratic colonialism may have been a more insidious form of colonialism because there was no one particular colonizer, but rather many who claimed a higher concealed 'boss.'[26] In some respects, that absence was almost disappointing as it would have been easier to isolate and replace them, and thereby rectify the system.

The two models described above are most fitting to events in Northern Saskatchewan. However, a limitation of both theories is that they are broadly conceived, and do not acknowledge the inconsistencies inherent in colonialism. The two state-focused models provide an important top-down explanation for events in Northern Saskatchewan, but they do not address the on-the-ground or bottom-up activities, such as nursing, that also influenced the region. Therefore, I focus on how the top-down process of internal/bureaucratic colonialism influenced the bottom-up or socialization process, which in turn expands our understanding of the complex forces that shape regions such as Northern Saskatchewan.

Nursing Stations in Northern Saskatchewan

To address the enormous social and economic discrepancies experienced by northern residents compared to those in the south, and to pave the way for exploitation of the region's natural resources, the provincial government delineated Northern Saskatchewan as a specific geographic space through the Natural Resources Act of 1944. Social renewal, particularly the integration of the primarily Aboriginal population into mainstream Canadian society, was premised on a development model in which the exploitation of natural resources would provide the wealth necessary for modernization of public services and result in improved living standards for people within the region.[27] To achieve these ends, changes were required to the way people lived in the vast, isolated, and under-serviced region. Therefore a variety of public institutions were introduced to not only provide education, health, and social services to residents but also to replace the traditional norms with modern customs.

One such institution was public health, a service provided by nurses located at nursing stations throughout Northern Saskatchewan. Nurses cared for the ill and injured, and introduced people to modern concepts of health care through preventative and educational programs.[28] Living and working among their patients made the nurses effective vehicles for promoting a way of life that corresponded with modernization theories where Western-based knowledge challenged traditional systems.[29]

The provincial government introduced the nursing outpost system in Northern Saskatchewan following the Second World War.[30] A provincial-run public health nursing station opened in Cumberland

Table 10.1 Medical facilities in Northern Saskatchewan (1957)

Community	Established	Jurisdiction
Ile a la Crosse	1927 (although the Sisters of Charity (Grey Nuns) began caring for people at the mission in 1860)	Erected by provincial and federal governments; administered by Oblates; operated by Grey Nuns of Roman Catholic Church
Cumberland House	1941 (1929)	Provincial
Gunnar	1944	Gunnar Mines
Buffalo Narrows	1947	Provincial
Sandy Bay	1948	Provincial
Snake Lake (Pinehouse)	1948	Provincial
Stony Rapids	1948	Provincial
La Loche	1951	Church (Roman Catholic)
Lac La Ronge	1951	Federal/provincial
Uranium City	1952 (relocated from Goldfields)	Community
Pelican Narrows	1955	Federal

Source: Government of Saskatchewan, Department of Public Health,
Saskatchewan Public Health Nursing Annual Report, 1957.

House in 1929, but the Depression and the war stalled any further expansion of the fledging health care system in the region. In 1944, when the CCF was elected, northern medical services consisted of a mission hospital at Ile a la Crosse, the outpost hospital at Cumberland House, infirmaries at La Loche and Green Lake, and nurses attached to residential schools at Beauval and Lac La Ronge.[31] By 1957, eleven nursing stations had been established (see table 1). Northern Saskatchewan was so sparsely settled and the population so dispersed that it was believed little more could be done than to provide basic care at the outpost facilities and transfer patients out to larger centres when necessary. Because of the distances involved and the lack of roads in the region, patients had to be flown out, prompting the creation in 1946 of the first air ambulance system in North America, designed specifically to provide back-up services for the nursing stations.

So Much To Do and So Few Nurses

The establishment of nursing stations in Northern Saskatchewan coincided with significant advances in medicine such as the development of vaccines and antibiotics. The nurses themselves expressed amazement at the "near miraculous wonders of penicillin and other antibiotics," noting "the little ones come in here so sick, and after a few treatments, make such a quick recovery."[32] Information in table 2, gleaned from Department of Public Health, Public Health Nursing Annual Reports, provides the annual total number of home and office visits reported by the nursing stations, and the number of nurses working at each outpost between 1947–53.

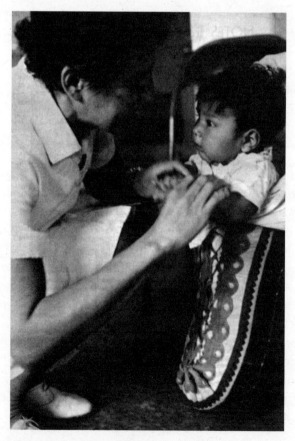

10.1 Northern nurse and baby.

Table 10.2 Numbers of home visits, office visits, and nurses, 1947–53

	1947	1948	1949	1950	1951	1952	1953
Total home visits	833	1,015	1,253	1,234	1,910	1,859	2,764
Total office visits	1,653	2,127	4,618	5,912	5,509	5,941	7,062
Total nurses	1	3+1 pt	3+1 pt	4+1 pt	5+2 pt	4+3 pt	6

Source: Government of Saskatchewan, Department of Public Health, Public Health Nursing Annual Reports, 1947–53. This summarizes statistics from nursing stations in Buffalo Narrows, Cumberland House, Goldfields, Lac La Ronge, Sandy Bay, Snake Lake (Pinehouse), Stony Rapids, and Uranium City. pt = part-time

The figures in the table can be construed in different ways, particularly the number of visits *to* the nursing station (office visits). One interpretation of the high number of office visits is that it illustrates that the community's traditional health care customs were replaced. And according to Scheper-Hughes and Morantz, such acquiescence to outside authority, whether voluntary or involuntary, is an indication of colonialism. However, I contend this was not the case in Northern Saskatchewan, that rather than capitulation, it was the adopting of new ideas related to health care, a response that made sense given the region's past.[33]

The people of Northern Saskatchewan had experienced more than their fair share of illnesses, diseases, and loss of life due to smallpox, tuberculosis, and typhoid.[34] With memories of disease sweeping through their communities, it is hardly surprising that people looked to the nurses for assistance with their health care concerns. The dread of diseases such as measles was stronger than even the fear of needles, and nurses reported that people attended immunization clinics willingly. Confidence in needles actually grew to the point where nurses complained that too many people believed that shots and pills were the answer to everything.[35] Lastly, Northern Saskatchewan, the hospital at Ile a la Crosse (established in 1860), Indian agents, priests, and Hudson's Bay Company managers had provided basic medical assistance for generations prior to the arrival of nursing stations. Therefore, the practice of seeking help was not new and Aboriginal peoples were aware of what Western medicine could offer them. Community leaders were also well aware that their population could benefit from advances in medicine and some lobbied to have nursing stations situated in their communities.[36]

Overall, it is difficult to determine the extent to which the population of Northern Saskatchewan benefited from Western medicine
because little data were collected about Aboriginal peoples prior to
1960.[37] Furthermore, what information may have been collected was
unreliable as people lived a traditional nomadic lifestyle (i.e., hunting,
trapping, fishing) that required moving about the region rather than
residing in permanent settlements. But visits to the nurses and nursing
stations did not diminish people's ability to make their own decisions,
and in some instances the Aboriginal population were reported as
"bold and demanding."[38] Moreover, "it would be arrogant to assume
that recipients were incapable of discriminating between those services
and ideas which were useful and those which were not."[39] This position gains additional support from Reiffel (1999) and Abel and Reiffel
(1996) whose work on American Indian reservations found that people played an active role in determining what advice and treatment were
accepted, rejected, or integrated with their traditional ways.[40]

Altering Northern Space

Not only were nursing stations new to the region but so also was the
idea of living year-round in permanent communities. The majority of
permanent northern settlements in the region were relatively young,
having been established after the Second World War when people
shifted from a nomadic hunting, fishing, and trapping lifestyle to a
sedentary way of living.[41] Residing in permanent communities was a
new way of living that required different sets of skills. Therefore, federal and provincial government programs were implemented to instill
in the population 'modern' notions of living, with the aim to assimi-
late Aboriginal peoples into mainstream society.

These programs had a history. For example, a field matron program was implemented in the United States between 1888 and 1938;
hundreds of white women were employed to live on reservations and
instruct Native American women about correct forms of domesticity.[42]
In Canada, Homemakers' Clubs were established, in some instances
by nurses, to encourage Indian women to adopt Western ideals of femininity and domesticity in hopes that these standards would subsequently ripple through Aboriginal society.

In Northern Saskatchewan, nurses established women's auxiliary clubs, new baby clubs, home craft clubs, girls and boys clubs, and so on. Nurses reported that the local women took great pride in participating in the clubs and were more than willing to support their local nursing station.[43] Ladies' clubs were formed for educational purposes and to raise funds for work to be done on children and adults to improve their health. The money collected through fundraising activities covered the cost for a dentist to visit the community and paid for toys and games to amuse the children so that the time in hospital would "not be so tedious for the wee ones."[44] The time and effort spent on organizing various clubs is commendable, but at the same time, the activities also served to socialize people with ideas of play and adult behavioural norms. The actions of nurses who lived and worked at outpost hospitals went beyond normal nursing practices and presented a means of changing the way the primarily Aboriginal population lived their lives. This serves as a fitting example of social engineering within Morantz's concept of bureaucratic colonialism.[45]

The 'appropriate' use of time was another aspect of life that some nurses tried to instill. As nurse Lyons stated, "In my estimation our biggest contribution to Public Health in this district is training the women and girls how to use their leisure time profitably."[46] As a result, sewing and hobby classes were held and became popular with younger children. Nurse Lewis remarked, "hobby classes are going to begin again, they proved so popular that the last season ended with even the small boys wanting to learn to crochet, as they were getting fed up with having nowhere to go in the evenings."[47] The lengths to which nurses went to socialize people varied, as did their techniques. Generally, instructional sessions were held at the outpost, but as the following demonstrates, in some instances, meeting at the nurses' home met with greater success. "I have found that the natives get very little out of planned lectures or demonstrations but have had wonderful results, especially from the school children and some mothers of allowing them to visit in our home. They are very observant and follow our habits readily ... I have been encouraging the native children to come to our home to visit hoping they may gain some knowledge of cleanliness and the ways of living properly."[48]

To convey their messages the nurses used a variety of methods, including filmstrips, slides, posters, and leaflets – all in English. It is significant to note that nurses never received any language instruction (nor any cultural training) and relied on interpreters to convey their messages. As the following demonstrates, however, the situation became complex at times. The nurse wrote: "It was amusing the other day – I was doing the dressing of a French priest who could speak "Chip" but little English. A "Chip" boy came in who could speak nothing else, so I asked Adrienne in English to ask the priest in French to ask the boy in "Chip" my questions, and so gradually I got some idea of his trouble – I'm not usually so fortunate."[49]

Generally, local women in the community provided translation services but when it became necessary for them to visit the nursing station up to three or four times in an afternoon, they tired of the inconvenience and started charging for their services, which was a very unpopular move.[50] As more people in the community came to speak English, demand for interpreters declined, although even today they remain essential in many northern communities in Saskatchewan. Interestingly, the nurses never mentioned the loss of language as an issue for Aboriginal peoples, leading one to assume that either the nurses were too busy to consider the question or they believed that the population would eventually become part of mainstream English-speaking Canadian life.[51]

Despite the language barriers, nurses covered a range of public health topics, including healthy eating, handwashing, dental care, sanitation, and preventing the spread of diseases such as tuberculosis and venereal disease. Child-rearing literature was also important and nurses relied on materials used in Canadian mainstream society, such as *Canadian Mother and Child*.[52] In other words, nurses were "envoys of middle class values ... teaching them the rules of 'scientific cleanliness' in order to combat ill health in the home and community at large."[53]

The nurses' notions of cleanliness, however, were not out of step with public health practices of the time, despite the position of Ehrenreich and English who claim that the obsession with cleanliness was little more than "busy work."[54] Tomes refutes this idea and points out that at a time when infectious diseases were the leading cause of death in the general population, the emphasis on cleanliness had some utility.[55] The situation for the people of Northern Saskatchewan was no different, but as most residences lacked appropriate infrastructure such as running water and sewage systems, it was difficult for residents to adopt the recommended hygiene practices. Being trained in public health, the nurses were well aware of the health hazards associated with the lack of potable water and appropriate waste disposal, and they tried to improve the situation by holding community meetings as well as raising their concerns with authorities in Regina.[56]

Influencing Northern Diets

As indicated in Lill's quotation at the beginning of this essay, promoting a diet based on Canada's Food Guide was an important, although unrealistic, objective. The nurses grew and canned much of the food for their own use and that of the outpost.[57] People in the community hunted, fished, and trapped and preserved food according to their own traditions, and some of the nurses preferred country food over that provided to them in annual shipments.[58]

But promoting a diet that included plenty of fresh fruits and vegetables was impractical given the northern lifestyle and personal tastes, not to mention the problems associated with growing gardens in sub-arctic conditions. Unless people planted their own gardens, they simply did not have the financial resources to purchase the recommended foods. In-patients at the outpost hospital were fed Euro-Canadian–style food, but relatives often took country food to their ill or injured family members as they considered it much more palatable and believed it would help with recovery. This caused no end of frustration for some nurses who did not see the nutritional value of country food. But perhaps the non-compliance was a source of irritation because it underscored the nurses' lack of power. In the end, there was little the nurses could do beyond complaining about their patient's behaviour to their supervisors.

Some nurses, rather than dismissing the traditional diet, sought ways to enhance people's existing food. For example, when low fish prices resulted in a particularly difficult economic situation, people were taught to make nourishing soups with ingredients on hand. They were also encouraged to ration their food rather than eating it all in one day then going without, which was considered "a very native habit."[59] Another nurse displayed a great deal of initiative by seeking advice from a nutritionist on ways to improve people's diet based on the foods they already used. As a result, people were encouraged to use whole-wheat flour when making bannock, and skim milk powder rather than evaporated milk because it was less expensive in the dry form and would keep without refrigeration. The nurse was praised for her efforts by the director of nursing services in Regina, whose statement captured the essence of the contradictory nature of northern nursing: "your approach to the nutrition problem in the north seems so wise. It seems so unreasonable to expect those people to accept our way of life. Much more sensible to improve their own way of life. It is too bad that more persons do not have your attitude."[60]

In spite of their efforts to change and/or enhance people's diet, the importance of traditional activities of hunting, fishing, trapping, and berry gathering – activities that sustained people in northern communities – were recognized. When caribou were plentiful, people had enough food to eat and they kept remarkably well. One year, a nurse remarked, "the natives that were in the north this year seem to have had a very good living, the babies were all very well and they certainly looked well cared for." The following year she again commented that "the Natives are all busy fishing now they have put up their dry meat and there was plenty of caribou for all so this should be a good year for them."[61] As mentioned earlier, the nurses also relied on country food due to either circumstances or personal choice.

However, when hunting was poor, people's health suffered. And when regulations were implemented to control access to the food supply, the hardship increased. Such was the case when the Indian agent who held the key for the community meat locker failed to make arrangements for opening the storeroom during his absence. In her letter, the nurse reported that she had been very busy with an outbreak of illness, which she attributed to the fact that without the key "the Natives were unable to get their meat from the freezer so they went hungry."[62] This event points to the increasing layers of bureaucratic power that northerners *and* the nurses had to contend with in Northern Saskatchewan.

The Nurses' Space: Homeplace and Workspace
Rolled into One

The hyacinths are really making the hospital look like a conservatory. There are three pots blooming in the living room and I have 5 more in the other windows being forced along. There are some daffodils and tulips I am hoping to have for February 14th. I will have enough bulbs to keep us in fresh flowers until the end of March ... I have never had so much luck and enjoyment with them on any previous attempts of growing these inspiring plants. The patients get so much pleasure out of watching them grow also.[63]

A unique feature of the nursing outposts was that they served as both the nurses' homeplace and workspace. The nurses' homeplaces served as examples of modern modes of living for the local population.[64] But as the outposts were the nurses' homes, it is not surprising that they tried to make their surroundings as comfortable as possible. The effort put into establishing a home setting is one of the most notable and consistent comments made by the nurses. Perhaps this is attributable to the fact that in the late 1940s and early 1950s, when the nursing stations were being established, Northern Saskatchewan was considered a frontier, and "little pieces of feminine comfort" were important to women who lived and worked in pioneer-like conditions.[65]

Conditions at the nursing stations were primitive to say the least, with some described as "deplorable, poorly equipped, and poorly furnished."[66] Some nurses came from rural areas of the country so were used to living without electricity, running water, and plumbing. Nevertheless, there were many requests for dishes, furniture, paint, and items to enhance their surroundings. At one outpost hospital the nurse reported that she had finished sewing curtains as the room looked so awful without them and the new colourful ones would look very nice for the rest of the summer. She also mentioned that the selection of pictures could wait until later, although "the walls, curtains and lamps were all light colours so I would think that pictures to give colour to the room might be quite nice."[67]

Ongoing efforts were also put into "freshening up" the nursing stations with floors and furniture being refinished and requests being submitted for items to make the outposts more comfortable for both

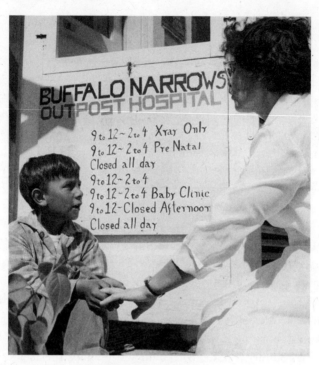

10.2 Buffalo Narrows Outpost Hospital.

nurses and patients.[68] Nurses also took pride in their flower gardens. There was considerable concern when an early frost or neglect left the flowers "a sorry sight and the window boxes absolutely dead."[69] Lastly, tending to large gardens and preserving fruits and vegetables were other time-consuming responsibilities; however, not only did this provide food for the nursing stations but the activities also served as an example for the local population.

But the work of producing much of their own food added to the already heavy workload of the nurses, and at times domestic duties seemed to take precedence over their professional duties. In a letter to her supervisor, one outpost nurse reported that although she was pleased to have preserved 136 quarts of blueberries and about 50 quarts of caribou, she needed someone to help with baking and canning as there was not enough time to do everything.[70]

Anther nurse protested outright, declaring, "I am a nurse and not a housekeeper!"[71] But it was a side of outpost nursing that supervisors did not necessarily want highlighted. For example, when asked to write an article for the *Canadian Nurse*, the nurse's supervisor replied, "Now about the article for the *Canadian Nurse*. I do not think it necessary that you write especially about your work in the north. Why not concentrate on the scenery and the life of the people there, the garden which Miss Lyons had at Buffalo Narrows and refer just quite briefly to the work of the nurse in such a settlement."[72]

In the subsequent article published in the *Canadian Nurse* (vol. 47 (9) September 1951), there was no reference whatsoever to the often-difficult working conditions encountered in the north. Later, in another letter to her supervisor, nurse Aylsworth reported lightheartedly, "you'd scarcely recognize Buffalo Narrows if you hear me describing it. You'd think it was the dawn of the golden age or something, to let me tell it. So if you hear of a group of people from Madoc district chartering a plane to Buffalo Narrows to have a look at that Utopia, don't be surprised."[73] Although efforts were made to downplay negative aspects of northern nursing, the lack of support and professional and personal isolation did not remain concealed.

Northern Nurses and Social Isolation

The personal and professional isolation encountered by the nurses resulted in an often-palpable loneliness. For example, one nurse pleaded with her supervisor not to leave the same day as she arrived because "the visit is far too hurried and there is not enough time to talk about anything."[74] In another instance, depression brought about by isolation and loneliness was cited as the reason for leaving the north. The nurse referred to the community as "a most lonesome depressing place" and wrote: "One needs something in a Native settlement to offset the every day happenings ... the beating of dogs and their incessant yelping. The drunks ki-yi ing at all hours. Children in the snow with bare seats. The starving horse that was driven until it dropped dead. I am rambling on and on but I want you to know how I feel. Up until this past year I have been happy in the north. I was disappointed when I came here, after the friendly people in Cumberland this was quite a shock ... I am proud of my outpost ... it does look nice and it was not without deep thought that I decided to leave."[75]

The nurse dismissed her feelings at the end of her letter by attributing her rather negative mood to the lack of someone to have a good laugh with rather than the conditions about which she had written. But attempts to end on an upbeat note could not mask the depth of her loneliness, even though her son lived with her in the community.

Socializing with local residents may have alleviated the nurses' feelings of isolation but social boundaries were clear between the (for the most part) white professionals (i.e., teachers, nurses, police) and the predominantly Aboriginal population of northern communities. The very nature of nursing work required a certain degree of professional distance between caregiver and patient, which isolated the nurses. But at the same time, nurses as "white women in uniforms, all enjoyed a privileged community status as recognized care-givers" which further set them apart from the local community.[76]

Nurses were criticized by local residents for their lack of participation in community events, but they defended themselves by pointing out that it was often not possible to socialize due to their extraordinary workload and being on call twenty-four hours a day, seven days a week. In a letter to her supervisor, the nurse claimed: "As for any lack of friendliness on my part in the settlement, I might mention that during the past 5 months, there has been scarcely a day without patients, and my time for social activities has been very limited. I have gone out a few times a week, usually for an hour or so … leaving a note on the door for anyone who might come looking for me."[77] In another instance, the nurse detailed the stress of being on duty twenty-four hours a day and having to face acute emergencies and make decisions concerning patients' lives. She went on to say that the increased tensions caused nurses to become irritated by things that would otherwise not bother them, producing a situation of "unfriendly relationships with patients and other members of the community."[78]

The social isolation experienced by nurses was compounded by gender and the fact that as women, they had less latitude in *how* they interacted with community members. When one nurse was seen "driving around with a man" she received a "little warning … in a spirit of well meaning in order that there would be no justification whatever for injury" to her good reputation.[79] The nurse replied that she was providing family counselling and was incensed to hear comments about her behaviour. She wrote: "As far as I am concerned it is only business and co-operation in our work, which I think should be. And furthermore I have helped a number of families by listening to them, instead of brushing them aside and putting them further into the gutter. I feel as a nurse that this is part of my work ... I have tried to help people in these difficulties and have been successful a number of times, that is there is now a happy family instead of a broken up home. And still my reputation is as good as ever in any place I have worked."[80]

The nurse originally threatened to resign her position, but after reassurances that the comments were not meant to offend her, the situation calmed down. However, in subsequent letters, reference to the event often resurfaced and relations between the nursing supervisor and the nurse never recovered. The situation became increasingly antagonistic, particularly as the nurse was constantly relocated, causing her considerable stress. As a subordinate, considerable pressure was put on the nurse to comply with whatever the director of nursing and medical health officer requested so she would not "fail to meet her great professional need."[81] The situation underscores the lack of power that northern nurses had within the bureaucratic structure of the Department of Public Health. Yet, at other times, the department imbued nurses with a sense of power in order to achieve certain results.

Nurses and Power

The physical presence of the outpost nursing stations and the nurses themselves were symbols of power. Although the Department of Public Health stood behind expenses incurred in the course of providing care, it looked for ways to encourage people into covering some of the costs. Nurses' attitudes about fee-for-service varied. Some believed strongly that those who had the resources should pay for professional nursing services, and those who did not were expected to pay by, for example, providing wood for the nursing station. However, one nurse felt that local people should be paid for the services that they provided, and therefore paid people for supplying her with fuel or transportation. The nurse who subsequently took over the nursing station was appalled when people "absolutely refused to take the 'nurse' anywhere unless they were paid" and sought direction from her supervisor about what to do.[82] The letter was passed on to the chief medical officer who replied that he was unhappy about the situation as it set a bad precedent. He thought that perhaps the local people were just testing out the new nurse and that with a bit of pressure, people might be shamed into paying.[83] But the nurse who had paid people for their services made it clear "that the precedent had been set and it was difficult, if not altogether impossible, to the change the attitude of the people."[84]

Given the dire economic conditions for many northern residents, nurses were often uncomfortable with being put in the position of having to deal with money matters. They requested that they not be put in a position of having to badger people for payment.[85] Nurses expressed their reluctance to become involved with financial issues and tried to deflect administration's requests by pointing out that people simply did not have the means to pay for much at all.

Nurses used their position in other ways to improve services for northern residents. They lobbied for dentists to visit communities, for tuberculosis screening to be conducted in all communities, and for children with special needs (i.e., deafness, physical deformities) to see specialists. They notified their supervisors about the lack of safe water supplies and improper sewage disposal and asked what could be done to help matters in the community. Advocating on behalf of their patients points out that health care workers were not simply tools of the state.[86] But there were limits to how far the nurses could go with their requests and, as the following example shows, if they overstepped certain boundaries there were repercussions.

In a letter to the chief medical officer, a nurse expressed her frustration that completion of the nursing station was taking too long, and after a year of improvising, she was fed up. She asked for a carpenter to be sent to finish the building as soon as possible and described what she felt were the priorities. The letter was sent to the director of nursing to be forwarded to the chief medical officer. However, the director of nursing did not forward the letter and returned it to the nurse with a warning that although the medical health officer "championed the cause of the nurses, he had complete control and could make life very unhappy and uncomfortable for us."[87] This response reinforces that although the nurses may have been perceived as important figures in northern communities, they actually held very little power, particularly when it came to dealing with the bureaucratic structures that they looked to for support.

+ + +

There is no doubt that the nurses' professional objectives were aimed at bettering people's health by changing customs and habits and providing them with medical care and treatments of the day. Through their daily routine, nurses tried to influence the way people lived in Northern Saskatchewan and were pleased when they gained the confidence of people and saw improvements in their health.[88] At the professional level, public health practices were effective in preventing loss of life and illness but they almost always entailed ending certain practices that were "sanctioned by centuries of tradition."[89] Nevertheless, people embraced, rejected, or adjusted to the lifestyle changes as they saw fit.

The actions of nurses are not those typically associated with colonization. For example, nurses were purveyors of benevolent not oppressive structures. However, as Memmi argues, colonization takes place on a number of levels with many dimensions of oppression involved in the subjugation of people.[90] Nurses represented the values of the state; they were employees of the provincial Department of Public Health and "as such had to conform to the rules, regulations and discipline of supervisors."[91] The socializing practices of the nurses altered the way in which people organized the knowledge of the world around them. Although subtle, the nurses as a collective were part of the colonization apparatus, but at the individual level, attitudes and approaches varied from nurse to nurse. In all likelihood government did not view nursing as a means to advance their agenda, because if they had, the nursing posts would have been better supported, rather than chronically underfunded. At the same time, as one of the few non-Aboriginal people in northern communities, the nurse represented authority, although in the end, local people made their own decisions about what was or was not good for them. For example, people appeared to comply with the nurses' 'ways' while in-patients at the hospital, but reverted to their own practices when discharged. When an unpopular suggestion was made to local women – that they should take up needlework while attending a program at the clinic – the women expressed their dissatisfaction by simply not going.[92] There was little the nurses could do in these situations except to adjust their approach, which they often did.

When it came to certain medical care and practices – particularly difficult maternity cases – the nurses, for good reason, were more assertive in trying to convince their patients to comply with their instructions. Nevertheless, nurses reported that even with difficult pregnancies they could hardly force their patients to go out to larger centres for care. Yet the responsibility of having women in the community when complications were likely was stressful. As one nurse reported, "If I had lost the mother and babe the other mothers-to-be would have lost confidence in me to say nothing of losing confidence in myself."[93]

As indicated in the opening quotation of this essay, some of the changes promoted by the nurses were inappropriate for northern communities. This is because the public health nursing model was introduced with little, if any, consultation with the communities. Many management decisions affecting the north during this time were made within government bureaucracies that had little knowledge or understanding of northern conditions.[94] But once confronted with the realities of life in remote northern communities, individual nurses did not necessarily agree with instructions that went beyond those required to improve people's health, forcing some nurses to question their own motives.

The nursing stations and nurses played a role in shaping Northern Saskatchewan as it emerged as a specific northern place within the provincial milieu. Nursing provided much-needed professional medical care for northerners but ongoing funding and support was often lacking and also shifted as interests and political agendas changed.

The theoretical models of colonization introduced by Quiring and Morantz go some way in describing development processes in Northern Saskatchewan.[95] Although attempts to modernize the region were perhaps well intended, resources and support for the institutions responsible for transforming the traditional way of life were sadly lacking. But in delving deeper into the various layers of institutions and individuals involved in the overarching colonial process, the picture becomes complex and untidy, which the broadly conceived models cannot address. Including the nurses' experiences from an on-the-ground perspective contributes another layer of explanation and thereby expands our understanding of colonialism

The nurses' position within the process of bureaucratic colonialism was contradictory. Although well intended, the nurses carried with them the ideas and practices of the dominant society; yet they were also sensitive to local cultural practices, advocating for the primarily Aboriginal population, and gaining their acceptance and appreciation. The nurses provided care to northerners but, at the same time, strongly encouraged them to adopt different ways of living, believing it would result in improved health. Unfortunately, the Aboriginal population was under considerable stress due to other changes in the region (i.e., increasing levels of bureaucracy) that both they and the nurses were ill equipped to handle. Despite the contradictory nature of their activities, the nurses played a role in shaping Northern Saskatchewan by mitigating the worst effects of the rapid change that took place in the region following the Second World War. However, regardless of the good intentions of the nurses and their sincere efforts to provide greatly needed health care to the people of Northern Saskatchewan, political, economic, and social structures became dominant factors in determining people's everyday experience. The nurses and the Department of Public Health may have "treated people with respect and decency, but the frameworks that enabled them even to decide what was dignified were powerfully defined by forces often outside of their control."[96]

To conclude, the nurses' contribution is perhaps best captured in the words of Jean Cuthand Goodwill (the first Aboriginal woman to graduate from nursing school in Saskatchewan), who stated that she "was amazed at how well the non-native nurses, with their high ideals, their curiosity, determination and strong sense of responsibility, managed to cope with the adversity they encountered in this setting ... to some extent the scenery, terrain, serenity and silence comforted the nurses trying to deal with the human devastation that resulted from the imposition of another way of life on Canada's Aboriginal people."[97]

NOTES

I would like to thank Myra Rutherdale for her inspiration to create this book and for staying the course to ensure its completion. Thank you to Dr Maureen Reed and members of my PhD Committee for their enthusiasm and direction, and to the SSHRC (Social Sciences and Humanities Research Council for the financial support that funded this research. Special recognition goes to the nurses, both past and present, whose experiences are the foundation of this research.

1 Wendy Lill, "The Occupation of Heather Rose." In Diane Bessai and Don Kerr, eds, NeWest Plays by Women (Edmonton: NeWest Press, 1987).

2 Diane Bessai and Don Kerr, eds., NeWest Plays by Women (Edmonton: NeWest Press, 1987).

3 Joy Duncan Frontier Nursing Collection, interview conducted with 'Yvonne,' 4 February 1976.

4 For a comprehensive discussion of outpost nursing in northern Manitoba and the Northwest Territories, see Corrine Hodgson, "Sitting on an Island: Nurses in the Canadian North," MA thesis (Hamilton: McMaster University, 1980); Corinne Hodgson, "Ambiguity and Paradox in Outpost Nursing" in International Nursing Review 29, 4 (1982): 108–17.

5 In this research the term state refers to the set of institutions (e.g., government agencies that provide public goods and services (R.J. Johnston, Derek Gregory, Geraldine Pratt, and Michael Watts, The Dictionary of Human Geography (Oxford: Blackwell Publishers, 2000): 788–9.).

6 Toby Morantz, The White Man's Gonna Getcha: The Colonial Challenges to the Crees in Quebec (Montreal & Kingston: McGill-Queen's University Press, 2002).

7 Morantz, The White Man's Gonna Getcha; David Quiring, "Battling Parish Priests, Bootleggers and Fur Sharks: CCF Colonialism in Northern Saskatchewan," PhD dissertation (Saskatoon: University of Saskatchewan, 2004).

8 Murray Dobbin, The One-and-a-Half Men (Regina: Gabriel Dumont Institute, 1981).

9 Ed Weick, A Socio-Economic Overview of Uranium Mining in Northern Saskatchewan (Ottawa: Environmental-Social Advisory Services (ESAS) Inc., 1992).

10 A.L. Swiderski, "Development Planning and Aboriginal Rights: The Case of Northern Canada" in Progress in Planning 27, 1 (1992): 1–82.

11 David E. Wilkins, "Modernization, Colonialism, Dependency: How Appropriate Are These Models for Providing an Explanation of North American Indian 'Underdevelopment'?" in Ethnic and Racial Studies 16, 3 (July 1993): 390–419.

12 Johnston et al., Dictionary of Human Geography, 93.

13 Ron F. Laliberte, Priscilla Settee, James B. Waldram, Rob Innes, Brenda Macdougall, Lesley McBain, and F. Laurie Barron, *Expressions in Canadian Native
   Studies* (Saskatoon: University of Saskatchewan Extension Press, 2000): 56.

14 Paul L. Knox, Sallie A. Marston, and Alan E. Nash, *Human Geography: Places
   and Regions in Global Context* (Toronto: Pearson/Prentice Hall, 2004): 55.

15 Wilkins, "Modernization, Colonialism, Dependency," 98.

16 Bruce Willems-Braun, "Buried Epistemologies: The Politics of Nature in (Post)
   Colonial British Columbia," in *Annals of the Association of American Geographers* 87, 1 (1997): 4.

17 Albert Memmi, *The Colonizer and the Colonized* (New York: Orion Press,
   1965); Iris Marion Young, *Justice and the Politics of Difference* (Princeton, New
   Jersey: Princeton University Press, 1990), 39–65.

18 Yuri Slezkine, *Arctic Mirrors: Russia and the Small Peoples of the North* (Ithaca:
   Cornell University, 1994).

19 James S. Frideres and René R. Gadacz, *Aboriginal Peoples in Canada*, 7th ed.
   (Toronto: Pearson Prentice Hall, 2005): 2.

20 Wilkins, "Modernization, Colonialism, Dependency."

21 Morantz, *White Man's Gonna Getcha*; Quiring 2004, *Battling Parish Priests*;
   Pamela White, "A Heartland-Hinterland Analysis of Images of Northern Canada
   as Frontier, Wilderness, and Homeland," MA thesis (Ottawa: Carleton University, 1979); Wilkins, "Modernization, Colonialism, Dependency."

22 Quiring, *Battling Parish Priests*; Morantz, *The White Man's Gonna Getcha*.

23 Quiring, *Battling Parish Priests*.

24 Ibid.

25 Morantz, *White Man's Gonna Getcha*.

26 Ibid., 242.

27 F. Laurie Barron, *Walking in Indian Moccasins: The Native Policies of Tommy
   Douglas and the CCF* (Vancouver: UBC Press, 1997).

28 David E. Smith, ed., *Building a Province: A History of Saskatchewan in Documents* (Saskatoon: Fifth House Publisher, 1992).

29 Modernization theory stressed the importance for societies to become more like
   modern Western societies and depended on the presence of social structures that
   were produced, promoted, and protected by the state. The premise of modernization theory was that once less-developed traditional societies shed their customs and modernized, their development was assured. The rather optimistic view
   did not last long though because the model did not take into account the diverse
   structure of various societies. Consequently, there was little confidence in the
   model and resistance to its universal application grew.

30 It is worthwhile to note that the marked shift that took place in the twentieth
century with respect to the welfare of the northern population coincided with increasing awareness of the region's rich natural resources, particularly forestry
and uranium deposits. As a result, the state's traditional laissez-faire policy toward the region was replaced with a level of involvement that within little more
than a decade made government the most important industry and major employer in the North.

31 C. Stabler, R.G. Beck, J.A. Warner, D. Russell, M.R. Olfert, S.M. Howard, and
A. Tuck, *Socio-Economic Saskatchewan* Final Report 25 (Saskatoon: Churchill
River Study – Missinipe Probe, 1975).

32 Saskatchewan Archives Board (SAB) Department of Public Health, Nursing Services Division (DPH, NSD), PH5, File 48, letters from Helen Janzen, Stony Rapids
to M.P. Edwards, Regina, 27 January 1954.

33 Nancy Scheper-Hughes, *Death Without Weeping: The Violence of Everyday Life
in Brazil* (Berkeley: University of California Press, 1992); Morantz, *White Man's
Gonna Getcha.*

34 For a discussion of (poor) health conditions of the general Canadian population at the time, see Janice P. McGinnis, "From Health To Welfare: Standards
of Public Health for Canadians 1919–1945," PhD dissertation (Edmonton: University of Alberta, 1980).

35 SAB File 46, letters from M.E. Lewis, Stony Rapids to Miss Smith, Regina, 29
March 1953; SAB File 48, letters from Helen Janzen, Stony Rapids to Miss
Smith, Regina, 7 October 1953.

36 Evelyn Linklater, Personal communication, Pelican Narrows, Saskatchewan,
June 2001.

   Further evidence of the awareness of medical care is provided in Treaty 6
(1876) where Indians negotiated the medicine chest clause. Indians in subsequent
treaties also requested the same terms. Treaty 6 encompasses a portion of Northern Saskatchewan.

37 Sally M. Weaver, *Making Canadian Indian Policy: The Hidden Agenda 1968–
1970* (Toronto: University of Toronto Press, 1981).

38 SAB File 1, letters from Helen Janzen, Buffalo Narrows to Miss M. Edwards,
Regina, 11 August 1954.

39 Margaret Jones, "Infant and Maternal Health Services in Ceylon, 1900–1948:
Imperialism or Welfare," in *The Society for the Social History of Medicine* 15,
2 (2002): 263–89.

40 Nancy Reiffel, "American Indian Views of Public Health Nursing, 1930–1950," in *American Indian Culture and Research Journal* 23, 3 (1999): 143–54; Emily K. Abel and Nancy Reiffel, "Interactions Between Public Health Nurses and Clients on American Indian Reservations During the 1930s," in *Social History of Medicine* 9, 1 (April 1996): 89–108.

41 John W. Elias, *Report to the Northern Inter-Tribal Health Authority on Mental Health Needs, Resources, Systemic Issues, and Ideas Concerning the Development of a More Responsive and Accountable Mental Health System* (Saskatoon: Elias and Associates Consulting Inc., 1999).

42 Mona Domosh and Joni Seager, *Putting Women in Place: Feminist Geographers Make Sense of the World* (New York: Guilford Press, 2001).

43 SAB File 50, letters from M.E. Pierce, Stony Rapids to Miss Smith, Regina, 22 January 1948.

44 SAB File 50, letters from Mary Lyons, Buffalo Narrows to Miss E. Smith, Regina, 19 October 1949.

45 Morantz, *White Man's Gonna Getcha.*

46 SAB File 3, letters from Mary Lyons, Buffalo Narrows to Dr C.R. Totten, Regina, 20 April 1949.

47 SAB File 46, letters from M.E. Lewis, Stony Rapids to Miss Smith, Regina, 24 November 1952.

48 SAB File 44, letters from Mrs Enid Broome, Snake Lake (Pinehouse Lake) to Miss E. Smith, Regina, 15 February 1950; SAB File 44, letters from Mrs Enid Broome, Snake Lake (Pinehouse Lake) to Miss E. Smith, Regina, 4 January 1951.

49 SAB File 49, letters from D.M. Glenny, Stony Rapids to Miss E. Smith, Regina, 1 August 1952.

50 SAB File 50, letters from M.E. Pierce, Stony Rapids to Miss Smith, Regina, 25 April 1948.

51 Douglas F. McArthur, "The Development of Northern Saskatchewan: Problems and Issues," a paper presented to Saskatchewan Science Council Meetings, Uranium City, 26 January 1978, points out that an element of government policy between 1869 and 1945 was the assimilation of Indian people through the use of English language, culture, and an emphasis on self-sufficiency.

52 SAB File 3, letters from Mary Lyons, Buffalo Narrows to Miss E. Smith, Regina, 18 August 1947.

53 Beverly Boutilier, "Helpers or Heroines? The National Council of Women, Nursing and 'Women's Work' in Late Victorian Canada." In Dianne Dodd and Deborah

Gorham, eds., Social Sciences Canadian Society, *Caring and Curing: Historical Perspectives on Women and Healing in Canada*, 38 (Ottawa: University of Ottawa Press, 1994).

54 Barbara Ehrenreich and Deidre English, *For Her Own Good: 150 Years of the Experts' Advice to Women* (New York: Anchor Books, 1979).

55 Nancy Tomes, "Spreading the Germ Theory: Sanitary Science and Home Economics 1880–1930." In Sarah Stage and Virginia B. Vencenti, eds., *Rethinking Home Economics* (New York: Cornell University Press. 1997).

56 SAB File 6, letters from Winnifred Lacy, Cumberland House to Miss Smith, Regina, 1 October 1953.

57 SAB File 14, letters from Isobel Scriver, Cumberland House to Miss Smith, Regina, 3 August 1946; SAB File 3, letters from Mary Lyons, Buffalo Narrows to Miss E. Smith, Regina, 3 August 1948; SAB File 50, letters from M.E. Pierce, Stony Rapids to Miss E. Smith, Regina, 11 August 1948.

58 SAB File 44, letters from Mrs Enid Broome to Miss E. Smith, Regina, 4 January 1951; SAB File 46, letters from M.E. Lewis, Stony Rapids to Miss Smith, Regina, 24 November 1952; SAB File 44, letters from Mrs Enid Broome, Snake Lake (Pinehouse Lake) to Miss E. Smith, Regina, 21 November 1954).

59 SAB File 44, letters from Enid Broome, Snake Lake (Pinehouse Lake) to Miss E. Smith, Regina, 21 January 1953.

60 SAB File 6, letters from Miss E. Smith, Regina to Miss W. Lacy, Cumberland House, 24 September 1953.

61 SAB File 6, letters from M.E. Lewis, Stony Rapids to Miss Smith, Regina, 2 May 1952; SAB File 46, letters from M.E. Lewis, Stony Rapids to Miss Smith, Regina, 24 May 1953.

62 SAB File 46, letters from M.E. Lewis, Stony Rapids to Miss Edwards, Regina, 30 July 1954.

63 SAB File 3, letters from Mary Lyons, Buffalo Narrows to Director of Nursing, Regina, 19 January 1948.

64 SAB File 44, letters from Mrs Enid Broome, Snake Lake (Pinehouse Lake) to Miss E. Smith, Regina, 4 January 1951; Laurie Meijer Drees and Lesley McBain, "Nursing and Native Peoples in Northern Saskatchewan: 1930s – 1950s," in *Canadian Bulletin of Medical History* 18 (2001): 43–65.

65 Domosh and Seager, *Putting Women in Place*.

66 SAB File 54, letters from C. Augener, Uranium City to Miss Edwards, Regina, 5 September 1954.

67 SAB File 50, letters from M.E. Pierce, Stony Rapids to Miss E. Smith, Regina, 14 August 1948.

68 SAB File 1, letters from Helen Janzen, Buffalo Narrows to Miss M. Edwards, Regina, 11 August 1954.

69 SAB File 2, letters from G. Aylsworth, Buffalo Narrows to Director of Nursing, Regina, 6 August 1952.

70 SAB File 46, letters from M.E. Lewis, Stony Rapids to Miss Smith, Regina, 24 November 1952.

71 SAB File 36, letters from C. Augener, Sandy Bay to M.P. Edwards, Regina, 25 November 1953.

72 SAB File 2, letters from Miss E. Smith, Regina to G. Aylsworth, Buffalo Narrows, 24 November 1950.

73 Ibid.

74 SAB File 36, letters from C. Augener, Sandy Bay to M.P. Edwards, Regina, November 25, 1953.

75 SAB File 3, letters from M.E. Mlazgar, Sandy Bay to Miss Smith, Regina, 3 February, 1951.

76 Kathryn McPherson and Meryn Stuart, "Writing Nursing History in Canada: Issues and Approaches," in *Canadian Bulletin of Medical History* 11 (1994): 5.

77 SAB File 2, letters from G. Aylsworth, Buffalo Narrows to Miss E. Smith, Regina, 7 February 1952.

78 SAB File 5, letters from M.P. Edwards, Regina to Mr G. Townshend, Regina, 4 February 1954.

79 SAB File 33, letters from Director of Nursing Services, Regina to J. Walz, Prince Albert, 14 December 1949.

80 SAB File 33, letters from J. Walz to Miss E. Smith, Regina, 10 December 1949.

81 SAB File 10, letters from Director of Nursing Services, Regina to J. Walz, Lagenburg, 18 January 1950.

82 SAB File 13, letters from M.E. Mlazgar, Cumberland House to Miss E. Smith, Regina, 7 November 1947.

83 SAB File 13, letters from C.R. Totten (MD) to Miss E. Smith, Regina, 13 November 1947.

84 SAB File 13, letters from Director of Nursing Services, Regina to M.E. Mlazgar, Cumberland House, 18 November 1947.

85 SAB File 13, letters from M.E. Pierce, Stony Rapids to Miss Smith, Regina, 23 February 1947.

86 Jones, "Infant and Maternal Health Services."

87 SAB File 3, letters from Director of Nursing, Regina to Miss M. Lyons, Buffalo Narrows, 13 October 1948

88 SAB File 44, letters from Mrs Enid Broome, Snake Lake (Pinehouse Lake) to Miss E. Smith, Regina, 4 January 1951.

89 Jones, "Infant and Maternal Health Services," 285.

90 Memmi, *Colonizer and the Colonized.*

91 Kathryn McPherson, *Bedside Matters* (Don Mills: Oxford University, 1996): 62.

92 Joy Duncan Frontier Nursing Collection, interview with 'Edna' taped by Edna herself and submitted to the Joy Duncan project, 1976.

93 SAB File 6, letters from Winnifred Lacy, Cumberland House to Miss Smith, Regina, 20 June 1953.

94 McArthur, "Development of Northern Saskatchewan."

95 Quiring, *Battling Parish Priests*; Morantz, *White Man's Gonna Getcha.*

96 Corey Dolgon, *The End of the Hamptons* (New York: New York University Press, 2005): 224–5.

97 Jean Cuthand Goodwill, "Nursing Canada's Indigenous People," in *The Canadian Nurse* 80, 1 (1984): 6.

11

+++++

Baby Rats and Canada's Food Rules: Nurses as Educators in Northern Communities

JUDITH BENDER ZELMANOVITS

In her November 1952 report, Department of National Health and Welfare (DNHW) nurse Mrs Raynor included a detailed and amusing account of six rats that played their part in the nutrition education program being launched at Norway House, an Aboriginal community in Manitoba. "Each pair," she explained, "is being fed according to prescribed diets: Set 1 – bannock and tea with sugar; Set 2 – cake, candy, soft drinks, white bread, jam and coffee; and Set 3 – according to Canada's Food Rules – particularly what's available at Norway House."[1] The experiment, intended to capture the interest of schoolchildren, drew many adult visitors as well, and according to archival records and the journal *Canadian Nurse*, it was used in many communities across the North.[2]

It is likely that this section of Mrs Raynor's report was reprinted in a regional newsletter for its entertaining and idea-sharing aspects. But her account also suggests several themes that are important in the discussion of northern nurses' role as public health educators in the communities to which they were assigned. First, nurses were hampered in their educational work by the paucity of effective and culturally appropriate teaching materials and the fact that they lacked the indigenous language skills necessary to provide public health education in the way that they would have done in southern communities. Second, despite the fact that DNHW emphasized public health as the cornerstone of nurses' work,[3] nurses themselves claimed that they had little time for teaching because of the demands of acute care and disease management. Thus much of their education occurred on an on-going ad hoc basis using non-traditional teaching methods and taking advantage of 'teachable moments.' Third, the experiment suggests the conflict that many nurses felt – at the time or in retrospect – about imposing 'southern' values on community members. In the case of nutrition, in spite of any reluctance they may have felt as they sought to alter the eating habits of schoolchildren and their families, they knew that poor nutrition led to or exacerbated disease. And, as the rat experiment shows, they were cognizant of the fact that poor or inadequate nutrition in communities was often a result of contact with outsiders, with one set of rats eating 'junk' food found on the shelves of the local store[4] and another set eating an Aboriginal diet lacking traditional meats and fish, which were at certain times and places in short supply.[5]

In the documents of the branches[6] of the DNHW charged with administering health care to northern Aboriginal communities and in journal articles where the work of northern nurses is detailed and described, tasks are usually divided into two broad categories: public health nursing (prevention) and primary care nursing (treatment).[7] It is in the realm of public health that most of the nurses' 'teaching' tasks are described and recorded (see appendix 1). In their oral and written accounts, nurses frequently make similar divisions; however, a close look at the day-to-day work of northern nurses reveals that where education is concerned, the dichotomy was an artificial one. In fact, nurses were educating in different ways on an ongoing basis. Education was, and is, an important part of the role of northern nurses; but, it is also a role that is contentious since it is here that we see most clearly the part nurses played in the assimilatory process of health care, as they consciously or subconsciously imposed the medical model of healing[8] and southern, urban notions of sanitation and nutrition on individuals and communities.

This chapter begins with a brief outline of the history of federally provided health care in Northern Aboriginal communities, then moves to a close examination of the work of northern nurses as educators in the area specifically defined as 'public health' and more broadly in their medical practice and community involvement. It explores the attitudes of nurses toward their role as educators and, in particular, their view of northern health care as a tool of the ongoing process of colonization both at the time of their service and in subsequent oral and written discussions. Although it cannot be denied that nurses were agents of the federal government's policy of internal colonization,[9] much of their work as educators was aimed at undoing or minimizing the wrongs of the past by halting the spread of infectious and other diseases introduced to isolated communities from the 'outside.' This, in turn, served some communities well, in the sense that disease detected early responds more quickly to treatment and fewer patients had to be sent 'out' for treatment of their illness. The nurses also helped patients to understand the reasons for the course of treatment and thus helped to reassure them.

Locating Southern Nurses in the North

In this exploration of the role played by non-Aboriginal 'southern' nurses as health educators in isolated Inuit and Indian communities in northern Canada in the decades following the Second World War (1945–85), the focus is on *station* or *outpost* nurses, those women who, alone or with another nurse,[10] were charged with providing primary care in nursing stations established and maintained by the DNHW. Some attention is paid as well to nurses who worked in the small hospitals established in the DNHW Zones[11] because they cared for Aboriginal patients who were evacuated from their communities and they also provided escort duty on 'medevac' missions[12] to transport ill or injured people from their remote communities to southern hospitals.[13] Although traditional research methods based on archival sources are used in this study, the insights of nurses, as recorded in unpublished sources such as diaries, letters, and field reports, published accounts including articles from professional journals and memoirs in book format, and recollections shared in personal and telephone interviews provide the centre of focus.[14] Their voices reflect their unique, personal stories, which differed according to training and experience, time frame and geographic location of their service to the DNHW, and personal world view. Perspectives differ also since some of their stories were written at the time of their sojourn in the North; others were filtered by time. All interviews took place after a lapse of time; for some, this was almost half a century. Many of the intervie-wees refreshed their memories by looking at slides, photos, souvenirs, and government correspondence and by rereading letters and diary entries, materials that were often shared with me at the time of the interview or subsequently. Although the narratives offer an incomplete story, shaped as they are by nostalgia, selection, and self-censorship, they point clearly to overriding commonalities of theme.

Nurses were posted to Canada's 'northern regions,' a vast territory that includes the Arctic and Subarctic. The arctic area extended from the 60th parallel north to Ellesmere Island and from Yukon Territory in the west to Baffin Island in the east[15] and the subarctic area consisted of the northern areas of the provinces, where communities were distant from provincial health facilities. Many of the settlements were – and are at present – accessible only by plane and by season. The majority of the inhabitants were Aboriginal peoples, but nurses also provided primary health care to non-Aboriginals, including teachers, RCMP, and store managers living in the communities.[16] In many cases, they made regular visits to small surrounding settlements that did not have a nurse. Although most of their patient care was done on an outpatient basis, the nursing stations in which they lived and worked included beds for short-term live-in patients such as parturient women or those newly diagnosed with tuberculosis. As will be shown in this essay, the role of region is important, as it shapes the work performed by the nurses. There is a strong body of critical literature that explores the class, race, and gendered dimensions of various types of public health work, including service to Indian reservations.[17] Although northern nurses are not public health nurses per se and, in fact, few among those included in this study had official training in public health when they accepted their initial posting, many of the themes that emerge from their accounts are similar to those in the public health literature. A major factor that differentiates their experience is the geographic and social isolation of the communities they served.[18] Their responsibility was significant as they were forced to make diagnostic and prescrip-tive decisions, often without benefit of advice from colleagues; they had to perform procedures that were outside their usual scope because transport of patients to the nearest hospital was not expedient; and they worked with little supervision since those they reported to were in distant offices in zone headquarters or Ottawa.

Responsibility for providing health care to Aboriginal peoples has historically been a controversial issue, as attested to in government documents dating back to Confederation in 1867. While the BNA Act charged the federal government with the responsibility for 'Indians and the lands reserved for Indians,' the government acknowledged a moral but not a legal or treaty[19] responsibility to provide health services. The Department of Indian Affairs (DIA) demonstrated little interest in the development of medical services, waiting until 1904 to appoint its first medical superintendent, then terminating the position in 1910. Between 1910 and 1927, the service was without a superintendent. Responsibility changed hands when the DIA was absorbed by the Department of Mines and Natural Resources in 1936 and its medical division, Indian and Northern Health Services (INHS), was subsequently transferred to the newly formed DNHW in 1945.[20] Dr Percy Moore, Director of INHS at the time of expansion, clearly expressed the position of the branch when he wrote in 1946, "Although neither law nor treaty imposes such a duty, the Federal government has, for humanitarian reasons, for self-protection, and to prevent spread of disease to the white population, accepted responsibility for health services to the native population."[21] At that time, service to the vast area of the northern regions consisted of twenty-seven full-time physicians and twenty-four field nurses whose professional care was supplemented by the work of part-time field matrons and dispensers, many of whom were without formal medical training.[22] Until the mid-1970s, there was a steady increase in the number of nursing stations,[23] which J.B. Waldram described as "the backbone" of the Medical Services Branch (MSB), which replaced INHS in 1962.[24]

State medical service to Inuit communities developed much more slowly than that provided to Indian communities. In their study of the Inuit people of Arctic Canada, Tester and Kulchyski refer to "an era of neglect of Inuit affairs on the part of the state"[25] in the first half of the twentieth century, which slowly began to change in the case of medical services when the federal government established its first nursing station at Port Harrison in the eastern Arctic in 1947. By the mid-1960s, there were twenty-five stations.[26]

Nurses' public health work tends to be underemphasized in their own written accounts, perhaps because, to them, it seemed more consistent with the work that they were doing in their jobs in the south.

In the North, work in acute care was, of necessity, their first priority
and it was often more dramatic and hence more memorable, as it
stretched the boundaries of their professional training and experience
in obvious and unexpected ways. For those intending to publish written accounts of their experiences, the description of a trip to provide
emergency care in communities ravaged by diphtheria was a useful device to capture the interest of potential readers. The prologue to Amy
Wilson's 1965 book, *No Man Stands Alone*, attests to this: "Risking
her life to save Indians caught by epidemic and accident in Canada's
sub-arctic, Nurse Amy Wilson's tour of duty was one of urgent drama."[27]
And recounting acute care experiences often served to emphasize the
excitement and adventure of their northern experience in letters to
families and friends back home.[28] This is particularly evident in the
early years examined in this study, when some young graduates were
eager to experience life beyond the professional, gendered, and social
restrictions of hospital schools of nursing. As Lois Chételat remarked
about her decision to apply for a position with MSB: "I thought of it
[working in the Arctic] as an adventure."[29] Her letters were enlivened
with stories of adventure such as her description of flying to a remote
area on a stormy morning to escort a woman in premature labour to
the hospital.[30] In comparison, the tasks subsumed under the broad
category of public health, as described in the accounts written by MSB
bureaucrats,[31] seemed not greatly different from the work of public
health nurses in rural communities further south. However, a closer
examination of this work, as reflected in interviews and in reports written by nurses to their employers, reveals that the demands of providing health care education in northern settlements greatly expanded the
'traditional' boundaries of public health and drew upon nurses' medical and non-medical skills in many unique ways, even for those nurses
with previous training or experience in public health.[32]

Northern Nurses as Public Health Providers

Prior to the DNHW's expansion of northern services, which began in
1945, the few medical personnel providing health care in the North
concentrated their efforts on treating injury and illness. Following
expansion, the MSB and its precursors began to emphasize public
health in policy and practice in many ways. This is evident in docu-

ments beginning in the early 1950s. Annual reports such as that of 1952 included variations of the following statement: "Public health education and practice has been the keynote of Indian Health Services, the avowed purpose being to forestall disease or detect it in the earliest stages."[33] The MSB sought to hire nurses with public health training, rewarded them with higher salaries, and offered financial incentives for employees to pursue public health training. For example, in 1952, nurses were graded and paid according to experience and special training. A nurse with public health training was placed in Grade 111 and earned the same salary as a charge nurse.[34] In the mid-1950s, the DNHW began providing leave of absence at half pay to nurses wanting to upgrade their public health skills.[35]

The public health mandate broadened over the next decade from a narrow focus on disease control to a wider public health goal of wellness promotion. Observations from the field confirmed that a gradual shift in emphasis was occurring. As Dr T.J. Orford, zone superintendent for Saskatchewan wrote in a 1958 newsletter: "The role of the field nurse ... is slowly changing – from treatment to prevention ... the treatment approach is too limited and we are now swinging to the broader concept – the promotion of good health, not good health just for an individual but the sum total of good health for families and the entire community."[36]

The departmental emphasis on public health coupled with the arbitrary division between public health and acute care was often a source of conflict for northern nurses. A recurring theme in discussions with nurses was their feeling that MSB's emphasis did not reflect the reality of their experience. As Kay Semple commented, "Our work was supposed to encompass 80% public health but in fact it was 80% clinical."[37] This could be frustrating for nurses, as Sue Pauhl explained: "I found that when you got into a settlement, everyone talked about how important Public Health was but you didn't have time to do the basics – like sick clinic, to take care of the sick people – to even think about getting into prevention programs. They kept saying 'our focus has to be public health.' Well, my goodness, you can't go out and do, say a workshop on "Stop Smoking" or "Healthy Eating" when the sick clinic was so full of people at times."[38]

Pauhl's complaint is a refrain in nurses' reports over the years. Twenty years earlier, nurse M.V. Peever wrote from Norway House: "On visits there [outlying communities] so much time is spent treating sickness that little time is left for teaching."[39] The time factor was crucial for much of the 'formal' public health teaching that nurses felt they should be doing.

Beyond the actual teaching time, they needed time to plan content and prepare materials. In the early post-war years, according to nurses, there was a paucity of audio and visual material in print or film form, a problem that was more prevalent in the more isolated communities. Although a variety of teaching materials was gradually developed and made available to nurses on a rotating basis, lack of materials continued to be an issue of concern in the 1970s. In 1973, Marcia Smith, MD, the consultant to the MSB on maternal and child health care, initiated an active campaign to identify "visual or audio visual aids for rental or purchase ... suitable for use with mothers of ethnic groups, Indians and Eskimos, in our northern areas."[40] In a subsequent letter to the health educator of the MSB Northern Region, Smith wrote: "I have a suspicion that we won't get very much and, in fact, we may need to think soon along the lines of developing our own video tapes. I would like to look into this possibility as I think we could do it inexpensively and have a product more suitable for the needs of the north."[41]

But access to useful materials was not the only problem nurses experienced, as Barbara Bromley pointed out. Working at their home base in Yellowknife, she and her co-workers had projectors and films for use in prenatal education, but when they went out to some of the satellite communities for which they were responsible, such as Dettah, there was no power available.[42] Problems like this were not limited to the early years of health service. In 1989, an Ontario NDP Task Force on Northern Health Issues referred to a culturally sensitive poster explaining the benefits of brushing teeth – but the community where it was displayed had no running water.[43] In the absence of 'official' teaching materials, some nurses drew upon their own creative skills. Anna Chan told of the apple-a-day nutrition awareness project she initiated in Arctic Bay. As one of the activities, she drew pieces of fruit, and then organized the schoolchildren to colour, cut, and paste them onto posters.[44]

Another issue of concern to field nurses and administrators was the cultural appropriateness and the relevance of teaching materials to the people in northern communities. A colonialist attitude, reflected in the lack of respect for indigenous language and oral culture shown by

NURSES AS EDUCATORS IN NORTHERN COMMUNITIES

some administrators and health care providers in the early post-war years, is demonstrated in a letter written by a doctor employed in northern Manitoba by IHS to Branch Superintendent Dr Moore in 1946. The writer makes reference to a circular in Cree 'Celabics.' [45] "I think it is a mistake to do anything to perpetuate this language. Any language that has not a literature is dead and the more we attempt to perpetuate it the more trouble we are making for ourselves,"[46] he wrote, in words reminiscent of Lord Durham reporting a century earlier to the British government about French spoken in Lower Canada.[47] By contrast, nurse Joyce Goodman regrets her lack of indigenous language skills in her 1952 report from Duck Lake. "It was rather difficult to do any real teaching among these people both because of the lack of a good interpreter and because of my limited knowledge of the Chipywans [sic] and their way of life."[48]

Many primary care nursing tasks could be carried out with a minimum amount of oral communication. However, the tasks of public health teaching as outlined in DNHW job descriptions[49] usually demanded reasonable language skills and, in many communities, a good interpreter.[50] There was no provision for language training for nurses before they took up their posts and there was no official training for the position of interpreter in Aboriginal settlements. In the hiring of nursing station staff from the community to work as handyman/driver or housekeeper/receptionist, those who spoke English were more likely to be chosen. Thus, they functioned also as interpreters for nurse and patient. In some homes, children of the family would fulfill this role as needed. Communication was further hampered by the fact that interpreting involved not only words and grammar but also the way these words were spoken and the body language that accompanied them. For example, certain phraseology that is appropriate in English may not be deemed respectful or culturally appropriate in particular Aboriginal languages or communities.[51]

Smith's approach also stands in sharp contrast to that of the doctor in northern Manitoba quoted above. In her search for suitable materials for use in northern areas, she borrowed textbooks on cultural anthropology and requested references from a professor at Trent University.[52] She reviewed books to use as reference texts at nursing stations and commented about one: "While it is an excellent book, particularly on the subject of breast feeding, I can't help but feel that

it's rather strongly oriented to white middle-class culture. This does
not invalidate the material in any way, but I think that the readers
should be aware that there are discrepancies, even among the different social groups of our own culture, and that there may be marked
differences between what is represented there and what one might find
in native culture."[53] Her comments, while progressive for the period,
do not go so far as to recognize or acknowledge the fact that the term
'native culture' encompasses many diverse groups.

While lack of time and lack of culturally appropriate teaching
materials often hindered nurses' efforts to mount the 'formal' public
health programs and health education classes that were advocated by
the MSB, nurses frequently carried out their teaching on an individual
basis as need and opportunity arose. And they made use of opportunities within the community. As nurse Welna reported from Onion
Lake nursing station in 1952: "Arrangements were made to have a
health film shown ... between two feature pictures on Saturday night.
For our first night we chose a Walt Disney picture on sanitation. I gave
a short introduction to the film ... We also showed the film at the local
school ... there is a value in having both children and parents seeing
the same film."[54] Welna's report points to northern nurses' use of a
strategy employed during the expansion of the public health movement
in southern urban areas of the country in the early twentieth century.
Public health officials set up school health programs in an attempt to
reduce communicable disease, to develop basic health habits, and perhaps to 'sell' their message to families through their children.[55]

In the early decades of health care under the jurisdiction of the
DNHW, nurses' responsibilities in the area of public health targeted two
major problems in Aboriginal communities: tuberculosis and infant/
child mortality. Their duties fell into several broad but interrelated and
overlapping categories: first, education concerning prevailing health
problems and the methods of preventing and controlling disease, including immunization against the major infectious diseases; second,
promotion of basic sanitation; third, provision of safe water; fourth,
advocacy of 'proper' nutrition, including provision of an adequate food
supply; and fifth, prenatal and postnatal education, which included
family planning. In all areas of this work, they functioned in different
capacities – not only as nurses but also as teachers, inspectors, enforcers
– tasks that were complicated both by language and cultural differences

and by the ambiguity of their position of power vis-à-vis members of the community, the medical team, and their employers. As well, they dealt with people in different sectors of the community, including settlement officials,[56] station employees, Hudson's Bay Company (HBC) and co-op store managers, Aboriginal healers, RCMP, and school-teachers. The next section of this essay examines nurses' work within these categories. Sanitation, water supply, and nutrition are addressed together with particular attention to their impact on maternal and child health. The section concludes with a brief discussion of the nurses' role in the family planning debate. It is important to note that conditions and challenges varied from community to community so that nurses were called upon to adapt their skills and knowledge to the settlement in which they were placed. Even within their area of responsibility, they might find different situations as they travelled from their home base to provide care in satellite communities.[57]

Sanitation, Water Supply, and Diet

In the early period of colonization, Aboriginal communities were ravaged by successive waves of virgin soil epidemics that occurred at first contact with 'outsiders' – usually traders, travellers, and missionaries from Europe.[58] In the sixteenth to eighteenth centuries, the most devastating of the diseases contracted by people without immunity was smallpox, while by the late nineteenth century, tuberculosis (TB) became the most prevalent.[59] At the turn of the century, it had become endemic in many communities even as it continued to spread to uninfected northerly areas. Native people themselves could be the source of infection when they returned to their communities after spending time in institutions such as residential schools[60] or correctional facilities[61] where communal living fostered the spread of contagious disease. One of the first to comment formally on the government's lack of attention to the increasing rate of TB in Aboriginal communities was the first director of medical services, Dr Peter Bryce, who was appointed in 1904, then re-assigned when the position was terminated in 1910. He waited until after he retired from the civil service to write his strong indictment. At the time of writing, Bryce had to make his comparison based on funding rather than mortality rates because the federal government did not begin counting Aboriginal deaths until 1925.[62] In *The Story of a National Crime*, published in 1922, Bryce claimed: "We find a sum of only $10 000 has been annually placed in the estimates to control tuberculosis amongst 105 000 Indians scattered over Canada in over 300 bands, while the City of Ottawa, with about the same population and having three general hospitals spent thereon in 1919 ... $33 364.70."[63]

Colonel E.L. Stone, appointed superintendent of the medical services division of the Department of Indian Affairs in 1927 following a seventeen-year hiatus without a director, intended to address the tuberculosis problem, but the cuts in funding and service because of the 1930s depression led him to order that no cases of pulmonary tuberculosis could be hospitalized.[64] During the war years, appropriation for TB treatment was increased regularly;[65] however, it was not until shortly after the end of the war, when the Department of National Health and Welfare assumed responsibility for INHS, that an aggressive policy to reduce the incidence of tuberculosis among Aboriginal people was introduced. Thus the campaign, which had been an important part of public health reform in southern communities in the early decades of the century,[66] came to the North. There were several obvious reasons for this: first, the oft-repeated statistical evidence that TB was the leading cause of mortality among Indians and Inuit in Canada;[67] second, the knowledge that federally generated morbidity and mortality figures indicated a disproportionately high rate of tuberculosis among members of the Aboriginal sector of the population when compared with the population of the country as a whole; third, the availability of increased funding for TB control;[68] and fourth, the discovery of the antibiotic streptomycin in the United States in the 1940s, which led to a new era in the treatment of tuberculosis. With the advent of 'wonder drugs,' the DNHW had no excuse for neglect of the problem. However, its policy was not altogether altruistic; in addition to the shame of the statistics related to TB in a country just recovering from the losses of the Second World War, there was an ongoing underlying fear of the spread of the disease to non-Aboriginal communities where rates of infection were much lower.[69]

In his 1946 submission to the joint Senate/House of Commons Committee to investigate the Indian Act, Brooke Claxton, minister of national health and welfare and joint chair of the submission, identified tuberculosis as the number one cause of death among the Aboriginal population and outlined proposals for extending and improving health services. His general recommendations included increasing the number of personnel and facilities and modernizing existing facilities; for the TB program in particular, he proposed that the DNHW intensify case finding and extend the use of BCG, the anti-TB vaccine discovered in the 1920s but not widely used in Canada until the late 1940s.[70] Claxton specifically notes that "provision of more field nurses with public health training is contemplated. This is in keeping with the proposal to extend the number of nursing stations."[71]

Claxton's report clearly points to fundamental structural problems beyond the jurisdiction of the DNHW.[72] He writes, "it is probable that the health conditions of the Indians [this term includes 'Eskimos' in his report] cannot be adequately remedied until their economic status and mode of life are greatly improved."[73] While it has been argued that the DIA did not take adequate measures to address Claxton's criticism, the DNHW attempted to treat the symptoms of the problem by acting upon many of the recommendations.[74] They completed construction of new hospitals at Sioux Lookout and Norway House in 1949 and at Moose Factory in 1950,[75] for example. Most of the beds in these facilities were occupied by patients with tuberculosis. Nurses were hired to provide extended services and many of these were key players in the campaign to reduce TB. Some worked to provide care in hospitals across the North; others worked in settlements. The tasks of station nurses in this effort were many and time-intensive, and included immunization, detection,[76] distribution and monitoring of medications,[77] caring for infected patients in the station until transfer to hospital, keeping records, monitoring 'old TB' patients,[78] explaining treatment procedures, and reassuring patient and family. Dealing with tuberculosis in northern communities was historically problematic. Before communities had nursing stations, many were visited annually or semi-annually by INHS X-ray and medical teams, who came into communities by plane or boat. Patients identified as having active TB were transported out of the community for treatment in distant hospitals.[79] When onset of disease occurred shortly after a visit, the patient would have to wait until the next appearance of the team for diagnosis and treatment. In the meantime, the untreated disease often worsened and could be transmitted to others in the family and community. Sicker patients

required longer periods of treatment and hence longer periods away
from family and community. There was also a problem with those who
feared the diagnostic procedures and course of treatment, especially
if they knew this meant evacuation from the community: they absented
themselves while the medical team was in the community. As Dr Otto
Schaefer, field officer of INHS in the Eastern Arctic, reported in 1959,
"difficulties [in the fight against TB] were augmented by the animosity
of natives to all medical equipment and in particular, roentgenograms.
[They] fled over the hills in some places when X-ray equipment was
landed."[80] A decade later, nurse Sharon Richardson, working as a
dispenser in the isolated community of Grise Fiord before the area was
assigned a nurse, reported similar reactions. "They [the residents] were
very leery ... because the way the government handled cases of positive sputum tests was to take the individual immediately on the
ice-breaker and remove them to the sanitorium in Montreal and historically, a number of them never came home and historically families lost children and never saw them again so it wasn't uncommon
when the ice-breaker would show up for the TB survey for individuals to disappear ... if they were unwilling to be shipped out. They really were at the mercy of the DNHW."[81]

Since it was accepted that the disease was spread by contact with
an infected person, isolation of the TB patient was central to the management of TB control. In urban areas, in the early decades of the century, this was sometimes accomplished without hospitalization. In
Toronto, for example, innovative tactics included erecting a tent for
the patient in the backyard of the family dwelling.[82] For the most part,
living facilities in many northern communities did not lend themselves
readily to isolation procedures. In communities where many members
left for perhaps three months at a time to work on the traplines or to
fish, there were periods when homes were sparsely populated. However, when all the members of the extended family were at home base,
dwellings often accommodated large numbers of people living in very
close quarters. And for those living in snow houses, which were
designed to keep heat in, there was little circulation of fresh air. Chan
described the lodging situation. "[In one room there is] a family – husband, wife, grandmother, grandfather, maybe four kids ... it's all the
space they can afford ... But half the time the men aren't at home and

the kids are in school or outside. But it's sleeping time [that is the prob-lem] ... and also they're sharing the same dishes."[83]

In a 1952 'informational' newsletter from the office of the Sask-atchewan regional superintendent's office addressing the topic, the writer points to problems that facilitated the transmission of conta-gious disease but he makes no attempt to conceal his disdain for and lack of understanding of the life conditions of the Inuit. "We must also remember the lack of hygiene in the igloo, the squallor [sic], sicken-ing at times, and the scarcity of water ... They all sleep together on the fur covered snow-bench, and they indiscriminately use cups that are seldom, if ever, washed. Try to isolate a contagious case! The Eskimo is a hardy type who has managed to survive and accustom himself to the country, in spite of unfavourable conditions. That he has done so is often a source of wonder to us."[84] While this voice is marked by its insensitivity, there was a general consensus that isolation was not pos-sible in the community; hence, patients must be evacuated from their homes and communities.

Evacuation was a policy that did not change over the early years covered in this study but the presence of a nursing station did make a difference in the management of TB by facilitating earlier diagnosis, effecting a shorter course of treatment, and hastening the eventual reduction in mortality rate. Some of the obvious benefits had to do with the medical management of the disease:[85] carefully organized and monitored program of vaccination of all members of the community, which involved extensive record keeping; earlier diagnosis of the dis-ease and hence earlier initiation of a chemotherapy regime; removal of the infected person to the nursing station to await hospitalization thus minimizing spread of the disease;[86] and close monitoring of patients returning to the community from a period of hospitalization to insure compliance with treatment and to detect any activity in old lesions. As directly observed therapy (DOTS) became the strategy of choice in tuberculosis management, nurses in communities assumed responsi-bility for administration of the program. For example, with the devel-opment of more advanced drugs, the most apparent symptoms of pulmonary TB – coughing and fever – were quickly reduced, leading some patients to stop their medication in the false belief that they had been cured.[87] To reduce this problem, nurses could advise patients and encourage compliance. As Jan Stirling explained: "Years ago we'd give them 30 days medication and they'd take their bottles home. But we never knew if they swallowed it or threw it out. And a lot of these people would be [TB] negative for a while but all of a sudden it would reoccur or their lesions weren't healing and it was because they weren't taking their medications or they weren't taking them properly. So now everybody that's on TB medications has to go to the health unit twice a week ... and you watch them swallow the medication."[88]

But where the course of TB was concerned, it was in their teaching and support of family members that nurses had the potential to make an important difference in the community. There was a consensus among interviewees and others writing on the topic that patients who understood the process of rehabilitation and the necessity of procedures such as taking medication regularly and eating a balanced diet were more likely to follow the prescribed regime. The ongoing presence of a nurse in a community offered the opportunity for the type of care that was not possible from teams moving in and out of settlements who had neither the time nor the personnel for educating patients and their families.

Chan ran regular classes on TB prevention in her nursing station. For her, explaining about the spread of infection was an important task. She encouraged people to avoid spitting on the ground, "I say 'when you cough, turn your face or use some toilet paper ... or use the old cigarette cans and when you finish, close and dispose of it. Also, use your own dishes if you don't feel well or if you're coughing.'"[89] Other nurses chose to teach within the family unit when one of their members was infected with TB.

In a 1952 report, nurse Joyce Goodman referred to a problem that was common to all communities and frequently mentioned in documents and interviews: the fear of leaving the community for treatment. Those infected with TB required particularly long periods of rehabilitation. She wrote:

They are rather sceptical about the length of time some of the patients stay out in Sanatorium. Although quite ready to send members out if necessary, they do not understand why treatment should take so long or why it has sometimes been unsuccessful. It seems that word of miracle drugs has been taken quite literally.

As much as possible was explained about tuberculosis, its treatment and the probable results, depending upon the stage of disease when treatment was begun. It was pointed out that with the annual X ray surveys there should not be as many far-advanced cases requiring such long and sometimes unsuccessful hospitalization. ALL ASKED FOR MORE FREQUENT WORD OF THEIR PEOPLE IN HOSPITAL. [emphasis is hers][90]

Nurses observed and expressed concern about the impact of long periods of evacuation on the patients and families of their communities. Nurse Kathleen Dier offered concrete examples of the disruption: "The really sad thing about TB treatment – it really disrupted families – a man resisted going, consented after requesting police to watch his wife. No sooner had his plane taken off when another man moved in with her. A child returned home after years in hospital unable to remember a word of his own language; he was sent to residential school since he was unable to fit back into his own community."[91] While nurses could do little more than observe the social dynamics of families as they attempted to cope with the absence of a family member, several mentioned that they tried to help by searching out information about the hospitalized patients and passing this along to those at home. Sometimes this meant informing them of the death of a loved one. They also visited hospitalized community members when they went 'out.' Thus, in many capacities, nurses played a vital role in the campaign to prevent and treat TB, leading to a decline in the rate of mortality and also in the incidence of infection.[92]

While TB has been the focus of this section, similar strategies were being applied to other infectious diseases such as measles, German measles (rubella), smallpox, diphtheria, and whooping cough.[93] And the prevention, detection, and treatment of sexually transmitted diseases gradually became an important part of the public health program.[94]

As Myra Rutherdale makes clear in chapter 6, a dramatic example of nurses' responses to the challenge of controlling infectious disease in the early days is that of the diphtheria epidemic that occurred in Halfway Valley in northern British Columbia in December/January 1949–50.[95] INHS nurse Amy Wilson, stationed at Whitehorse, travelled by plane, radio-equipped power wagon, horseback, single horse cutter, and on foot to administer antitoxin and antibiotics to those in the stricken communities. After being joined by her provincial counterpart, the two nurses travelled over 1,000 miles in a ten-day period to inoculate 947 persons living within travelling distance of the Alaskan Highway. This feat led the BC government to present the women with medals.[96]

Infant Mortality

In DNHW reports justifying the expansion of health services in the North in the mid-1940s, government officials cited high rates of tuberculosis as one of two key factors for concern. The other main factor was a high rate of infant mortality.[97] Although there is some slippage in the way this term is defined in the sources of the time, in general, and for the purposes of the present discussion, it referred to deaths occurring in the perinatal period and in early childhood – usually up to the age of two. The published reports focussed on mortality rates; however, it is understood that morbidity rates among northern Aboriginal peoples were also higher than those in the overall popula-tion. Statistics indicated that the most common afflictions of the young were gastroenteritis and respiratory infections, maladies that were caused or exacerbated by poor sanitation in the home or community,[98] poor nutrition, and insufficient or polluted water supplies. Hence, nurses' attention to the domestic hygiene, nutritional habits, and safe water supply in their communities was an important part of their public health mandate. Furthermore, this focus was supported by their professional knowledge and training and their personal beliefs, whether or not they were trained in public health.

In their approach to public health problems in their communities, nurses faced constant challenge and some, inevitably, were unrealistic in their expectations and patronizing in their attitudes toward their community members, using the tools of public health to attempt to impose southern ideals of health and hygiene. For the most part, how-ever, it seems that they were reasonable and focussed in their choice of issues. Many developed strategies that were practical and culturally appropriate to their communities and some took on causes not listed in the rigidly prescriptive "Duties of a Public Health Nurse" distrib-

uted by the DNHW. In so doing, they served as advocates for community members. Their written and oral reports, whether intended or not,
frequently offered a critique of the outside influences, including government policy, which precipitated or aggravated health problems in
the communities where they served.

Archival records indicate that, particularly in the early years
included in this study, some nurses were overzealous in their attempts
to impose their standards on northern households. In a poem penned
by a nurse in 1956, "Indian Woman's Lament," the woman of the title
lists a litany of health and social problems that nurses encountered
when they visited homes in their communities (see appendix 2). In referring to the "hound[ing] and dig[ging] and scold[ing] and prod[ding]"
(by the nurse) and asking "when is it all going to stop?" the poem
points to the tension between nurses, who were in a position of power
based on their specialized professional knowledge to treat or cure, and
women of Aboriginal households. In a suitably ironic twist, the author
puts the thoughts that troubled many nurses into words spoken by the
Indian woman in her retort, "All this [cleaning] was intended for white
Men, NOT for the Indian race." The words point clearly to the conflict, deeply felt by many nurses, about imposing southern, urban notions of hygiene on northern communities.

Pauhl, speaking of her experience at Rankin Inlet in the 1970s and
80s, shared the sentiments of the poet as she expressed her criticism of
the unrealistic expectations on the part of the MSB. "That's imposing
our standards and three-quarters of the world live more like that [the
Inuit community] than we [southerners] do in our sterile little houses,
the shower once a day. Most of the world doesn't live like that and
they do very well," she asserted.[99]

Another theme emerges from the poem, whether the author intended it or not. It is clear that inadequate infrastructure resulting from
insufficient governmental funding contributed greatly to health problems in northern communities. However, in the eyes of the employer,
both the nurse, who failed to 'convert' the Indian woman to southern
standards of hygiene, and the Indian woman, who failed to comply
with the nurse's dictates could be blamed for lack of improvement in
health statistics in certain communities. Hence they, as individuals,
served as scapegoats for a government that chronically neglected
northern communities.

Nurses employed different approaches in dealing with the problems they encountered as illustrated in two reports submitted in the 1950s. Glenna Robinson wrote from Fort Norman nursing station in 1957: "For the past month I had been treating the ... children for sores without much success. They were very dirty and had no proper clothing to wear ... The house was also very dirty. So the Welfare teacher and I decided to take action. On November 17th we went to clean the house ... We then went to the Bay and outfitted the children with necessary clothing ... The children were brought to the Nursing Station and bathed."[100] While a frustrated Robinson did the work she deemed necessary herself, nurse Welna, in her 1958 article from Onion Lake, outlined the effectiveness of teaching by example. "Show [her emphasis] the mother how to bathe her baby, treat impetigo," she wrote, adding that nurses can set an example. "When we enter a home and before we leave, handwashing is a habit everyone can expect of us."[101]

Nurse Welna's example of handwashing may have been effective in her community but water was not always a readily available commodity in northern communities. As nurse T. Fortin wrote in a lengthy report from the Payne Bay area of Ungava Bay, "It is easy, indeed very easy, for the nurse to teach the Eskimos the importance of daily washing, teeth brushing, regular laundering. Very easy teaching for the nurse – difficult of practice for the Eskimos." She was troubled also by the gender implications of the water problem. "The water supply is essentially a woman's problem; whatever their condition or state of health, they have to go a long way to find this precious water."[102] Her community was fortunate enough to have access to a river, but other communities collected their water from icebergs[103] or from polluted ponds.[104]

Diet

Nurses in all communities encouraged mothers to breastfeed their babies: an unreliable water source was one of the key reasons.[105] Thus, when the government policy increased pressure to send parturient mothers 'out' to deliver their babies, nurses such as Richardson were concerned. As she explained: "Bottles [in Grise Fiord] were out. In fact that was one of the reasons for not sending women out to the hospital in Frobisher because invariably they'd come back with the baby on a bottle which was not healthy and we had no assured water supply. Our water came from icebergs that ran aground off shore. So no iceberg, no water. So that's not a very good environment for bottle feeding." She offered further reasons for advocating breastfeeding: "my observation was that infants who continued to be breast-fed – and most of them were breast-fed for one year – had far fewer respiratory infections. It was when they began to eat that there were problems."[106]

Nurses were well aware of the relationship between diet and disease and noted, for example, that those families who received the tuberculosis ration showed improved health.[107] Like bottle-feeding, poor nutrition was related to contact with outsiders. Dietary imbalance fell into two broad categories. In some communities, the food supply was affected by poor catches in the camps. The problem was aggravated in certain areas by government relocation of Inuit settlements – a process that placed people who relied on caribou in areas where they were expected to rely on fish[108] – and by encroachment of southerners exploiting natural resources of the North and, in the process, disturbing fishing grounds and patterns of animal migration.[109] Chan worked with the women in her community of Arctic Bay to ameliorate this problem. She noted that they were particularly affected when the community went off to the camps as they stayed at the base camp and had to find food for themselves while the men were away hunting or fishing. So Chan made a list of foods such as dried eggs and tinned vegetables that they could buy at the HBC store and take with them to supplement their diet.[110]

According to nurses, the other main cause of dietary imbalance was decreasing reliance on traditional foods and increased consumption of processed and 'junk' foods brought into the communities by southerners, a change that resulted in increased incidence of dental caries[111] and sometimes in vitamin deficiencies[112] and anemia.[113] Pauhl's description of the store in Rankin Inlet was typical of the critique offered by nurses of HBC stores in their communities: "Consider ... the store had 4 aisles; 2 of the 4 had pop and candy; the third had cleaning supplies. Not much space for food."[114] So they advocated on behalf of the community for the HBC to bring in fresh food when possible and to reduce the amount of junk food on the shelves.

Archival materials reveal that INHS attempted to address dietary imbalance by searching for solutions that could be applied broadly in

Aboriginal communities across the country. One example was the search for a special infant food – a type of precooked cereal mixture, "cheaper than pablum"[115] that could be mixed with powered skim milk.[116] They also closely supervised the spending of the family allowance by placing the cheque with the local trader.[117] Further, INHS attempted to coerce and cajole families through letters such as the following, which was translated into "Eskimo syllabics."

> "To all Mothers with small children"
> Our King has made a law that all mothers of children will get
> help in seeing that these children grow up to be strong and
> healthy. One way this help will be given is by bringing to them
> good baby foods. All the traders will have these foods at the
> stores and will let you have them. These foods are for small
> children up to three years old.[118]

Nurses, by contrast, worked at the grassroots level to improve nutrition within their communities. In schools, they encouraged children to decrease pop drinking[119] and they organized school lunch programs.[120] In homes, they advised mothers to breastfeed their babies and they taught the women how to prevent botulism, which could result from eating raw meat.[121] Sometimes their suggestions were as basic as putting a handful of currants or raisins in bannock when a poor hunt threatened to result in iron deficiency.[122] And they encouraged HBC store managers to increase the amount of nutritious food on their shelves. In doing so they were promoting wellness in their communities and carrying out their public health mandate on a day-to-day basis.

Pregnancy and Birth

Advice on domestic sanitation, clean water, and dietary balance was an integral part of the prenatal and postnatal programs that were offered widely in northern communities. Whether they taught these programs to groups with the assistance of an interpreter or provided individual instruction, nurses were enthusiastic about this aspect of their job.[123] This teaching fostered positive relationships between the nurses and the women of their communities.[124] The main topics covered included healthy pregnancy, childbirth, postnatal care, and infant care. Since many of the women were sent out of the settlement to deliver, nurses tried to prepare them for what would take place on admission to hospital and during their labour and delivery, in hopes of making the experience less intimidating and stressful for them.

The related topic of family planning was absent from nurses' 'official' list of duties and little discussed in the first two decades dealt with in this study, which is not surprising since providing birth control information and supplies was illegal under the Criminal Code of Canada until 1969.[125] However it is clear that, prior to this time, the MSB was counting on the fact that "no law enforcement agency in Canada [was] anxious to enforce [this law].[126] In a reply to a query in early 1956, Dr Moore, Director of INHS, agreed that contraceptive materials should be supplied "when ordered by a medical officer." He further stated, "I think this policy can be defended if necessary,"[127] but his defence was not linked to reducing the high infant mortality rate, as suggested in some documents.[128]

The distribution of birth control devices across the North was uneven as shown in correspondence between the director general and the zones. The superintendent of the Quebec Zone was "sceptical" when a more intensive program to encourage birth control was suggested. He replied, "Our opinion might change if the criminal code was amended and if uncomplicated methods could be devised that were at the same time accepted by the various churches."[129] The Saskatchewan regional director wrote, "Under no circumstances do I consider the drug should be indiscriminately supplied to single females for strictly contraceptive reasons."[130] As a result of the lack of policy, some women who wanted to control their fertility did not have access to the means or information to do so and other women who did not want to use artificial means of birth control had it imposed on them. Even after 1969, access was unequal as church and medical personnel imposed their beliefs on communities.[131]

Nurses were supposed to dispense pills only on the order of a doctor, but it was their responsibility to "keep patients under observation," which included teaching the proper use of pills and devices[132] and ensuring compliance.[133] Further, when the MSB proposed doing a study in 1966 "to determine knowledge of the native population of reproduction and means for its control or timing," it was suggested that nurses would gather the information.[134] Some nurses said that they were not involved in discussion or distribution until 1969.[135] Richardson, however, reported that although she was never apprised of any policy, she was well aware that birth control prescription was going on. According to her, "when women were sent out to the hospital, there was usually an attempt made by the attending physician to get them on some type of birth control if they were multi-parips and they didn't like it. So in my experience – it was inappropriate for their role in the Inuit community … Women were highly valued … for their contribution to the ongoing life of the community."[136] She cited a specific example of a woman who had an IUD inserted before she came back to the settlement. She asked Richardson to remove it but this could not be done until some months later when a physician visited the community.[137] When women asked her advice about the pill, she tried to explain how it worked but assured them that it was their choice to take it or not. Thus, although there was no official policy in place, nurses were involved, by their employer, in a task that was illegal and that, in their opinion, was imposed upon some women against their will.[138] In the absence of government policy, they, for the most part, supported the needs of the women in their communities on an individual basis.[139] In so doing, they helped to minimize problems occurring as a result of contact with outsiders and they provided women with some measure of reproductive choice.

+++

Northern nurses' work as educators in the area of public health appears to be well documented in official records – what they were expected to do and what they did. However, when nurses speak or write about this work, their perspective is somewhat different. Although they claimed they did not have adequate time, materials, or indigenous language skills to follow the prescribed program of public health education, they were educating in different ways on an ongoing basis and the education that they provided was, as a result, more relevant to the needs of the people of their communities. Whether this education meant taking advantage of a teachable moment or advocating for the community in relations with other 'outsiders' or the MSB, they were serving their community better than if they interpreted their job description literally. And, in spite of the fact that health teaching was an instrument of colonization, much of what nurses did was aimed at undoing or minimizing the wrongs of past and present. Further, there was much in their public health teaching that encouraged Aboriginal peoples to take responsibility for health issues, given that, in many areas, diseases and ill health resulting from contact with outsiders were already established.

Appendix One

Educational and Informational Newsletter, LAC RG29
v 2697 file 802-2-2 pt 1, 1947–51

Duties of a Public Health Nurse [PHN]
The PHN is primarily concerned with preventive medicine and to do this must spend a large portion of her time in close contact with the individual family. She is directly responsible to the Medical officer and must look to him for instructions and guidance in her duties.

These duties would include:

1 Home visits in which she should check on sanitary arrangements and cleanliness of the homes and demonstrate the proper methods of hygiene.

2 Inspections of children for various infectious diseases and arrange that any needing medical attention should receive it.

3 Instructing the housewife in Pre and Post natal care where necessary.

4 Instructing the mother in infant care, preparation of formulas, etc.

5 Arranging for immunization of pre-school children

Then in general she should be responsible for the arranging of various surveys and clinics, such as

1 immunization

2 T.B. surveys

3 dental clinics

4 other necessary clinics

Records
She should be responsible to see that records are kept up-to-date.

Drug requisitions
In some locations it will also be necessary for the nurse to take charge
of Departmental drugs, requisitions for new supplies and do minor
dressing and dispensing.

If a car is supplied the Public Health Nurse, it will be necessary to
use her services and the car in some instances in the transportation of
patients.

Appendix Two

"Indian Woman's Lament," as it appeared in Regional
Superintendent's Newsletter 48, November 1956

Field Nurses are my greatest curse, a fever for work they spread,
It's wash the baby, clean the house, make up that dirty bed.
Now – I dont mind the talking, the drinking tea, or time,
But it's an awful lot of effort, to get my wash out on the line.

Over my babies they fret and bother, with routines, schedules
 and such,
Now, I dont mind the resting, it's the work I dont like too much.
The formulas and the bathing, Infantol once a day,
The moss bag is far less trouble, and I like it better that way.

Oke – so my nose is runny, my bugs are dug in to the root,
I dont mind the itching, I could'nt give a hoot,
My house can be dirty, my baby underfed,
Live, die, or save me, – enough has been said.

I'll scrub the floor tomorrow, or maybe the day hence,
But a cup of tea and sitting, makes far more sense.
Now – I dont have no pleasures, to – why all the woes,

And please send no more nurses, to keep me on my toes.
I'm cleaning, scouring, scrubbing, until I'm blue in the face,
All this was intended for White Men, NOT for the Indian Race
But hound and dig and scold me, prodding me on till I drop,
Just who invented Nurses?
And when is it all going to stop?

NOTES

The research for this essay was supported in part by the Kitty Lundy Memorial Grant.

1 Regional Superintendent's Newsletter #32, 1952, Library and Archives Canada (LAC) RG29 v2697 file 802-2-2 pt. 2.

2 In some cases, only two pairs of rats were used and the diets varied somewhat.

3 DNHW *Annual Report* 1952, "Public health education and practice has been the keynote of Indian Health Services, the avowed purpose being to forestall disease or detect it in the earliest stages."

4 Interview with Sue Pauhl, 15 August 2001.

5 Frank James Tester and Peter Kulchyski, *Tammarniit (Mistakes): Inuit Relocation in the Eastern Arctic 1939–63* (Vancouver: UBC Press, 1994), 72–84.

6 1945: Indian Health Services (IHS); 1955: Indian and Northern Health Services (INHS); 1962: Medical Services Branch (MSB)

7 In 1971 a project was set up and sponsored by MSB in co-operation with University Schools of Nursing and the Canadian Nurses' Association to "help promote recruitment and retention of well-qualified nursing personnel" to MSB and to "help improve and expand the educational level of nurses to meet Canadian needs." For purposes of the project, field activities at nursing station were divided into the two usual categories, Treatment Program (primary care nursing) and Health Program (public health tasks), and a third was added, "Involvement in Confinement."

8 Lesley Malloch examines the key similarities and differences between the medical model and traditional Indian healing practices in "Indian Medicine, Indian Health: Study Between Red and White Medicine," in *Canadian Woman Studies* 10, 1 and 2 (Summer/Fall, 1989).

9 This concept is explained in J.D. O'Neill, "The Politics of Health in the Fourth World: A Northern Canadian Example," in *Human Organization* 45, 2 (1986): 119–28. "Structured as internal colonies in relation to the larger nation-state,

Fourth World situations exist within First (e.g., American Indians and Australian Aboriginals) World context. These situations are better characterized as Fourth World rather than as ethnic minorities because the populations involved are the original inhabitants of the area whose lands have been expropriated and who have become subordinate politically and economically to an immigrant population. Fourth World peoples generally inhabit marginal geographic regions relative to central metropolitan areas, and their resources have historically been exploited by the dominant group without local consultation."

10 Ideally, there were usually two nurses at a station, but INHS was chronically short-staffed, so a nurse was often on her own. This occurred even if there were two nurses at the station because one nurse would have to make visits to satellite communities, or go out on medevac or leave.

11 Such hospitals were located, for example, in Frobisher Bay (now Iqaluit) in the Eastern Arctic, Moose Factory in northeastern Ontario, Sioux Lookout in northwestern Ontario, and Yellowknife and Inuvik in the Northwest Territories.

12 'Medevac' is the term used for medical evacuation missions. A nurse accompanied the pilot of a small plane to airlift the patient(s) to a Zone hospital.

13 Lois Chételat recounted the story of her trip between Fort McPherson and Inuvik seated on the floor of a small, draughty Beaver aircraft beside a woman who was in premature labour and about to deliver a baby in a footling breech position. Telephone interview, 24 August 1999.

14 Testimonies from Aboriginal women are limited to proceedings of a 1988 workshop funded by a branch of DNHW as reported in John D. O'Neil and Penny Gilbert, eds., *Childbirth in the Canadian North: Epidemiological, Clinical and Cultural Perspectives* (Winnipeg: Northern Health Research Unit, University of Manitoba, Monograph Series #2, 1990). This is an area that would benefit from further research.

15 Since 1988, health services to communities in the NWT have been provided through the government of the NWT in Yellowknife.

16 For example, in stations such as Resolute Bay where she was posted in the late 1970s, nurse Kay Semple looked after the medical needs of researchers working at the nearby meteorological station. Interview with Kay Semple, 19 July 2000.

17 This essay builds on studies such as: Kari Dehli, "Health Scouts for the State? School and Public Health Nurses in Early 20th Century Toronto." in *Historical Studies in Education* 2, 2 (Fall 1990): 247–64; Kathryn McPherson, *Bedside Matters: The Transformation of Canadian Nursing, 1900–1990* (Don Mills, ON: Oxford University Press, 1996), 57–63; Susan L. Smith, *Sick and Tired of Being*

Sick and Tired: Black Women's Health Activism in America, 1890–1950 (Philadelphia: U of Penn Press, 1995), chap. 5, "The Public Health Work of Poor Rural Women"; Emily K. Abel and Nancy Reifel, "Interactions Between Public Health Nurses and Clients on American Indian Reservations During the 1930s." In J. Walzer Leavitt, ed., *Women and Health in America: Historical Readings*, 2nd ed., 489–506 (Madison, WI: University of Wisconsin Press. 1999).

18 The impact of psycho-social isolation is discussed in the work of Brenda Canitz, "A Study of Turnover in Northern Nurses: Isolation, Control and Burnout," MSc thesis (Toronto: University of Toronto, 1991.

19 This statement appeared in annual reports written by all the superintendents from Dr Bryce to Dr Moore. However, as noted in James B. Waldram, D. Ann Herring, T. Kue Young, *Aboriginal Health in Canada* (Toronto: University of Toronto Press, 1995), 146, certain Indian organizations have claimed that medical services are a treaty right but court challenges have upheld the position of the federal government.

20 All other aspects of Indian administration remained with Indian Affairs Branch [IAB] and were transferred to newly created Department of Indian Affairs and Northern Development [DIAND] in 1966. Analysts of Aboriginal health policy claim that this split in jurisdiction did not serve Aboriginal people well.

21 Percy Moore, "Indian Health Services," in *Canadian Journal of Public Health* (1946): 37.

22 In many communities, the Indian agent, priest or the RCMP officer served as dispenser.

23 In the post-war expansion of services, the government was able to set up facilities on abandoned military sites.

24 Waldram et al., *Aboriginal Health in Canada*, 164.

25 Tester and Kulchyski, *Tammarniit (Mistakes)*, 5.

26 Waldram. *Aboriginal Health in Canada*, 172. The nursing stations were supported by hospitals in Inuvik and Frobisher Bay (now Iqaluit).

27 Amy V. Wilson, RN, *No Man Stands Alone* (Sidney, BC: Gray's Publishing, 1965). (reprinted in 1966 as *A Nurse in the Yukon*.)

28 Interview with Lois Chételat, 11 September 2001.

29 Chételat explained that she was influenced in her decision by the work of Dr Tom Dooley in the organization Medico. She subsequently volunteered with CUSO in India. Interview, 11 September 2001.

30 Lois James Chételat, *Alice's Daughters: A Social History of Three Generations of Women in One Family*, unpublished manuscript, 1999, chap. 11, 24.

31 Appendix 1.

32 Until the program to train northern nurses opened at Dalhousie University in 1967, public health nursing programs did not consider the special challenges of northern health care. "Clinical Training of Medical Services' Nurses working in areas not served by physicians," 25 May 1970, LAC RG29 V 2741 file 820-2-24.

33 DNHW Annual Report 1952.

34 Department of National Health and Welfare, Indian Health Services, *Regional Superintendent's Letter*, 1 October 1952, 2.

35 Interview with Irene Culver, outpost nurse at Fort George who went to University of Toronto for ten months in 1956 to earn a public health certificate. Manitoulin Island, 8 July 1998.

36 T.J. Orford, MD, zone superintendent, North Battleford, SK, "A Change in Emphasis," in *Newsletter* (October 1958).

37 Interview with Kay Semple, 9 June 1999.

38 Interview with Susan Pauhl, 15 August 2001.

39 Report by Nurse Peever, November 1952, LAC RG29 v2697 file 802-2-2 pt. 2.

40 Marcia Smith, Various letters to companies and organizations such as Heinz, Gerber, Canadian Diabetes Association, 1973, LAC RG29 file 351-1-6 pt. 2a.

41 Marcia Smith. Letter to Hope Spencer, health educator of MSB Northern Region, 3 July 1973, LAC RG29 file 851-1-6 pt 2a.

42 Interview with Barbara Bromley, 10 January 2000.

43 *New Democrats' Task Force on Northern Health Issues: First Come, Last Served: Native Health in Northern Ontario* (Toronto: New Democratic Party of Ontario, 1989).

44 Interview with Anna Chan, 30 August 2001.

45 This word is generally written as 'syllabics.'

46 Dr Cameron Corrigan, Norway House, Manitoba to Dr P. Moore, Superintendent IHS, DNHW, 4 March 1946, LAC RG29 file 851-6-2.

47 Gerald M. Craig, ed., *Lord Durham's Report: An Abridgement of Report on the Affairs of British North America* (Toronto: McClelland & Stewart, 1963), 150-1.

48 Report from Miss Joyce Goodman, RN, Duck Lake, 1952, LAC RG29 v2697 file 802-2-2 pt. 2.

49 Appendix 1.

50 This is probably one reason why nurses liked using the rat experiment – little oral communication was required to make the project accessible to all members of the community.

51 Nancy Cummins, locum physiotherapist in a community in the Oji-Cree region

of northwestern Ontario, shared the following story with me. A woman who was partially paralyzed as a result of a stroke reported that she had burned herself on the stove. The therapist suggested that she shouldn't use the stove as it was dangerous. When the therapist and the community health representative (CHR) who was serving as interpreter left the house, the CHR gently explained that saying "Don't cook" was seen as disrespectful and left the woman no alternatives. A culturally appropriate response would have been "It worries me when you cook," a response that passed the power to the patient to understand that the therapist was saying she shouldn't cook.

52 Smith, Various letters to companies, 7 August 1973.

53 Smith, Various letters to companies, 5 November 1973.

54 Report from Mrs I.M. Welna, RN, Onion Lake Nursing Station, 1952, LAC RG29 v2697 file 802-2-2.

55 Heather MacDougall, *Activists and Advocates: Toronto's Health Department 1883–1983* (Toronto: Dundurn Press, 1990), chap. 9; Neil Sutherland, *Children in English Canadian Society: Framing the Twentieth Century Consensus* (Toronto: University of Toronto Press, 1976).

56 Including Band Councils and Elders.

57 Yellowknife is a prime example. Nurses such as Nancy Menagh, Barb Bromley, and Jan Stirling stationed at the health unit in Yellowknife all commented on the different sorts of issues that they might be called upon to deal with when they went into small settlements. Interviews, 20 September 1999, 10 January 2000, 23 July 2001.

58 See for example, Waldram et al., *Aboriginal Health in Canada* ; T. Kue Young, *Health Care and Cultural Change: The Indian Experience in the Central Subarctic* (Toronto: University of Toronto Press, 1988); Susan Johnston, "Epidemies: The Forgotten Factor in Seventeenth Century Native Warfare in the St Lawrence Region." In Bruce Alden Cox, ed., *Native People, Native Lands: Canadian Indians, Inuit and Métis* (Ottawa: Carleton University Press, 1992).

59 It should be noted that Aboriginal peoples contracted different types of tuberculosis: pulmonary, glandular, bone, and joint. The following sources, in addition to archival materials, provide background for the section on tuberculosis: Brooke Claxton, "Submission to the Special Joint Committee ... to Examine and Consider the Indian Act. By the ... Minister of National Health and Welfare" in Canada, Parliament Joint Senate/House of Commons Committee to Investigate the Indian Act, *Minutes of Evidence and Proceedings* No. 3 (6 June 1946): 61–98; P.E. Moore, "Indian Health Services," in *Canadian Journal of Public Health* 37 (1946): 140–2; P.E. Moore, "Medical Care of Canada's Indians and

Eskimos," in *Canadian Journal of Public Health* 47, 6 (1956): 227–33; P.E.
Moore, "No Longer Captain: A History of Tuberculosis and Its Control
Amongst Canadian Indians," in *CMAJ* 84 (1961):1012–16; C.R. Maundrell,
"Indian Health: 1867–1940," MA dissertation (Kingston: Queen's University,
1941); Robert G. Ferguson, *Studies in Tuberculosis* (Toronto: University of
Toronto Press, 1955); Dr George Graham-Cumming,"Health of the Original
Canadians, 1867–1967," in *Medical Services Journal, Canada* February 1967:
115–66; H.B. Hawthorne, "The Politics of Indian Affairs." In Ian A.L. Getty and
Antoine S. Lussier, eds., *As Long as the Sun Shines and Water Flows: A Reader
in Canadian Native Studies*, Nakota Institute Occasional Paper No. 1 (Vancouver: UBC Press, 1983); M. Matas, "Tuberculosis Programmes of the Medical
Services Branch, Department of National Health and Welfare," in *Medical Services Journal of Canada* 22 (1966): 878–83; LAC RG10, v3957, file 140754;
Arthur J. Ray, "Diffusion of Diseases in the Western Interior of Canada, 1830–
1850." In S.E.D. Shortt, ed., *Medicine in Canadian Society: Historical Perspectives* (Montreal & Kingston: McGill-Queen's University Press, 1981).
60 Olive Patricia Dickason, *Canada's First Nations: A History of Founding Peoples
from Earliest Times*, 2nd ed. (Toronto: Oxford University Press, 1997), 310.
61 Walter Vanast has chronicled in articles and film the 1929–31 story of the Inuit
in Coppermine whose community was decimated when TB was introduced by
a returning community member who had contracted the disease while incarcer-
ated in Edmonton for murder. "The death of Jennie Kanajuq: Tuberculosis,
religious competition and cultural conflict in Coppermine, 1929–31," in *Études/
Inuit/Studies* 15, 1 (1991): 75–104.
62 John D. O'Neil, "Aboriginal Health Policy for the Next Century." In *Royal
Commission on Aboriginal Peoples: The Path to Healing* (Ottawa: Ministry of
Supply and Services, 1993).
63 Peter Henderson Bryce, *The Story of A National Crime: Being An Appeal for
Justice to the Indians of Canada* (Ottawa: James Hope and Sons, 1922)
64 Claxton, "Submission to the Special Joint Committee," 9; George J. Wherrett,
The Miracle of the Empty Beds: A History of Tuberculosis in Canada (Toronto:
University of Toronto Press, 1977), 10–12. In a 1937 directive to all Indian
Agents, Harold W. McGill, director of Indian affairs, stated in section 5, "There
will be no funds for tuberculosis surveys; treatment in sanatoria or hospitals of
chronic tuberculosis." Full text of directive reprinted in Wherrett.
65 Wherrett, *The Miracle of the Empty Beds*, 114.
66 MacDougall, *Activists and Advocates*, 126–35.

67 Graham-Cumming states that this was true until 1952. In 1953, it dropped to third place and by 1967, at the time he was writing, "it is now a relatively insignificant cause of death." Dr Moore, director of INHS services, stated that the rate of death from TB among Canadian Indians was "about 15 times that of the white population." Moore, *Indian Health Services*, 140.

68 Moore, "No Longer Captain," 1012–16.

69 Moore, *Indian Health Services*.

70 Bacillus Calmette-Guerin was developed in France by Dr Albert Guerin and Dr Albert Calmette as a vaccine against tuberculosis.

71 Claxton, "Submission to the Special Joint Committee."

72 As a result of a split in jurisdiction in 1946, DNHW assumed responsibility for health matters of Aboriginal people while DIA continued to have responsibility for other aspects of governance such as social services, education, housing – a situation which did not always serve the constituents well.

73 Claxton. "Submission to the Special Joint Committee."

74 A notable exception is Claxton's recommendation to "make every effort to train Indians as doctors, nurses and sick attendants wherever this is possible. It is felt that the true interests of the Indians will best be served when they are taking an active part in looking after their own people." This seems to have been largely ignored by DNHW in its subsequent policies.

75 Noted in Annual Reports.

76 Various detection and monitoring methods were used over the years including X-ray, Mantoux skin test, sputum-smear microscopy.

77 DOTS, directly observed treatment short-term, became and continues to be the most successful strategy. Sometimes referred to as direct observation therapy.

78 Term refers to patients whose TB was inactive but whose lesions could become active at any time.

79 Field officers preferred to hospitalize patients as close to home as possible. As Dr Otto Schaeffer wrote, "For patients being evacuated, rehabilitation is usually much more difficult after returning from the south than after comparable periods in local mission hospitals." O. Schaeffer, "Medical Observations and Problems in the Canadian Arctic,' in *CMAJ* 81 (1959): 248–93.

80 Ibid., 249.

81 Interview with Sharon Richardson, 10 June 1999. Residents of Grise Fiord had reason to be leery. The federal government moved Inuit from Port Harrison in Arctic Quebec and Pond Inlet on Baffin Island to Grise Fiord, created as an artificial community in the 1950s to ensure the sovereignty of Ellesmere Island,

which previously had no permanent habitation. For a discussion of the re-colonization of the Arctic Islands, see Frank James Tester and Peter Kulchyski, *Tammarniit (Mistakes)*, 7 and 138–204.

82 See photos in MacDougall, *Activists and Advocates*, 127 and 129; and in Wherrett, *The Miracle of the Empty Beds*.

83 Interview with Anna Chan, 30 August 2001.

84 Regional Superintendent's Newsletter, 1952, LAC RG29 V2697, file 802-2-2 pt. 2.

85 Sanitation manuals that outlined the protocols were placed in the stations. Copies of sections of the manuals were shown to me by nurse interviewees Kay Semple and Sheila Clark.

86 As Kathleen Dier noted "After the Xray team moved along the coast, it was a difficult time. At one time we had 14 active TB patients in the nursing station [Cambridge Bay, 1957] waiting for transport to Edmonton," in "Early Days in Cambridge Bay NWT," in *Canadian Nurse* 80 (1 January 1984).

87 Interviews with various nurses.

88 Interview with Jan Stirling, 29 November 1999.

89 Interview with Anna Chan, 30 August 2001.

90 Report from Miss Joyce Goodman, RN, Duck Lake, 1952. LAC RG29 V2697, file 802-2-2 pt. 2.

91 Dier, "Early Days," 19.

92 Moore, "No Longer Captain"; Matas, "Tuberculosis Programmes"; Graham-Cumming, "Health of the Original Canadians"; Waldram et al., *Aboriginal Health in Canada*. Unfortunately, there is currently a resurgence of TB in northern communities and this is an antibiotic-resistant strain. While an increase in incidence of the disease is occurring in other areas of the country, recent statistics indicate that in Nunavut, the rate of infection is ten times the national average. Accessed at http://hc-sc.gc.ca on 8 December 2004.

93 Regional Superintendent's Newsletter, W.J. Wood, IHS (Manitoba and NW Ontario area), undated but stamped 10 November 1952; LAC RG29 V2697, file 802-2-2 pt 2.

94 Interview with Anna Chan who said that when the first group of men who went out to do repair work on the Pan Arctic pipeline returned to Arctic Bay, half of them required treatment for VD.

95 Letter to director, IHS from E.L. Stone, regional superintendent IHS on 31 March 1950. Attached is a report from Amy Wilson, a parody of the poem "The Highwayman" entitled "Operation Toxoid," LAC RG29 V2697 802-2-2 pt. 1.

96 "Diamond-Studded Medals Presented to Nurses Who Saved Indian Village,"

Victoria Daily Colonist, 14 April 1950. Copy of article in LAC RG29 v2697, file 802-2-2 pt 1.

97 Annual Reports.

98 Miss Craig reported from Nelson House that she was trying to get some of the boys, aged ten to fifteen, interested in cleaning up the garbage in the community. "I buried 1500 old tin cans last week and some of them I am sure have been around for at least 15 years. To tell the truth if one were to walk from here to the "Bay" store they wouldn't know I'd lifted one can." 1947, LAC RG29 v2697, file 802-2-2 pt 1.

99 Interview with Sue Pauhl.

100 Glenna Robinson, "Housecleaning is Part of the Job," in *INHS Newsletter* Autumn 1957.

101 I. Welna, "Teaching by Example," in *INHS Newsletter* December 1958. Emphasis is in the original.

102 J. Fortin, "Never a Dull Moment around Payne Bay," in *Indian Health Newsletter* Autumn 1957.

103 Interview with Sharon Richardson.

104 Interview with Kay Semple who told how people in the community of Rae Edzo emptied their "honey buckets" into the snow outside their doors every day. During thaw, the sludge drained into the pond from which they drew their water.

105 Other reasons included increased immunity to communicable diseases and other maladies such as otitis media and safety factors as explained to Dr Moore by nurse Gilda Graves. "Indian mothers have no place to store formula, nor sufficient utensils to make up a whole days [sic] supply," 20 December 1952, LAC RG29 file 851-6-2.

106 Interview with Sharon Richardson.

107 Nurse Peever, writing in a report from Norway House. *IHS Newsletter* November 1952, LAC v2697 file 802-2-2 pt. 2." The TB supplemental ration goes a long way towards keeping these patients in generally good condition, besides teaching entire families to appreciate the use of milk and other nourishing foods."

108 Tester and Kulchyski report how attempts to integrate Inuit of the Eastern Arctic resulted in the relocation of people who relied on caribou to areas where they were expected to rely on fish, *Tammarniit (Mistakes)*, 8.

109 Anna Chan spoke about workers on the Pan Arctic pipeline in Ellesmere Island and Grise Fiord.

110 Interview with Anna Chan.

111 Interview with Sharon Richardson.

112 J.H. Wiebe, MD, and Heather P. McDonald, "Work Among the Indian and

Eskimo People of Eastern Canada," in *Canadian Nurse* (June 1963): 540. "[The 'Eskimo'] is encouraged to adopt new foods, often to the exclusion of native ones. Dietary imbalance is almost inevitable under these circumstances and avitaminoses, rarely seen on a native diet of raw meats and the vegetable matter from the stomach of game, are beginning to occur."

113 Dr Jean Webb, chief, Child and Maternal Health Division, in a letter to Dr Moore, 19 July 1957, speaks to memo on nutritional anaemia among mother and young children in Indian population, LAC RG29 file 851-6-2.

114 Interview with Susan Pauhl.

115 22 January 1948, LAC RG29 v2846 file 850-3-12 pt. 1.

116 One of the suggestions advanced was to buy rejected Muffets from Quaker Oats. The plan to mix the material with powdered skim milk did not take into consideration the problems with water supplies in some communities. The search for the 'special food' is mentioned in archival records from the 1940s to the 1960s.

117 Ivy Maison, "Nursing on Canada's Rooftop," in *Canadian Nurse* 46 (August 1950): 622.

118 2 April 1947, LAC RG29 file 851-6-2.

119 Interview with Sue Pauhl.

120 Interview with Kay Semple.

121 Ibid.

122 Interview with Sue Pauhl.

123 Maison, "Nursing on Canada's Rooftop," 621, stated "Prenatal and well-baby clinics are pet projects of the nurse."

124 In Arctic Bay, the midwife trusted Anna and sent women to talk to the nurse when they were pregnant. Interview with Anna Chan.

125 1954–69, LAC RG29 v2869 file 851-1-6 pt 1a, provides information about family planning programs directed at Aboriginal peoples in the period prior to decriminalization. [27 June 1969] Before I was permitted to read the file, many items were removed under exemption 23 – not open to the public. From the mid-1950s, INHS/MSB searched for economical means of birth control: IUDS [15 June 1965]; pills Enovid and Ortho-novum [13 August 1962, 15 December 1964] In the early 1960s, Dr Moore received several letters from industrialist and eugenicist A.R. Kaufman who founded the Parents Information Bureau in the 1930s. [See Diane Dodd, "Hamilton Birth Control Clinic," in *Ontario History* March 1983.] Kaufmann offered to provide birth control literature for the government to distribute to 'Eskimo' families and also advocated vasectomy to control the 'population explosion.' Moore, careful to avoid any suggestion of

population control, replied that "our Eskimo people ... as Canadian citizens, are entitled to have as many [children] as they wish."

126 H.A. Proctor, director general MSB, 19 April 1966.

127 3 January 1956, LAC RG29 v2869 file 851-1-6, memo from Dr Blake, DNHW.

128 6 December 1963, Moore wrote to Kaufman "I do not think the issue of contraceptive literature would help us in reducing the high infant mortality rate."

129 21 September 1965, LAC RG29 v2869 file 851-1-6, Letter from Superintendent, Quebec Zone.

130 18 March 1966, LAC RG29 v2869 file 851-1-6, Letter to Director General from Regional Director, Saskatchewan.

131 Interview with Sue Pauhl.

132 IUDs and cervical coils were the devices used.

133 10 September 1962, LAC v2869 file 851-1-6 pt 1a, memo from Moore to all regional superintendents. He was responding to reports of toxic reactions to the drug Enovid.

134 Jean L. Webb, chief, Child and Maternal Health Division to H.A. Proctor, director general MSB, 3 August 1966.

135 Interview with Barb Bromley.

136 Interview with Sharon Richardson.

137 Interview with Sharon Richardson. The nurse was reluctant to remove the device as she didn't know what type it was and was concerned about causing damage to the woman.

138 In 1966, Dr H.A. Proctor, director of MSB, described the questions of family planning as a "political hot potato."

139 When I asked Sharon Richardson if she had any directive from MSB regarding birth control, she replied: "I was never apprised of any policy and I wouldn't have paid any attention to it anyway."

Contributors

HEIDI COOMBS-THORNE is a PhD candidate in history at the University of New Brunswick. Her dissertation explores class identity and the transformative nature of nursing at the Grenfell Mission in northern Newfoundland and Labrador, 1939–81. She is the recipient of several awards, including a general scholarship from the Hannah Institute for the History of Medicine and a Hugh John Flemming Graduate Scholarship from the University of New Brunswick. Her research has also contributed to the large, interdisciplinary research project Coasts Under Stress, funded by SSHRC and NSERC.

ELIZABETH DOMM obtained her diploma in nursing from Regina Grey Nun's School of Nursing, her baccalaureate in nursing from the University of Saskatchewan, her Master of Science in Nursing from the University of Mary, in Bismarck, North Dakota, and is currently completing her doctorate in nursing at the University of Alberta. Her research interests include the history and practice of nursing. She is currently an assistant professor with the University of Saskatchewan, College of Nursing.

JAYNE ELLIOTT is the research facilitator and administrator of the Associated Medical Services Nursing History Research Unit in the School of Nursing at the University of Ottawa. Her doctoral research examined the Red Cross outpost hospitals in Ontario and she continues to focus her research on the history of nursing and medical care in rural and remote regions of Canada. She is co-editor with Meryn Stuart and Cynthia Toman of *Place and Practice in Canadian Nursing History*.

MARLENE EPP is associate professor of history and peace and conflict studies at Conrad Grebel University College at the University of Waterloo. She is the author of *Women without Men: Mennonite Refugees of the Second World War* and *Mennonite Women in Canada: A History*, and chief editor (with Franca Iacovetta and Frances Swyripa) of *Sisters or Strangers?: Immigrant, Ethnic, and Racialized Women in Canadian History*.

LINDA KEALEY is a professor in the Department of History at the University of New Brunswick (UNB). Her research is supported by a CURA (Community-University Research Alliance) grant, 2005–10, funded by the Social Sciences and Humanities Research Council of Canada. She is also the academic convenor of Congress 2011, the annual meeting co-sponsored by the Canadian Federation of the Humanities and Social Sciences with a single university or several co-located universities in Canada. UNB and St Thomas University, both located in Fredericton, New Brunswick, are co-sponsoring Congress 2011.

MARY-ELLEN KELM holds a Canada Research Chair in the Department of History at Simon Fraser University. She is the author of *Colonizing Bodies: Aboriginal Health and Healing in British Columbia*. She is co-editor of *In the Days of Our Grandmothers: A Reader in Aboriginal Women's History in Canada* and editor of *The Letters of Margaret Butcher: Missionary Imperialism on the North Pacific Coast*.

LESLEY MCBAIN is a faculty member at First Nations University of Canada. The stories of nurses who worked in remote communities continue to intrigue her. Their experiences also inform her ongoing research into the delivery of health care services to people living in rural, remote, and reserve communities in Canada.

LAURIE MEIJER DREES is a regular faculty member in the First Nations Studies Department at Vancouver Island University (VIU), and a teaching scholar in Indigenous knowledge and Aboriginal education at the VIU Teaching and Learning Centre. She has also been on faculty at the University of Alaska-Fairbanks, the First Nations University of Canada, and the University of Saskatchewan.

MYRA RUTHERDALE is an associate professor in the Department of History at York University. She is the author of *Women and the White Man's God: Gender and Race in the Canadian Mission Field* and co-editor of *Contact Zones: Aboriginal and Settler Women in Canada's Colonial Past*. Her research on northern health care has been generously supported by the Social Sciences and Humanities Research Council.

JUDITH YOUNG completed a Master of Arts in history from York University and is an emeritus faculty member from the University of Toronto School of Nursing. She has also been an instrumental member of the Canadian Association for the History of Nursing (CAHN).

JUDITH BENDER ZELMANOVITS taught in the School of Women's Studies and the Faculty of Education at York University. Her interest in northern health services stems from her early work as a physiotherapist at a hospital that maintained an outpost in Iqaluit. She is currently involved in local history projects in Prince Edward County, Ontario.

Index

Abel, Emily K., 258–9, 288

Aboriginal children: Butcher and, 136; educators of, 150; teaching of gendered sphere to, 140. *See also* Aboriginal girls

Aboriginal communities: assertion of authority over, 6; bureaucratic colonialism of, 283; childbirth in, 63; colonialism and, 17; dispossession of land, 17; epidemics in, 319–20; federal nurses in, 248; health and welfare committees in, 199; interrelationships with white community, 146–7; and isolation, 5; learning from Western medicine, 18; modernization of, 279; nursing in, 198; outpost nursing and, 235n4, 258–9, 301; tuberculosis in, 319–25; whiteness vs. Englishness and, 70

Aboriginal girls: and landscape, 141–2; as nursing aides, 191, 195; as practical nurses, 197; teaching of domestic arts to, 139; as ward aides, 193 fig. *See also* Aboriginal children

Aboriginal health care workers, 19, 182; federal government and, 184–5; as former IHS hospital patients, 197; in hierarchy of health care, 202; in IHS facilities, 188–9, 202–3; as interface between IHS and communities, 203; recruitment of, 198

Aboriginal health care worker training, 22, 185, 196–7; community development and, 199; and community health, 199–201, 202; federal attitudes toward, 203; IHS and, 189, 198, 199; mission hospitals and, 189, 192; and public health, 202; tuberculosis and, 198. *See also* Aboriginal nurse training

Aboriginal Health in Canada (Waldram, Herring, Young), 182, 185, 337n19

integrationism. *See* assimilation

Inuit: birthing practices, 165–6; diet of, 329; and hygiene, 328; state medical service to, 313; training as ward aides, 193 fig; tuberculosis among, 323, 340n61; women as public health nurses, 19

Inuvik hospital, NT, 336n11, 337n26

Isaak, Frieda, 71, 72 fig

isolated/remote areas: Daniel's Harbour as, 94–5; and death in childbirth, 75–6; midwives in, 71; neighbour-midwives in, 70; nursing stations in, 187 (*see also* nursing stations); Ontario Red Cross and, 247; public health education in, 312; research into characteristics of nurses practising in, 269; research into history of nursing in, 182. *See also headings beginning* outport *and* outpost; northern Canada; northern Saskatchewan; rural areas

isolation, 5; colonialism and, 5; Mennonite settlement patterns and, 69; northern nurses and, 295–7; physicians and, 232–3; power relations and, 5; of station nurses, 233, 248

isolation hospitals, 38

Jasen, Patricia, 165–6

Jellicoe outpost, ON, 254

Johnson, William, 37

Johnston, R.J., 281

Jupp, Dorothy: about, 234–5n1; on childbirths, 220; in hospital vs. station nursing, 226, 227; and independence, 20, 224, 225, 227; Paddon and, 210–11, 224–8, 230,

231, 234; and physicians' lack of respect for nurses' abilities, 229; professional self-confidence of, 234

Kakabeka Falls, ON, 253

Kaufman, A.R., 344n125

Kealey, Linda, 12, 14, 15, 63, 67

Kelm, Mary-Ellen, 16–17, 70; *Colonizing Bodies*, 182

Kergin, Fanny, 134

Kiriline, Louise de, 250

Kitamaat, BC, 16–17, 128–50

Klassen, Pamela E., 77

Knox, Paul L., 281

Kulchyski, Peter, 313, 343n108

Labrador. *See* Newfoundland and Labrador

Lac La Ronge, SK: nursing station, 20, 191, 195; residential school, 285

Ladd-Taylor, Molly, *Women, Health and Nation*, 7

ladies' nurses, 34, 40–1, 42, 51

Lady Willingdon Hospital, ON, 189, 190, 199

Laliberte, Ron F., 281

La Loche infirmary, SK, 285

land/landscape: Aboriginal peoples and, 17, 129, 141–2; Butcher and, 141–2; Englishness of, 132; Wilson on northern, 172

Langford, Nanci, 75, 164

LaSalle, Dr, 97–8

Laurie, General, 119, 121

Lawrence, Karen R., 159

Lawrence, Mary, 164

Leipert, Beverly, 182–3